# Medication-Induced Movement Disorders

# Medication-Induced Movement Disorders

Edited by

**Joseph H. Friedman**
Butler Hospital and Department of Neurology at the Alpert Medical School of Brown University, Providence, RI,
and School of Pharmacy at the University of Rhode Island. Kingston, RI, USA

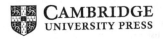

**CAMBRIDGE**
UNIVERSITY PRESS

# CAMBRIDGE
## UNIVERSITY PRESS

University Printing House, Cambridge CB2 8BS, United Kingdom

One Liberty Plaza, 20th Floor, New York, NY 10006, USA

477 Williamstown Road, Port Melbourne, VIC 3207, Australia

314-321, 3rd Floor, Plot 3, Splendor Forum, Jasola District Centre, New Delhi - 110025, India

79 Anson Road, #06-04/06, Singapore 079906

Cambridge University Press is part of the University of Cambridge.

It furthers the University's mission by disseminating knowledge in the pursuit of education, learning and research at the highest international levels of excellence.

www.cambridge.org
Information on this title: www.cambridge.org/9781316636817

First published 2015
First paperback edition 2020

*A catalogue record for this publication is available from the British Library*

*Library of Congress Cataloging in Publication data*
Medication-induced movement disorders / edited by Joseph H. Friedman.
    p.  ;  cm.
Includes bibliographical references and index.
ISBN 978-1-107-06600-7 (hardback)
I. Friedman, Joseph H., editor.
[DNLM:  1. Movement Disorders – etiology.   2. Neurotoxicity
Syndromes – diagnosis.   3. Movement Disorders – therapy.
4. Neurotoxicity Syndromes – therapy. WL 390]
RC376.5
616.8´3–dc23

2015008283

ISBN  978-1-107-06600-7  Hardback
ISBN  978-1-316-63681-7  Paperback

This book is dedicated to the memory of Stanley M. Aronson, MD, MPH, distinguished neuropathologist, founding dean of the Program in Medicine at Brown University, dean emeritus of the Alpert School of Medicine of Brown University, mentor and role model to generations, both in and outside the medical community.

# Contents

# Contributors

**Roongroj Bhidayasiri**
Chulalongkorn Center of Excellence on
Parkinson Disease & Related Disorders,
Department of Medicine, Faculty of Medicine,
Chulalongkorn University and King Chulalongkorn
Memorial Hospital, Thai Red Cross Society,
Bangkok, Thailand; Department of Neurology,
David Geffen School of Medicine at UCLA, Los
Angeles, CA, USA

**Kelvin L. Chou, MD**
Thomas H. and Susan C. Brown Early Career
Professor at the Department of Neurology, University
of Michigan, Ann Arbor, MI, USA

**Rob M.A. de Bie, MD PhD**
Neurologist at the Academic Medical Center,
University of Amsterdam, Amsterdam, the
Netherlands

**Atbin Djamashidian**
Department of Molecular Neuroscience and Reta Lila
Weston Institute for Neurological Studies, University
of London, London, UK

**Mark J. Edwards**
Sobell Department of Motor Neuroscience and
Movement Disorders, UCL Institute of Neurology,
University College London, UK

**Stewart A. Factor, DO**
Emory University, Department of Neurology,
Movement Disorder Program, Atlanta, GA, USA

**Gilles Fénelon, MD PhD**
AP-HP, Service de neurologie, Hôpital Henri
Mondor, Créteil, France; INSERM U955 E01, neu-
ropsychologie interventionnelle, Créteil, France;
Institut d'Etudes Cognitives, Ecole Normale
Supérieure (ENS), Paris, France

**Hubert H. Fernandez, MD**
Professor of Medicine (Neurology), Cleveland Clinic
Lerner College of Medicine, Head of Movement
Disorders, Center for Neurological Restoration,
Cleveland Clinic, OH, USA

**Joseph H. Friedman, MD**
The Stanley Aronson Chair in Neurodegenerative
Disorders at Butler Hospital, professor of Neurology
and chief of the division of Movement Disorders in
the Department of Neurology at the Alpert Medical
School of Brown University, Providence, RI; adjunct
professor in the School of Pharmacy at the University
of Rhode Island, Kingston, RI, USA

**Oscar S. Gershanik, MD**
Movement Disorders Unit, Institute of Neuroscience,
Favaloro Foundation University Hospital, Buenos
Aires, Argentina

**Israt Jahan, MD**
University of South Florida, Department of
Neurology, Parkinson's Disease and Movement
Disorder Center, James A. Haley Veteran's
Administration, Tampa, FL, USA

**Joseph Jankovic, MD**
Professor of Neurology, Distinguished Chair in
Movement Disorders, Director of Parkinson's Disease
Center, and Movement Disorders Clinic, Department
of Neurology, Baylor College of Medicine, Houston,
Texas

**Danna Jennings**
Institute for Neurodegenerative Disorders, New
Haven, CT, USA

**Tracy M. Jones, BSN ARNP**
University of South Florida, Department of
Neurology, Parkinson's Disease and Movement

Disorder Center, James A. Haley Veteran's Administration, Tampa, FL, USA

**Drew S. Kern, MD MSc**
Toronto Western Hospital, Morton and Gloria Shulman Movement Disorders Clinic and the Edmond J. Safra Program in Parkinson's Disease, Toronto, ON, Canada

**T.E. Kimber, MBBS [Hons] PhD FRACP**
Discipline of Medicine, The University of Adelaide; Department of Neurology, Royal Adelaide Hospital, Australia

**T.J. Kleinig, MBBS [Hons] BA PhD FRACP**
Discipline of Medicine, The University of Adelaide; Department of Neurology, Royal Adelaide Hospital, Australia

**Anthony E. Lang, OC MD FRCPC FAAN FCAHS FRSC**
Toronto Western Hospital, Morton and Gloria Shulman Movement Disorders Clinic and the Edmond J. Safra Program in Parkinson's Disease, Toronto, ON, Canada

**Peter A. Lewitt, MD MMedSc**
Departments of Neurology, Wayne State University School of Medicine, and Henry Ford Hospital, West Bloomfield, MI, USA

**Anne Marthe Meppelink**
Sobell Department of Motor Neuroscience and Movement Disorders, UCL Institute of Neurology, University College London, UK; Department of Neurology, University Medical Centre Groningen, Groningen, the Netherlands

**Dimitrios A. Nacopoulos, MD**
Fellow in Movement Disorders, Center for Neurological Restoration, Cleveland Clinic, OH, USA

**Sean S. O'Sullivan**
Department of Neurology, Cork University Hospital, University College, Cork, Ireland

**Pattamon Panyakaew**
Chulalongkorn Center of Excellence on Parkinson Disease & Related Disorders, Department of Medicine, Faculty of Medicine, Chulalongkorn University and King Chulalongkorn Memorial Hospital, Thai Red Cross Society, Bangkok, Thailand

**Raminder Parihar, MD**
Fellow in Movement Disorders, Department of Neurology, Beth Israel Deaconess Medical Center, Boston, MA, USA

**Juan Ramirez-Castaneda, MD**
Parkinson's Disease Center and Movement Disorders Clinic, Department of Neurology, Baylor College of Medicine, Houston, Texas

**Bernardo Rodrigues, MD**
Movement Disorders Fellow at the Department of Neurology, University of Michigan, Ann Arbor, MI, USA

**Marina Sanchez Abraham, MD**
Movement Disorders Unit, Institute of Neuroscience, Favaloro Foundation University Hospital, Buenos Aires, Argentina

**Michael R. Silver, MD**
Assistant Professor of Neurology at Emory University Hospital, Atlanta, GA, USA

**Daniel Tarsy, MD**
Professor in Neurology, Harvard Medical School, Director, Parkinson's Disease & Movement Disorders Center, Department of Neurology, Beth Israel Deaconess Medical Center, Boston, MA, USA

**P. D. Thompson, MBBS PhD FRACP**
Professor of Neurology, The University of Adelaide; Head, Department of Neurology, Royal Adelaide Hospital, Australia

**Theresa A. Zesiewicz, MD FAAN**
University of South Florida, Department of Neurology, Parkinson's Disease and Movement Disorder Center, James A. Haley Veteran's Administration, Tampa, FL, USA

# Introduction: medication-induced movement disorders

Joseph H. Friedman

Adverse drug events (ADE) are, unfortunately, very common events (Jha AK; Davey et al. 2008). They constituted over 2% of pediatric emergency visits to a Canadian hospital and 1.4% of admissions to a US hospital. ADE may be defined as an unwanted effect of the medication, whether anticipated or not, which is not due to a medical error.

Ascribing an ADE to a drug exposure is often difficult, especially in the setting of a rare reaction. A temporal relationship between starting a medication and experiencing a rare syndrome does not mean that the two are related. Nor does a seeming lack of temporal relationship indicate a lack of causality, as some effects may take weeks to months to appear. Ideally, one can follow the postulates Koch espoused for determining infectious etiologies: identify a syndrome, isolate the presumed causal agent, and demonstrate that this agent causes the same syndrome in other hosts. That, of course, is not always feasible, possible, or ethical.

Sometimes in the field of movement disorders the connection between drug and movement is straight-forward: lithium causes tremor, anticonvulsants cause ataxia, clozapine causes asterixis, etc. In some cases this has been less straightforward, as the history of the recognition of the tardive syndromes makes clear. Many years elapsed before the connection between neuroleptics and tardive dyskinesia was made, partly because, unlike other movement disorder adverse effects, this did not resolve when the offending medication was stopped. More unusual was the obser-vation that the movements typically got worse when the dose was reduced and improved when the dose was increased, which seemed paradoxical for an ADE. Compounding the difficulty was the longstanding association between psychotic behaviors and

movement disorders, that long predated the use of antipsychotic drugs.

Movement disorder side effects may go unnoticed, as is often the case with parkinsonism or tardive dyskinesia, but usually the side effects are perceived and are often troublesome. Some disorders are flagrant and life threatening, as with neuroleptic malignant syndrome and serotonin syndrome, while some are functionally disabling, although not "medically" serious, as is often the case with tremor. In middle aged and older patients, the development of a parkinsonian syndrome, perhaps from psychiatric or gastrointestinal motility drugs, raises the always worrisome concern about the unmasking of idiopathic PD. These issues are often important, first requiring recognition, then appropriate evaluation and treatment, when possible.

ADEs have a special place in the field of movement disorders. The field of movement disorders really began in the 1970s, and initially focused primarily on two major problems, Parkinson's disease and neuroleptic-induced movement disorders. There was a mirror image symmetry between the disciplines of neurology and psychiatry with these disorders, for the treatment of motor problems in Parkinson's disease caused the psychotic symptoms of hallucinations and delusions, while the treatment of hallucinations and delusions in psychotic patients caused motor signs that exactly replicated those of idiopathic Parkinson's disease. In addition, chronic treatment of PD with L-Dopa induced dyskinesias, which were often quite similar to the tardive syndromes induced by longstanding use of dopamine receptor antago-nists. And the early approaches to the treatment of PD and schizophrenia developed in parallel as well, with some neurologists advocating titrating doses of

L-Dopa until dyskinesias appeared, then reducing slightly, while some psychiatrists advocated increasing doses of neuroleptics until parkinsonism appeared. Both approaches now are considered outdated, and the appearance of parkinsonism is no longer viewed as a goal, since its occurrence was clearly divorced from antipsychotic effects with the development of clozapine.

It is not rare for patients to have suffered with movement disorders for years before the connection with a chronic medication was recognized. Certainly the number of lawsuits based on excessively long use of metoclopramide and prochlorperazine supports this unfortunate connection. This book will hopefully help reduce these problems. It is not always possible to follow the first commandment of medical practice, primum non nocere, but certainly we can always be alert to identifying and then reducing that harm.

Acknowledgements to Drs. M.S. Abraham and O. Gershanik for their helpful suggestions.

## References

1. Naranjo CA, Busto U, Sellers EM, Sandor P, Ruiz I, et al. A method for estimating the probability of adverse drug reactions. *Clin Pharacol Ther* 1981; **30**:239–45.

2. Meyboom RHB, Royer RJ. Causality classification in pharmacovigilance centres in the European Community. *Pharmacoepidemiol Drug Saf* 1992; **1**:87–97.

**Chapter**

**1**

# Acute akathisia

Drew S. Kern and Anthony E. Lang

## Introduction

Akathisia, a term coined by Ladislav Haksovec in 1901 from the Greek meaning "not to sit," is an inner sensation of restlessness that is alleviated by movement.[1] It was first described in patients with Parkinson's disease (PD); however, it is more commonly considered an adverse effect of antipsychotics (neuroleptics). Akathisia is the most common and distressing symptom in patients administered antipsychotics.

## Clinical presentation

Patients with akathisia commonly develop both subjective and objective symptoms. The recently revised Diagnostic and Statistical Manual of Mental Disorders, Fifth Edition (DSM-V) defines medication-induced akathisia as a syndrome with subjective symptoms often accompanied by objective findings.[2] Subjective symptoms are described as an inner tension, anxiety, irritability, discomfort, restlessness, or sleeplessness. The objective findings include movements that are semivolitional, purposeful and suppressible, repetitive, complex, and stereotypical. Patients with akathisia are unable to remain motionless and present as restless. These movements are most commonly evident in the legs, seen as crossing and uncrossing, swinging one leg lateral to medial or anterior to posterior, or pacing. Other movements include rubbing the scalp or anterior thighs, rocking while sitting, swaying while standing, swinging arms, and changing positions from sitting to standing. Forty percent of patients notice improvement in the supine position and worsening when standing compared with sitting.[3]

Typically the symptoms of akathisia are generalized; however, there are rare case reports of focal akathisia. An unusual presentation of akathisia affecting the oral and genital regions described as extremely uncomfortable and with burning pain has also been reported.[4] In addition, patients may make noises, including moaning and grunting. It is debatable whether these vocalizations are due to discomfort or are a component of akathisia with the purpose of providing subjective relief.

Akathisia is a distressing and disabling condition affecting an individual's quality of life. Acute akathisia often will result in noncompliance and may be associated with new onset suicidal ideation. It is possible that patients with underlying psychiatric disease are less able to cope with the distressing symptoms of akathisia, increasing the potential for suicide. However, there are rare reports of suicidal thoughts manifesting in patients with no history of mental illness. Consequently, clinicians need to be aware of this potential risk and monitor patients diligently.

## Diagnosis

Accurate diagnosis of akathisia is challenging and the disorder is likely underdiagnosed. Some patients, especially those with mental illness or dementia, and children, may lack the ability to communicate subjective symptoms of akathisia effectively. Symptoms may also be minimal, not reaching a threshold of concern by the patient to warrant discussion with the physician. In addition, akathisia severity can vary greatly and symptoms may be delayed, intermittent, or suppressed. This may result in objective symptoms being minimal or absent during a physician appointment. In research studies designed to evaluate effectiveness of treatment, potential adverse effects may not be fully evaluated. Therefore, in a brief examination, when other concerns and symptoms are evaluated, it is

*Medication-Induced Movement Disorders*, ed. Joseph H. Friedman. Published by Cambridge University Press.
© Cambridge University Press 2015.

possible to not recognize akathisia and the true prevalence may be underreported.

Patients with mental illness including bipolar disorder, depression, and schizophrenia may present with psychosis mimicking akathisia. Distinguishing akathisia from underlying psychiatric symptoms is difficult and misinterpretation may result in inappropriate medical management. For example, a patient with acute akathisia misinterpreted as having worsening of psychosis may be prescribed higher dosages of antipsychotics with resultant worsening of symptoms due to escalation of the offending medication. Akathisia may also overlap with psychiatric symptoms, making distinguishing between them nearly impossible. Akathisia may be associated with other "extrapyramidal" side effects including parkinsonism and tardive dyskinesias, though it has been reported to be less commonly present with oral tardive dyskinesias. Finally, recreational drugs such as cocaine may induce symptoms that appear to be akathitic in nature but other symptoms not consistent with akathisia also manifest, including psychomotor agitation and an altered level of consciousness.

It remains unclear whether the "jitteriness/anxiety syndrome" and akathisia are separate entities or part of a spectrum. Jitteriness/anxiety syndrome is a poorly characterized syndrome described in patients treated with selective serotonin reuptake inhibitors (SSRI) and tricyclic antidepressants. There is great variation in symptoms, including insomnia, anxiety, irritability, hypomania, and restlessness, that may also cause the urge to move. There is also variability in onset of presentation with the majority of symptoms occurring within two weeks of the start of antidepressants. Some authors have even incorporated akathisia as an essential component of the definition of jitteriness/anxiety syndrome.

Additionally, there are a number of movement disorders that mimic akathisia, including restless leg syndrome (RLS), stereotypies, tics, paradoxical dystonia (dystonia relieved with movement), punding, and withdrawal syndromes. RLS is characterized by an urge to move and unpleasant sensations in the legs predominately occurring in the evening and in repose. Relief is obtained by moving the affected limbs. In comparison, akathisia is much more generalized, does not have a diurnal component, and is often less in the lying position. Stereotypies are involuntary, typically continuous and repetitive non–goal directed movements that often begin prior to the age of two years.

Examples include hand waving, head nodding, head banging, covering of ears, chewing movements, and pacing. This disorder is most often seen in patients with developmental disorders including autism and Rett syndrome. Tics can be simple or complex, motor or phonic, often brought on by an urge to perform gestures with relief upon making them. In comparison, akathisia has a more restless feature to the movements. Punding is a compulsive behavior of repetitive, purposeless movements often involving mechanical tasks including shuffling, sorting, arranging and re-organizing environments, disassembly and assembly of items, and collecting objects. Patients with punding do not express an inner sense of restlessness as occurs in akathisia.

There is no universally held consensus on the diagnosis of akathisia. Diagnosis is most accurately made using both subjective and objective findings and a classification system of akathisia has been proposed based upon these.[5] Medication-induced akathisia is categorized into subtypes including acute, tardive, and withdrawal tardive. Acute akathisia is commonly defined as subjective and objective restlessness of $\leq$ 6 months duration often coinciding with the onset of starting, increasing, or changing to a more potent medication. Medication-induced acute akathisia decreases with drug reduction. In contrast, tardive akathisia occurs late in the treatment course without any provocation. An arbitrary duration is commonly considered as greater than three months. Analogous to tardive dyskinesias, tardive akathisia may worsen with abrupt drug withdrawal (in contrast to acute akathisia) and is challenging to treat. Withdrawal tardive akathisia is subjective, and objective restlessness presents within days to weeks after drug reduction or withdrawal. An arbitrary cutoff is 6 weeks. Chronic akathisia is not a distinct subtype. This refers to the duration of symptoms being more prolonged, typically greater than three months. It may have an acute, tardive, or withdrawal onset; however, the literature is inconsistent, often combining tardive, chronic, and withdrawal akathisia. "Pseudoakathisia" is a term used to describe motor restlessness unaccompanied by subjective symptoms and may be a symptom on a spectrum of akathisia or, in many patients, is probably a form of tardive dyskinesia, sometimes called "tardive stereotypy." The pathophysiology of the akathisia subtypes likely differs based upon variability of treatment effects and symptomatology. Most cases of akathisia are acute. The severity of subjective symptoms in acute akathisia may not significantly differ compared with tardive (chronic) akathisia. However, it is claimed that objective motor findings are more severe in acute akathisia although many patients with tardive akathisia can have very striking clinical features.[6] Therefore, clear definitions are needed for our current and future understanding akathisia.

There are several scales used to measure akathisia and the response to treatment.[7] The Barnes Akathisia Rating Scale (BARS) is an assessment composed of subjective, objective, and distress aspects of akathisia and has a high inter-rater reliability. The total score ranges from 0 to 9 with higher scores representing more severe akathisia. The Prince Henry Hospital Rating Scale of Akathisia (PHH) is a comprehensive diagnostic and grading instrument using duration and intensity of akathisia in rating. An abridged version of the PHH has also been developed with a 100% sensitivity and 99% specificity to PHH.[8] The Hillside-Akathisia-Scale (HAS) was designed to evaluate the frequency and severity of akathisia in clinical psychopharmacological research. There is no consensus on the best scale to use, although the BARS is the most commonly applied.

# Pathogenesis

Despite longstanding recognition of akathisia, its pathophysiology is not fully understood. It is likely that multiple complex pathways are involved and that more than one pathophysiological mechanism can result in akathisia. Since akathisia is predominately induced by antipsychotics and it often occurs in association with other "extrapyramidal" symptoms, much research has focused on the dopaminergic system either directly or indirectly.

Blockade of dopamine D2 receptors is believed to be a major factor in the pathophysiology of akathisia. Antipsychotics are potent D2 antagonists and are associated with the greatest risk of akathisia. Studies using positron emission tomography (PET) imaging have demonstrated that akathisia is associated with high degrees of antagonism of D2 receptors in the basal ganglia.[9] In patients with schizophrenia, D2 occupancy of greater than 78% was associated with extrapyramidal symptoms including haloperidol-induced akathisia.[10] However, this theory fails to explain other causes of akathisia, including antidepressants, dopamine depleting drugs, and PD. Furthermore, antipsychotics with low D2 potency, including clozapine and quetiapine,

are also known to induce akathisia. Consequently, other theories need to be considered.

Akathisia also may involve antagonism of two dopaminergic pathways originating in the midbrain: the mesocortical system with projections from the ventral tegmental area (VTA) to the frontal lobes, and the mesolimbic pathway with connections from the VTA to the nucleus accumbens.[11] In animal models, bilateral lesions of the VTA result in locomotor hyperactivity.[12] Furthermore, haloperidol administration produces an increase of neuronal activation determined by increased Fos (the protein produced from the immediate early gene *c-fos* and marker to visualize the pattern on neuronal activity in the CNS) neuronal expression in regions with high D2 expression, including the prefrontal cortex, striatum, nucleus accumbens, lateral septal nucleus, and dorsolateral striatum. Pretreatment with propranolol (an effective treatment for akathisia; see treatment section below) reduced the number of Fos-positive nuclei within the cortex, piriform cortex, and parietal cortex.[13] The nucleus accumbens is composed of two regions: the core and surface portions. Akathisia may result as a consequence of an imbalance between these two. The surface portion is involved in unconditional defense behaviors and receives noradrenergic input from the locus coeruleus. Reduced dopaminergic input from the VTA to the core portion permits unopposed stimulation of the surface portion from the locus coeruleus. Consequently, beta blockers may act by inhibiting this input. Theoretically, the mesocortical pathway may also be hyperactive due to impaired feedback mechanisms, as D1 receptors that predominate in the cortex, especially the orbitofrontal cortex, are less inhibited by antipsychotics. The orbitofrontal cortex also stimulates the locus coeruleus, further increasing noradrenergic input to the surface portion of the nucleus accumbens (see Figure 1.1). However, direct evidence for impairment of this system is lacking, and it fails to explain akathisia occurring with SSRIs and in PD.

The existence of SSRI-induced akathisia suggests that the serotoninergic system is also involved. The role of 5-HT2 receptors in the pathophysiology of akathisia is supported by the presence of these receptors in the VTA, the response of akathisia to 5HT2A antagonists, and treatment failure of buspiron, a 5-HT1a partial agonist, and granisetron, a 5-HT3 receptor antagonist (see treatment section below).[14,15] The dorsal raphe nucleus has serotonergic projections directly to

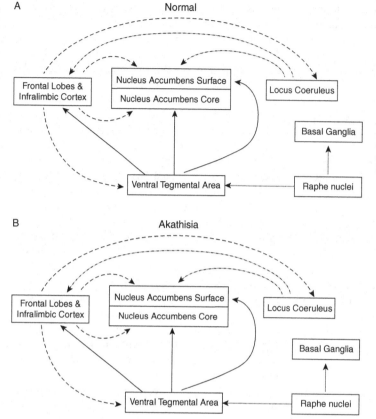

**Figure 1.1** Schematic proposal of pathways comparing normal (A) to akathisia (B). Reduced dopaminergic stimulation from the ventral tegmental area (VTA) may create unopposed stimulation of the pathway from the locus coeruleus to the surface portion of the nucleus accumbens. Thickness of arrows represent strength of input. Increased thickness of the serotonin input in bottom right corner of figure (B) exclusively relates to possible explanation of selective serotonin reuptake inhibitors (SSRI)-induced akathisia. Blue arrows = noradrenergic, Green arrows = glutamatergic, Red arrows = serotonergic, Black arrows = dopaminergic. Figure adapted from 11,86.

the basal ganglia inhibiting dopaminergic neurons, potentially via 5-HT2 receptors. The midbrain raphe nuclei also projects inhibitory serotonergic input to the VTA and substantia nigra. Studies evaluating SSRI-induced inhibition of the dopamine system have provided inconsistent results. This may relate to the varying distribution of different serotonin receptors in the midbrain and basal ganglia.

## Etiologies

Akathisia is most often iatrogenic, caused by antipsychotic medications, but also by SSRI antidepressants. Medication-induced acute akathisia typically begins within hours of administering the offending drug but may be delayed up to several days after initiation, during escalation of treatment, or upon switching to a more potent dopamine receptor blocking agent. There are several other etiologies of acute akathisia that have also been reported (see Table 1.1).

## Antipsychotics

Antipsychotics have been classified into two categories: first generation (typical) and second generation (atypical) antipsychotics. This classification system was originally developed partially by the pharmaceutical industry with the expectation that newer developed antipsychotics created in the 1990s would have less extrapyramidal adverse effects compared with the traditional first generation antipsychotics developed in the 1950s. First generation antipsychotics are potent dopamine D2 antagonists. In contrast, second generation antipsychotics, which are also D2 antagonists, are characterized by relatively low-affinity or rapid dissociation from D2 receptors and are potent antagonists of serotonin 5HT2A receptors (see Table 1.2).

Second generation antipsychotics are thought to be less prone to cause extrapyramidal symptoms, including akathisia, due to lower affinity for D2 receptors, although clinical evidence is conflicting. However, they do have more antimuscarinic and antiadrenergic activity, resulting in greater sedation and hypotension compared with first generation antipsychotics. For example, the risk of akathisia with haloperidol, a first generation antipsychotic, may be as high as 75%, while it is approximately 5% with clozapine, a second generation antipsychotic.[16] In a three arm double blind 8-week treatment study, akathisia developed in 19% and 22% of patients treated with second generation antipsychotics, olanzapine and risperidone, respectively, in comparison to 45% of patients treated with the first generation agent, molindone, with 18% of patients in this treatment arm reporting moderate to severe symptoms.[17] Furthermore, in comparing medications within the second generation class, those with higher D2 affinity are more likely to cause akathisia. Certain D2 receptor blockers are used as antiemetics, particularly chlorpromazine and prochlorperazine. In the emergency department, the incidence of akathisia with these medications has been reported to be 44%.[18]

Acute akathisia is the most common important adverse effect of antipsychotics. The reported incidence of antipsychotic-induced akathisia (AIA) ranges greatly, from 8%–76%, but more conservative estimates utilizing clear subjective and objective findings report an incidence of 20%–30%.[19] As noted above, accurate epidemiological data comes from studies using validated rating scales that include subjective and objective findings to consistently diagnose akathisia. Other causes of inaccurate prevalence estimates include the facts that patients are less inclined to spontaneously report milder

**Table 1.1** Etiologies of acute akathisia

Medications:
Antipsychotics (including metoclopramide, prochlorperazine & droperidol)
SSRI antidepressants
Mood stabilizers (lithium)
Catecholamine-depleting agents (tetrabenazine & reserpine)
Antiepileptics (carbamazepine, ethosuximide, gabapentin & pregabalin*)
Calcium channel blockers and antihistamines (flunarizine, cinnarizine)
Calcium channel blocker (diltiazem)*

Toxic:
Central stimulants (amphetamine and cocaine)*

Neurodegenerative:
Parkinson's disease
Spinocerebellar ataxia 3*
Wilson's disease*

Structural
Traumatic brain injury*
Encephalitis*
Stroke*

* Case reports or series

**Table 1.2** D2 receptor affinity of commonly used first and second generation antipsychotic medications divided into low, medium, and high potency

| First Generation | | Second Generation | | |
| --- | --- | --- | --- | --- |
| Low (8–16) | High (1–4) | Low (126–380) | Medium (20) | High (2–6) |
| Chlorpromazine | Haloperidol | Clozapine | Olanzapine | Risperidone |
| Levomepromazine | Fluphenazine | Quetiapine | | Paliperidone |
| Mesoridazine | Loxapine | | | Aripiprazole * |
| Periciazine | Molindone | | | Ziprasidone |
| Pipamperone | Perphenazine | | | Amisulpride |
| Thioridazine | Pimozide | | | Lurasidone |
| | Thiothixene | | | Iloperidone |
| | Zuclopenthixol | | | Cariprazine * |

Ranges reported as Ki. * denominate agonists

symptoms to care providers, and symptoms of akathisia may be misinterpreted as psychiatric symptoms. In a study of 100 patients taking antipsychotics for two weeks, 40% developed mild akathisia that did not require a change in therapy. Moderate to severe symptoms necessitating change or reduction of medication were evident in 21% of patients.[20]

The CATIE (Clinical Antipsychotic Trials of Intervention Effectiveness) study included 1493 patients with schizophrenia randomly assigned to receive ziprasidone (40–160mg/day), olanzapine (7.5–30mg/day), perphenazine (8–32mg/day), quetiapine (200–800mg/day), or risperidone (1.5–6mg/day) for up to 18 months. Surprisingly, this study did not demonstrate significant difference in the incidence of akathisia among the various treatment groups, which ranged from 5%–9%.[21] The lack of difference between first and second generation antipsychotics in this study may partially be the effect of underreporting of mild symptoms (BARS score of ≥ 3) or maybe the fact that all subjects had been taking neuroleptics for long periods of time with only a short washout before enrolling in the study.

Several potential risks factors for the development of AIA have been reported. As previously noted, one of the greatest risks is increasing dosage or switching to more potent medications with greater D2 affinity. A number of studies have also identified an association between other extrapyramidal symptoms and the development of akathisia, indicating that they often occur together; but one does not necessarily predict the occurrence of the other. Patients with bipolar disorder may have twice the risk of developing AIA as patients with schizophrenia.[22] Homozygosity for the Ser9Gly variant of the dopamine D3 receptor (DRD3) gene has been identified in eight of nine patients with schizophrenia and AIA.[23] Interestingly, DRD3 receptors are mainly localized in mesolimbic brain regions and therefore may play a role in the pathogenesis of acute akathisia. In addition, the TaqI_D polymorphism in the DRD2 gene was significantly associated with akathisia in patients treated on antipsychotics. For each extra C-allele a 2.3% times higher risk of having akathisia was found.[24]

Results are inconsistent with respect to several other reported risk factors. Smoking tobacco has been proposed to be protective against akathisia; however, a study of 250 patients with schizophrenia failed to demonstrate any association between akathisia and heavy smoking.[25] There is conflicting data regarding women having a potentially increased risk of AIA. Sandyk and Kay (1990) reported in schizophrenic hospitalized patients that akathisia was more common in women compared with men, although they did not separate acute and tardive akathisia.[26] However, most epidemiology studies have failed to identify any significant gender difference in the occurrence of AIA. Age and race are not associated with akathisia.[20] It is possible that low iron stores increase the risk of AIA. Several studies have been performed supporting this finding. Serum iron and ferritin levels were compared in 33 patients with AIA and 23 patients on antipsychotics without akathisia. Patients with AIA had significantly lower serum ferritin levels, although the differences were small and levels were within a normal range. There was no correlation between serum iron or ferritin levels and akathisia ratings.[27] However, other studies contradict these findings. Two prospective studies failed to demonstrate any differences in serum iron and transferrin levels between patients with and without AIA.[28]

Below we will provide more detail on selected commonly prescribed second generation agents. Table 1.3 summarizes information on AIA induced by other second generation medications not discussed below.

**Clozapine** – There are relatively few reports of AIA induced by clozapine. In one, hospitalized schizophrenic patients were enrolled in a double blind multicenter study aimed at comparing treatment with clozapine (N=75) to chlorpromazine (N=76). Akathisia occurred in comparable numbers of clozapine and chlorpromazine treated patients, 5 and 4, respectively. However, other extrapyramidal symptoms including rigidity, tremor, and dystonia were much less common in the clozapine treated group.[29] In a nonrandomized, nonblinded study of patients with a variety of psychiatric disorders the prevalence of akathisia was 39% with clozapine compared with 45% in patients treated with miscellaneous antipsychotics. A greater number of patients taking first generation antipsychotics had severe akathisia.[30] Selection bias was a limitation, as those treated with clozapine had more severe mental illness and often had previously failed conventional medications. In addition, the dose of clozapine was higher from other studies reporting a 7% incidence of akathisia.[31] The majority of patients treated with clozapine had been previously tried on other antipsychotics and it is unclear whether this past exposure increases the risk of developing AIA.

**Table 1.3** Summary miscellaneous second generation antipsychotic-induced akathisia

| Medication | Study Design | Dosage | Incidence | Reference |
|---|---|---|---|---|
| Paliperidone | Case Report | 37.5mg biweekly | – | 64 |
| Aripiprazole | RCT and case reports | 2–24mg/day | 23% | 42,65,66 |
| Ziprasidone | RCT and case reports | 80–160mg/day | 36% | 67,68 |
| Amisulpride | Prospective studies and case reports | ~ 400mg/day | 11% | 69,70 |
| Lurasidone | RCT | 20–120mg/day | 11–24% | 71,72 |
| Iloperidone | RCT | 4–24mg/day | 1–9% | 73 |
| Cariprazine | RCT | 1.5–4.5mg/day | 10% | 74 |

RCT = Randomized controlled trial

**Quetiapine** – Overall, similar to clozapine, quetiapine is generally well tolerated with only case reports of akathisia that typically have resolved with reduction of dosage. Data combined from four randomized double blind 3-week to 12-week studies of 1003 patients with bipolar disorder indicated that extrapyramidal symptoms, including akathisia, were comparable between quetiapine and placebo.[32] Furthermore, patients with AIA who switched from conventional antipsychotics to quetiapine (400–800mg/day) have reported resolution of symptoms.[20]

**Olanzapine** – A pooled analysis from four randomized, open label, parallel trials of 6 weeks in patients with schizophrenia compared olanzapine 5–20mg/day (N=77) to chlorpromazine 200–800mg/day (N=32). Akathisia was reported in 2.4% in the olanzapine and 10% of the chlorpromazine groups.[33] Similar results were reported from a 12-week study comparing olanzapine monotherapy with the combination of olanzapine and other antipsychotics, antidepressants, or mood stabilizers. Three percent of patients in the olanzapine monotherapy group experienced akathisia compared to twice this in the combination medication group.[34] Similar to oral formulations, intramuscular olanzapine injections were also well tolerated with low risk of akathisia.

**Risperidone** – In a comparison double blind 8-week study involving 296 patients, akathisia was reported in 26% treated with risperidone compared with 32% receiving haloperidol at similar strengths.[16] Risperidone appears to carry a slightly higher risk of developing severe akathisia necessitating medication adjustments compared with second generation antipsychotics with less D2 receptor affinity.[35]

## Other Dopamine Antagonists

Antiemetics are also a cause of akathisia. Metoclopramide is a presynaptic D2 antagonist prescribed as an antiemetic and intestinal prokinetic. There are several reports of metoclopramide-induced akathisia. It remains unclear if the rate of infusion is associated with risk of akathisia. A randomized double blind study comparing slow intravenous infusion of metoclopramide at 20mg over 15 min (N=102) compared with a bolus of 20mg (N=103) found no difference in development of akathisia (12% in both groups).[36] In contrast, another randomized prospective double blind study of 10mg metoclopramide in bolus (N=36) or slow infusion over 15 minutes (N=32) reported an incidence of 11% in the bolus treated group while none of the patients in the slow infusion group experienced akathisia.[37] Droperidol, an antidopaminergic used as an antiemetic, but more often for induction of anesthesia and sedation, has also been reported to result in acute dystonia and akathisia.[38]

## Antidepressants

Selective serotonin reuptake inhibitors (SSRI) including fluoxetine, paroxetine, sertraline, fluvoxamine, and citalopram are associated with akathisia. Fluoxetine is reported to have the greatest risk of akathisia among the SSRIs with an incidence of 9.8%–25%. It is possible that the incidence with newer SSRIs will increase as we gain experience. Similar to antipsychotics, the onset of SSRI-related akathisia typically occurs within 1 week of starting medication. Risk factors for the development of akathisia include simultaneous use of antipsychotics and higher SSRI dosages. Individuals with variant alleles in the CYP450 gene (involved in the metabolism of antidepressants) may be at increased risk of violent behavior when they develop akathisia.[39]

Other antidepressants and mood stabilizers have also been associated with akathisia. Atomoxetine, a selective norepinephrine reuptake inhibitor used in the treatment of attention-deficit/hyperactivity disorder (ADHD), has been reported to cause akathisia in a patient receiving a dose of 18 mg/day.[40] Venlafaxine has serotonergic properties at low dose and noradrenergic effects at higher doses. Akathisia was reported in a single patient treated with venlafaxine XR 150mg/day with resolution of symptoms in response to biperidin 4 mg/day.[41] Lithium has been reported to be associated with akathisia. In a double blind 52-week study comparing lithium to aripiprazole, nine of 159 patients treated with lithium experienced akathisia compared with 24 of 154 with aripiprazole.[42]

## Miscellaneous Medications

Cinnarizine and flunarizine (calcium channel blockers and antihistamines) have been reported to cause akathisia as well as concurrent dystonia, orofacial tremor, parkinsonism, and even acute dystonic reactions, possibly supporting a dopamine antagonist effect.[43] There are rare case reports of diltiazem, a calcium channel blocker, inducing akathisia. Tetrabenazine (often used in the treatment of tardive akathisia) and reserpine, catecholamine-depleting medications, have also been associated with akathisia with an estimated incidence of 7%–15%.[44] Finally, gabapentin and pregabalin (GABA analogs) have been reported to be associated with akathisia in case reports.[45]

## Treatment

As in the other section of this chapter, we will limit our discussion on treatment to the management of acute akathisia. The treatment of chronic tardive akathisia is distinctly different and generally similar to that of other tardive syndromes, which are covered elsewhere in this volume. There are two main treatment strategies for medication-induced acute akathisia: modification of the drug regimen and the addition of antiakathitic medications. The first treatment strategy should be to identify the offending medication and to withdraw this if possible. In situations where this is not possible, a dose reduction or switching to a less potent D2 blocking agent is recommended.

Unlike tardive akathisia, acute akathisia typically responds well to this approach. However, in severe acute akathisia or where drug adjustments are not possible, it may be necessary to treat with medication. The most commonly used medications in the treatment of AIA are antiadrenergics (β-adrenergic antagonists and α-2-agonists) and anticholinergics, while other treatments have also been investigated (see Table 1.4). A problem in the literature regarding treatment of AIA is that the majority of studies are small with short duration of follow-up and often combine akathisia subtypes. Studies are open-labeled, and given the marked response these patients have to placebo, interpretation must be made cautiously. We have summarized many studies on AIA treatment in Table 1.4.

**Antiadrenergics** – β-blockers are the most widely used treatment for akathisia. These medications are classified based on the type of β-receptors antagonized (selective β-1 or β-2 and nonselective blocking both types) and lipophilicity with more lipophilic medications having greater blood-brain barrier penetration. Propranolol, a lipophilic nonselective β-blocker, has been used as a first-line antiakathisia agent for more than two decades with approximately 70% positive response rate. Symptomatic improvement may be seen within 24 hours of starting; the typical dosage range is 60–120mg/day divided twice daily.[46,47] The duration of benefit is unknown but sustained effects of several months have been reported. Pindolol, a lipophilic nonselective β-blocker and partial 5HT1A receptor antagonist, has been reported to be efficacious in 4 of 9 patients with drug-induced akathisia.[48] In those who did not respond, benefit was obtained with propranolol. Metoprolol (75m/day) and betaxolol (5–20mg), lipophilic selective β-1 antagonists, are effective treatments with comparable results to propranolol. A specific lipophilic β-2 antagonist that was subsequently withdrawn from production, ICI 118,551, demonstrated significant improvement of AIA compared to placebo in a double blind study. In contrast to lipophilic β-blockers, the hydrophilic selective and nonselective β-antagonists, including nadolol, sotalolol, and atenolol, are less effective.[46,47]

**α2 adrenergic agonist** – A number of reports have indicated that clonidine, a central acting α-2 receptor agonist, may be effective in treating akathisia. Maximal beneficial effects are noted within 48 hours of starting medication with dosages ranging from 0.15–0.8 mg/day titrated to beneficial effects.[46] The use of clonidine

**Table 1.4** Summary of treatment studies of acute akathisia

| Medication | Study Design (number of studies) | N | Mean Dose (mg/day) | Outcome | Ref. |
|---|---|---|---|---|---|
| *Antiadrenergics* | | | | | |
| Propranolol | Double blind placebo crossover studies (2) | 32 | 20–60 | All patients noted improvement | 46,47 |
| | Double blind crossover & unblinded parallel D-propranolol & placebo study | 11 | D-propranolol 80 and D/L-propranolol 80 | No improvement in D-propranolol and placebo but 8 patients subsequently treated with D/L-propranolol noted significant improvement of symptoms | 46,47 |
| | Single blind crossover lorazepam (2mg) & placebo study | 6 | 20–30 | All patients demonstrated benefit | 46,47 |
| | Open studies (4) | 46 | 30–160 | All studies reported patients responded with a combined response rate of 81% | 46,47 |
| Pindolol | Open study | 9 | 5 | 4 patients with benefit | 46,47 |
| Metoprolol | Single blinded crossover propranolol (60mg) study | 8 | 75 | 6 patients had equivalent benefit with either β-blocker | 46,47 |
| | Unblinded crossover study with propranolol (15–80mg) | 5 | 200–400 | All patients demonstrated benefit comparable to propranolol | 46,47 |
| | Open study | 9 | 50–100 | All patients noted benefit | 46,47 |
| Betaxolol | Double blind crossover with propranolol (20–40mg) | 19 | 10 | Equivalent beneficial results to propranolol | 46,47 |
| | Open crossover with propranolol (60mg) | 8 | 5 | Equivalent beneficial results to propranolol | 46,47 |
| | Unblinded open study | 16 | 10–20 | Improvement in 10 of 16 patients | 46,47 |

**Table 1.4** (cont.)

| Medication | Study Design (number of studies) | N | Mean Dose (mg/day) | Outcome | Ref. |
|---|---|---|---|---|---|
| *α2 adrenergic agonist* | | | | | |
| Clonidine | Single blind trials (2) | 12 | 0.15–0.8 | Noted benefit but sedation reported as an adverse effect | 46,47 |
| *Anticholinergics* | | | | | |
| Benztropine | Double blind crossover propranolol (1mg iv) & placebo study | 6 | 2 mg iv | Greatest benefit evident in subjective findings | 46,47 |
| | Open studies (2) | 16 | 1.5–6 | Mixed results of minimal to significant improvement | 46,47 |
| | Open study including trihexyphenidyl (<15mg/day) | 32 | <8 | 14 of 32 patients with complete resolution | 46,47 |
| | Double blind vs benztropine (N=11) vs amantadine (N=13; 200mg) study | 11 | 2–8 | Improvement in all patients in both treatment groups | 46,47 |
| | Unblinded co-administration propranolol (30–60mg) trial in mixed subtype akathisia (9 AIA) | 19 | 2–4 im | Improvement in subjective and objective assessments | 75 |
| | Unblinded benztropine (N=8) and propranolol (N=9; 40–80mg) parallel study | 8 | 1.5–4 | 50% improvement in assessments of akathisia in both groups | 46,47 |
| Biperiden | Double blind biperiden (N=15) vs placebo (N=15) controlled study | 15 | 10 im | No significant difference between placebo, 7 patients in the biperiden and 5 in the placebo group responded | 49 |
| | Open study | 23 | 5 | All patients had complete resolution of akathisia | 76 |
| | Case report | 1 | 10 | Resolution of symptoms | 77 |

**Benzodiazepines**

| | | | | | |
|---|---|---|---|---|---|
| Diazepam | Open clinical trials (2) | 31 | 5 iv & 15 po | Overall effect of 75% | 46,47 |
| | Double blind diazepam (N=9) vs diphenhydramine (N=11; 50mg) study | 9 | 5 | Mean ratings significantly improved for both treatments | 46,47 |
| | Case report | 1 | 15 | Resolution of symptoms | 46,47 |
| Lorazepam | Case report | 1 | 2 | Resolution of symptoms | 46,47 |
| | Open study | 16 | 2–3 | 14 patients had benefit | 46,47 |
| Clonazepam | Double blind clonazepam (N=7) vs placebo (N=7) controlled study | 7 | 1 | All patients in the clonazepam group had significant improvement of akathisia and 4 of the 7 patients in the placebo cohort subsequently treated in an open trial of clonazepam obtained marked benefit | 46,47,78 |
| | Double blind clonazepam (N=6) vs placebo (N=6) controlled study | 12 | 0.5–2.5 | 71% improvement in rating scales in clonazepam treated patients | 78 |
| | Double blind clonazepam (N=8) vs trihexyphenidyl or promethazine (N=6) | 8 | 1.5 | All patients in the clonazepam treated cohort demonstrated improvement | 78 |
| | Open studies (2) | 31 | 0.5–3 | Significant improvement in akathisia | 46,47, 78 |
| | Case report co-administered baclofen (15mg) | 1 | 1.5 | Marked improvement in subjective and objective symptoms | 78 |
| Midazolam | Double blind midazolam (N=28) vs diphenhydramine (N=28; 20mg) metoclopramide-induced akathisia parallel study | 28 | 2 iv | Midazolam improved symptoms within 15 min while diphenhydramine took 60 min | 52 |

**Table 1.4** (cont.)

| Medication | Study Design (number of studies) | N | Mean Dose (mg/day) | Outcome | Ref. |
|---|---|---|---|---|---|
| | Double blind midazolam (N=75) vs diphenhydramine (N=75; 20mg) & placebo (N=75) prophylactic metoclopramide-induced akathisia trial | 75 | 1.5 iv | Midazolam reduced the risk of akathisia while diphenhydramine and placebo did not | 55 |
| *Serotonin 2a agonists* | | | | | |
| Cyproheptadine | Double blind cyproheptadine (N=18) vs propranolol (N=12; 80mg) study | 18 | 16 | Equivalent improvement between both treatments | 79 |
| | Open study | 17 | 16 | All patients demonstrated improvement | 80 |
| Ritanserin | Single blind trial | 10 | 13.5 | Effective treatment in 8 of 10 patients | 81 |
| Mianserin | Double blind mianserin (N=15) placebo (N=15) controlled study | 15 | 15 | Objective and subjective improvement | 82 |
| | Double blind mianserin (N=20) vs placebo (N=17) & vitamin B6 (N=23; 1200mg/day) controlled study | 20 | 15 | Only subjective improvements reported in treatment groups | 83 |
| Mirtazapine | Double blind mirtazapine (N=13) vs placebo (N=13) controlled study | 13 | 15 | 7 of 13 patients responded to treatment with 5 of them reporting complete resolution of symptoms | 84 |
| | Double blind mirtazapine (N=30) vs propranolol (N=30; 80mg) & placebo (N=30) controlled trial | 30 | 15 | 13 mirtazapine and 9 propranolol treated patients improved | 85 |

may be limited by well-known adverse effects including hypotension and sedation.

**Anticholinergics** – Despite the presumptive benefit and wide use of anticholinergics as a treatment for akathisia, there are few randomized controlled studies clearly demonstrating efficacy. Furthermore, coadministration of anticholinergics with antipsychotic medication is a common strategy used to prevent potential extrapyramidal symptoms, especially dystonia; however, the efficacy of this strategy in prevention of akathisia is unknown. Potential adverse effects, especially in older patients, including cognitive impairment and sedation, need to be considered. Efficacy of benztropine, procyclidine, biperiden, trihexyphenidyl, and benztropine has been reported. However, benztropine has been reported in other studies to improve only subjective measures, and biperiden was not efficacious in a randomized double blind placebo controlled study.[49]

**Benzodiazepines** – The most commonly used benzodiazepines are diazepam, lorazepam, clonazepam, and midazolam. The majority of studies demonstrating efficacy are small and open-labeled. Symptomatic improvement when evident may take 1 week to occur. In addition, reappearance of akathisia within 24 hours of intravenous administration has been reported.[50]

**Serotonin 2a (5-HT2A) Antagonists** – There are three 5-HT2A antagonists available: cyproheptadine, ritanserin, and mianserin. All three have shown efficacy in treating AIA. These effects may be related to establishing a better dopamine/5-HT balance. Mirtazapine is a widely used antidepressant. It has multiple effects, including being a potent presynaptic α-2 antagonist and 5-HT2A/2 c antagonist, and a 5-HT3 and histamine H1 postsynaptic receptor antagonist. Beneficial effects have been noted, although there are rare case reports of akathisia induced by mirtazapine. Trazodone is a weak inhibitor of 5-HT reuptake and a potent antagonist of postsynaptic 5-HT2A receptors. Beneficial effects were demonstrated on AIA in a double blind placebo controlled crossover study of only 6 days in 13 patients with schizophrenia or schizoaffective disorder, and this response has been supported by subsequent case reports.[51]

**Other Medications** – A number of other drugs have been tried for the treatment of AIA. Diphenhydramine has demonstrated mixed results. One randomized comparative trial found complete resolution of AIA within 60 minutes of diphenhydramine compared to 15 minutes with midazolam.[52] An open label study reported improvement of AIA within 30 minutes in 87 of 102 patients.[53] However, diphenhydramine was not found to be effective in preventing acute akathisia in two large double blind studies.[54,55] In one of these, midazolam did demonstrate significant efficacy assessed up to 1 hour from the time of administration.[55] Zolmitriptan is a selective 5-HT1D presynaptic receptor agonist used in the treatment of migraine. A double blind study comparing zolmitriptan 7.5mg (N=8) to propranolol 120mg/day (N=14) in the treatment of AIA found that both treatments had comparable beneficial effects.[56] In addition, an open label study of eight patients with acute or tardive AIA reported marked reduction of akathisia in response to zolmitriptan.[57] Interestingly, sumatriptan, a highly selective 5-HT1-like and 5-HT1B/D agonist, was reported to cause acute akathisia in five antipsychotic naïve patients.[58] Like anticholinergics, amantadine has also been widely used to prevent antipsychotic extrapyramidal side effects. Its efficacy in prevention and treating AIA is not certain. In a randomized double blind study comparing amantadine to benztropine, all patients with akathisia noted improvement with nearly complete resolution of symptoms in both groups within 28 days of treatment.[59] However, early tolerance has been reported in some patients.[60] Significant reduction of acute akathisia was obtained with 14mg nicotine patches in 15 of 16 nonsmoking patients in a single blind 3-day study.[61] In a blinded observational videotaped examination of five patients with acute or tardive AIA treated with propoxyphene or acetaminophen with codeine for two weeks, all patients demonstrated improvement, with the greatest response evident in those with acute AIA.[62] Amitriptyline has been shown to be efficacious in a single case report.[63]

## Conclusion

Akathisia is a challenging symptom to diagnose and is most often associated with antipsychotic use. The pathophysiology of akathisia remains elusive, although several theories have been proposed. Treatment starts with identifying the cause of akathisia. In medication-induced akathisia, withdrawal of the offending medication or reduction of the drug should be attempted. Several medications have been tried for akathisia with variable results. In the future, advances in our understanding of the pathophysiology of akathisia will hopefully provide better options for prevention and treatment.

# References

1. Haskovec L. Akathisie. *Arch Bohemes Med Clin.* 1902; 3:193–200.

2. Association AP. The Diagnostic and statistical manual of mental disorders (5th ed.; DSM-5). 5 ed. Arlington, VA: American Psychiatric Publishing, 2013.

3. Gibb WR, Lees AJ. The clinical phenomenon of akathisia. *J Neurol Neurosurg Psychiatry.* 1986; 49(8): 861–866.

4. Ford B, Greene P, Fahn S. Oral and genital tardive pain syndromes. *Neurology.* 1994; 44(11): 2115–2119.

5. Lang AE, Johnson K. Akathisia in idiopathic Parkinson's disease. *Neurology.* 1987; 37(3): 477–481.

6. Kim J-H, Jin Y-H, Kang UG, Ahn YM, Ha K-S, Kim YS. Neuroleptic-induced acute and chronic akathisia: a clinical comparison. *Mov Disord.* 2005; 20(12): 1667–1670.

7. Sachdev P. A rating scale for acute drug-induced akathisia: development, reliability, and validity. *Biol Psychiatry.* 1994; 35(4): 263–271.

8. Vinson DR. Development of a simplified instrument for the diagnosis and grading of akathisia in a cohort of patients receiving prochlorperazine. *J Emerg Med.* 2006; 31(2): 139–145.

9. Farde L. Selective D1- and D2-dopamine receptor blockade both induces akathisia in humans-a PET study with [11 C]SCH 23390 and [11 C]raclopride. *Psychopharmacology (Berl).* 1992; 107(1): 23–29.

10. Kapur S, Zipursky R, Jones C, Remington G, Houle S. Relationship between dopamine D(2) occupancy, clinical response, and side effects: a double-blind PET study of first-episode schizophrenia. *Am J Psychiatry.* 2000; 157(4): 514–520.

11. Loonen AJM, Stahl SM. The Mechanism of Drug-induced Akathisia. *CNS Spectr.* 2012; 16(01): 7–10.

12. Tassin JP, Stinus L, Simon H, et al. Relationship between the locomotor hyperactivity induced by A10 lesions and the destruction of the fronto-cortical dopaminergic innervation in the rat. *Brain Res.* 1978; 141(2): 267–281.

13. Ohashi K, Hamamura T, Lee Y, Fujiwara Y, Kuroda S. Propranolol attenuates haloperidol-induced Fos expression in discrete regions of rat brain: possible brain regions responsible for akathisia. *Brain Res.* 1998; 802(1–2): 134–140.

14. Poyurovsky M, Weizman A. Lack of efficacy of the 5-HT3 receptor antagonist granisetron in the treatment of acute neuroleptic-induced akathisia. *Int Clin Psychopharmacol.* 1999; 14(6): 357–360.

15. Poyurovsky M, Weizman A. Serotonergic agents in the treatment of acute neuroleptic-induced akathisia: open-label study of buspirone and mianserin. *Int Clin Psychopharmacol.* 1997; 12(5): 263–268.

16. Zhang J-P, Gallego JA, Robinson DG, Malhotra AK, Kane JM, Correll CU. Efficacy and safety of individual second-generation vs. first-generation antipsychotics in first-episode psychosis: a systematic review and meta-analysis. *Int J Neuropsychopharm.* 2012; 16(06): 1205–1218.

17. Sikich L, Frazier JA, McClellan J, et al. Double-blind comparison of first- and second-generation antipsychotics in early-onset schizophrenia and schizo-affective disorder: findings from the treatment of early-onset schizophrenia spectrum disorders (TEOSS) study. *Am J Psychiatry.* 2008; 165(11): 1420–1431.

18. Drotts DL, Vinson DR. Prochlorperazine induces akathisia in emergency patients. *Ann Emerg Med.* 1999; 34(4 Pt 1): 469–475.

19. Sachdev P. The epidemiology of drug-induced akathisia: Part I. *Acute akathisia. Schizophr Bull.* 1995; 21(3): 431–449.

20. Sachdev P, Kruk J. Clinical characteristics and predisposing factors in acute drug-induced akathisia. *Arch Gen Psychiatry.* 1994; 51(12): 963–974.

21. Lieberman JA, Stroup TS, McEvoy JP, et al. Effectiveness of antipsychotic drugs in patients with chronic schizophrenia. *N Engl J Med.* 2005; 353(12): 1209–1223.

22. Gao K, Kemp DE, Ganocy SJ, Gajwani P, Xia G, Calabrese JR. Antipsychotic-induced extrapyramidal side effects in bipolar disorder and schizophrenia: a systematic review. *J Clin Psychopharmacol.* 2008; 28(2): 203–209.

23. Eichhammer P1, Albus M, Borrmann-Hassenbach M, et al. Association of dopamine D3-receptor gene variants with neuroleptic induced akathisia in schizophrenic patients: a generalization of Steen's study on DRD3 and tardive dyskinesia. *Am J Med Genet.* 2000; 96(2): 187–91.

24. Koning JP, Vehof J, Burger H, et al. Association of two DRD2 gene polymorphisms with acute and tardive antipsychotic-induced movement disorders in young Caucasian patients. *Psychopharmacology (Berl).* 2012; 219(3): 727–736.

25. de Leon J, Diaz FJ, Aguilar MC, Jurado D, Gurpegui M. Does smoking reduce akathisia? Testing a narrow version of the self-medication hypothesis. *Schizophr Res.* 2006; 86(1–3): 256–268.

26. Sandyk R, Kay SR. Relationship of neuroleptic-induced akathisia to drug-induced parkinsonism. *Ital J Neurol Sci.* 1990; 11(5): 439–442.

27. Hofmann M, Seifritz E, Botschev C, Krauchi K, Muller-Spahn F. Serum iron and ferritin in acute neuroleptic akathisia. *Psychiatry Res.* 2000; 93(3): 201–207.

28. Gold R, Lenox RH. Is there a rationale for iron supplementation in the treatment of akathisia? A review of the evidence. *J Clin Psychiatry.* 1995; 56(10): 476–483.

29. Claghorn J, Honigfeld G, Abuzzahab FSS, et al. The risks and benefits of clozapine versus chlorpromazine. *J Clin Psychopharmacol*. 2006; **7**(6): 377–384.

30. Cohen BM, Keck PE, Satlin A, Cole JO. Prevalence and severity of akathisia in patients on clozapine. *Biol Psychiatry*. 1991; **29**(12): 1215–1219.

31. Miller CH, Mohr F, Umbricht D, Woerner M, Fleischhacker WW, Lieberman JA. The prevalence of acute extrapyramidal signs and symptoms in patients treated with clozapine, risperidone, and conventional antipsychotics. *J Clin Psychiatry*. 1998; **59**(2):69–75.

32. Nasrallah HA, Brecher M, Paulsson B. Placebo-level incidence of extrapyramidal symptoms (EPS) with quetiapine in controlled studies of patients with bipolar mania. *Bipolar Disord*. 2006; **8**(5 Pt 1): 467–474.

33. Dossenbach M, Treuer T, Kryzhanovskaya L, Saylan M, Dominguez S, Huang X. Olanzapine versus chlorpromazine in the treatment of schizophrenia: a pooled analysis of four 6-week, randomized, open-label studies in the Middle East and North Africa. *J Clin Psychopharmacol*. 2007; **27**(4): 329–337.

34. Vieta E, Panicali F, Goetz I, Reed C, Comes M, Tohen M. Olanzapine monotherapy and olanzapine combination therapy in the treatment of mania: 12-week results from the European Mania in Bipolar Longitudinal Evaluation of Medication (EMBLEM) observational study. *J Affect Disord*. 2008; **106**(1–2): 63–72.

35. Kumar R, Sachdev PS. Akathisia and second-generation antipsychotic drugs. *Curr Opin Psychiatry*. 2009; **22**(3): 293–299.

36. Egerton-Warburton D, Povey K. Administration of metoclopramide by infusion or bolus does not affect the incidence of drug-induced akathisia. *Emerg Med Australas*. 2013; **25**(3): 207–212.

37. Regan LA, Hoffman RS, Nelson LS. Slower infusion of metoclopramide decreases the rate of akathisia. *Am J Emerg Med*. 2009; **27**(4): 475–480.

38. Berna F, Timbolschi ID, Diemunsch P, Vidailhet P. Acute dystonia and akathisia following droperidol administration misdiagnosed as psychiatric disorders. *J Anesth*. 2013;**27**(5): 803–804.

39. Lucire Y, Crotty C. Antidepressant-induced akathisia-related homicides associated with diminishing mutations in metabolizing genes of the CYP450 family. *PGPM*. 2011; **4**: 65–81.

40. Baweja R, Petrovic-Dovat L. A Case of severe akathisia with atomoxetine. *J Child Adolesc Psychopharmacol*. 2013; **23**(6): 426–427.

41. Lai C-H. Venlafaxine-related akathisia side-effects and management in a depressed patient. *Psychiatry Clin Neurosci*. 2013; **67**(2): 127–128.

42. El-Mallakh RS, Marcus R, Baudelet C, McQuade R, Carson WH, Owen R. A 40-week double-blind aripiprazole versus lithium follow-up of a 12-week acute phase study (total 52 weeks) in bipolar I disorder. *J Affect Disord*. 2012; **136**(3): 258–266.

43. Fabiani G, Pastro PC, Froehner C. Parkinsonism and other movement disorders in outpatients in chronic use of cinnarizine and flunarizine. *Arq Neuro-Psiquiatr*. 2004; **62**(3B): 784–788.

44. Huntington Study Group. Tetrabenazine as antichorea therapy in Huntington disease: a randomized controlled trial. *Neurology*. 2006; **66**(3): 366–372.

45. Dag E, Gokee B, Buturak SV, Duygu T, Erdemoglu AK. Pregabalin-induced akathisia. *Ann Pharmacother*. 2013; **47**(4): 592–593.

46. Adler LA, Rotrosen J. Acute drug-induced akathisia. 2nd ed. In: Factor SA, Lang AE, Weiner WJ, editors. *Drug Induced Movement Disorders*. Malden: Blackwell Publishing; 2007; 140–173.

47. Sachdev P. *Akathisia and Restless Legs*. Cambridge: Cambridge University Press; 1995; 251–291.

48. Adler LA, Reiter S, Angrist B, Rotrosen J. Pindolol and propranolol in akathisia. *Am J Psychiatry*. 1987; **144**:1241–1242.

49. Baskak B, Atbasoglu EC, Ozguven HD, Saka MC, Gogus AK. The Effectiveness of intramuscular biperiden in acute akathisia. *J Clin Psychopharmacol*. 2007; **27**(3): 289–294.

50. Hirose S, Ashby CR. Immediate effect of intravenous diazepam in neuroleptic-induced acute akathisia: an open-label study. *J Clin Psychiatry*. 2002; **63**(6): 524–527.

51. Stryjer R, Rosenzcwaig S, Bar F, Ulman AM, Weizman A, Spivak B. Trazodone for the treatment of neuroleptic-induced acute akathisia: a placebo-controlled, double-blind, crossover study. *Clin Neuropharmacol*. 2010; **3**(5): 219–222.

52. Parlak I, Erdur B, Parlak M, et al. Midazolam vs. diphenhydramine for the treatment of metoclopramide-induced akathisia: a randomized controlled trial. *Acad Emerg Med*. 2007; **14**(8): 715–721.

53. Vinson DR. Diphenhydramine in the treatment of akathisia induced by prochlorperazine. *J Emerg Med*. 2004; **26**(3): 265–270.

54. Friedman BW, Bender B, Davitt M, et al. A randomized trial of diphenhydramine as prophylaxis against metoclopramide-induced akathisia in nauseated emergency department patients. *Ann Emerg Med*. 2009; **53**(3): 379–385.

55. Erdur B, Tura P, Aydin B, et al. A trial of midazolam vs diphenhydramine in prophylaxis of metoclopramide-induced akathisia. *Am J Emerg Med*. 2012; **30**(1): 84–91.

56. Avital A, Gross-Isseroff R, Stryjer R, Hermesh H, Weizman A, Shiloh R. Zolmitriptan compared to propranolol in the treatment of acute

neuroleptic-induced akathisia: a comparative double-blind study. *Eur Neuropsychopharmacol.* 2009; **19**(7): 476–482.

57. Gross-Isseroff R, Magen A, Shiloh R, Hermesh H, Weizman A. The 5-HT1D receptor agonist zolmitriptan for neuroleptic-induced akathisia: an open label preliminary study. *Int Clin Psychopharmacol.* 2005; **20**(1): 23–25.

58. Lopez-Alemany M, Ferrer-Tuset C, Bernacer-Alpera B. Akathisia and acute dystonia induced by sumatriptan. *J Neurol.* 1997; **244**(2): 131–132.

59. DiMascio A, Bernardo DL, Greenblatt DJ, Marder JE. A controlled trial of amantadine in drug-induced extrapyramidal disorders. *Arch Gen Psychiatry.* 1976; **33**(5): 599–602.

60. Zubenko GS, Barreira P, Lipinski JFJ. Development of tolerance to the therapeutic effect of amantadine on akathisia. *J Clin Psychopharmacol.* 1984; **4**(4): 218–220.

61. Anfang MK, Pope HGJ. Treatment of neuroleptic-induced akathisia with nicotine patches. *Psychopharmacology (Berl).* 1997; **134**(2): 153–156.

62. Walters A, Hening W, Chokroverty S, Fahn S. Opioid responsiveness in patients with neuroleptic-induced akathisia. *Mov Disord.* 1986; **1**(2): 119–127.

63. Danel T, Servant D, Goudemand M. Amitriptyline in the treatment of neuroleptic-induced akathisia. *Biol Psychiatry.* 1988; **23**(2): 186–188.

64. Ustohal L, Prikryl R, Hublova V, et al. Severe acute dystonia/akathisia after paliperidone palmitate application – a case study. *Int J Neuropsychopharmacol.* 2014; **17**(2): 341–342.

65. Kanba S, Kawasaki H, Ishigooka J, Sakamoto K, Kinoshita T, Kuroki T. A placebo-controlled, double-blind study of the efficacy and safety of aripiprazole for the treatment of acute manic or mixed episodes in Asian patients with bipolar I disorder (the AMAZE study). *World J Biol Psychiatry.* 2012; **15**(2): 113–121.

66. Berman RM, Marcus RN, Swanink R, et al. The efficacy and safety of aripiprazole as adjunctive therapy in major depressive disorder: a multicenter, randomized, double-blind, placebo-controlled study. *J Clin Psychiatry.* 2007; **68**(6): 843–853.

67. Zhang H, Li H, Shu L, et al. Double-blind comparison of ziprasidone and risperidone in the treatment of Chinese patients with acute exacerbation of schizophrenia. *Neuropsychiatr Dis Treat.* 2011; **7**: 77–85.

68. Penders T, Rohaidy R, Agarwal S. Persistent akathisia masquerading as agitated depression after use of ziprasidone in the treatment of bipolar depression. *Neuropsychiatr Dis Treat.* 2013; **9**: 463–465.

69. Atmaca M, Korkmaz S. Delayed-onset akathisia due to amisulpride. *Indian J Pharmacol.* 2011; **43**(4): 460–462.

70. Lim H-K, Pae C-U, Lee C, Lee C-U. Amisulpride versus risperidone treatment for behavioral and psychological symptoms in patients with dementia of the Alzheimer type: a randomized, open, prospective study. *Neuropsychobiology.* 2006; **54**(4): 247–251.

71. Nasrallah HA, Silva R, Phillips D, et al. Lurasidone for the treatment of acutely psychotic patients with schizophrenia: a 6-week, randomized, placebo-controlled study. *J Psychiatr Res.* 2013; **47**(5): 670–677.

72. Loebel A, Cucchiaro J, Sarma K, et al. Efficacy and safety of lurasidone 80 mg/day and 160 mg/day in the treatment of schizophrenia: a randomized, double-blind, placebo- and active-controlled trial. *Schizophr Res.* 2014; **145**(1–3): 101–109.

73. Dargani NV, Malhotra AK. Safety profile of iloperidone in the treatment of schizophrenia. *Expert Opin Drug Saf.* 2014; **13**(2): 241–246.

74. Citrome L. Cariprazine in schizophrenia: clinical efficacy, tolerability, and place in therapy. *Adv Ther.* 2013; **30**(2): 114–126.

75. Duncan EJ, Adler LA, Stephanides M, Sanfilipo M, Angrist B. Akathisia and exacerbation of psychopathology: a preliminary report. *Clin Neuropharmacol.* 2000; **23**(3): 169–173.

76. Hirose S, Ashby CR. Intravenous biperiden in akathisia: an open pilot study. *Int J Psychiatry Med.* 2000; **30**(2): 185–194.

77. Sunakawa Y, Wada M, Nishida T, et al. A case of respiratory akathisia in a cancer patient: a case report. *Palliat Support Care.* 2008; **6**(1): 79–81.

78. Pujalte D, Bottai T, Hue B, et al. A double-blind comparison of clonazepam and placebo in the treatment of neuroleptic-induced akathisia. *Clin Neuropharmacol.* 1994; **17**(3): 236–242.

79. Fischel T, Hermesh H, Aizenberg D, et al. Cyproheptadine versus propranolol for the treatment of acute neuroleptic-induced akathisia: a comparative double-blind study. *J Clin Psychopharmacol.* 2001; **21**(6): 612–615.

80. Weiss D, Aizenberg D, Hermesh H, et al. Cyproheptadine treatment in neuroleptic-induced akathisia. *Br J Psychiatry.* 1995; **167**(4): 483–486.

81. Miller CH, Fleischhacker WW, Ehrmann H, Kane JM. Treatment of neuroleptic induced akathisia with the 5-HT2 antagonist ritanserin. *Psychopharmacol Bull.* 1990; **26**(3): 373–376.

82. Poyurovsky M, Shardorodsky M, Fuchs C, Schneidman M, Weizman A. Treatment of neuroleptic-induced akathisia with the 5-HT2 antagonist mianserin. Double-blind, placebo-controlled study. *Br J Psychiatry.* 1999; **174**: 238–242.

83. Miodownik C, Lerner V, Statsenko N, et al. Vitamin B6 versus mianserin and placebo in acute neuroleptic-induced akathisia: a randomized, double-blind, controlled study. *Clin Neuropharmacol.* 2006; **29**(2): 68–72.

84. Poyurovsky M, Fuchs C, Weizman A. Efficacy of low-dose mirtazapine in neuroleptic-induced akathisia: a double-blind randomized placebo-controlled pilot study. *J Clin Psychopharmacol.* 2003; **23**: 305–308.

85. Poyurovsky M, Pashinian A, Weizman R, Fuchs C, Weizman A. Low-dose mirtazapine: a new option in the treatment of antipsychotic-induced akathisia. A randomized, double-blind, placebo- and propranolol-controlled trial. *Biol Psychiatry.* 2006; **59**(11): 1071–1077.

86. Dalley JW, Mar AC, Economidou D, Robbins TW. Neurobehavioral mechanisms of impulsivity: fronto-striatal systems and functional neurochemistry. *Pharmacol Biochem Behav.* 2008; **90**(2): 250–260.

# Acute dystonia

Anne Marthe Meppelink and Mark J. Edwards

## Introduction

Movement disorders can occur as a side effect of many different pharmacological agents, including antidepressants, antiepileptics, and cholinesterase inhibitors. Most commonly, these "extrapyramidal" side effects occur after exposure to dopamine receptor blocking drugs, including antipsychotics, antiemetics, and gastrointestinal promotility agents. Extrapyramidal side effects can be broadly divided into four categories: parkinsonism, akathisia, acute dystonic reactions, and tardive dyskinesia. While drug-induced parkinsonism and akathisia commonly occur after weeks to months of treatment with antipsychotics, and tardive dyskinesia after months to years, acute dystonic reactions to medications usually present within the first few days of treatment, often after a single dose [42]. In this chapter, we discuss the phenomenology and prevalence of acute dystonic reactions, their association with various medications and their possible underlying pathophysiology.

## Phenomenology

Acute dystonia is the earliest drug-induced movement disorder syndrome to appear and may arise after taking just a single dose of medication. Almost all drug reactions that fit within this category arise within the first 5 days of treatment [6], [65]. The fairly rapid disappearance of acute dystonic reactions on withdrawal of the offending drug is also one of its essential clinical features [20].

Acute dystonic reactions are characterized by abrupt onset of involuntary movements that most commonly involve the face and neck, but can also or only involve the trunk and extremities. Involvement of the face manifests as oculogyric crises, blepharospasm, trismus, forced jaw-opening, grimacing, protrusion, or twisting of the tongue and distortions of the lips. Neck and throat involvement includes laryngeal or pharyngeal dystonia, torticollis, or retrocollis. Dysarthria, dysphagia, jaw dislocation, and respiratory stridor may result [42]. In severe cases, acute laryngeal dystonia can lead to life-threatening respiratory distress following partial or complete obstruction of the upper airway [12]. Involvement of the trunk may give rise to scoliosis, lordosis, opisthotonos, tortipelvis, and a characteristic dystonic gait [42]. The acute dystonia and dyskinesias are distressing, frightening, and may be painful.

## Individual susceptibility

Acute dystonic reactions occur in only a proportion of people exposed to relevant medications. Some factors contributing to increased susceptibility to acute dystonic reactions have been delineated. Younger patients seem to be more susceptible to develop acute dystonic reactions, while older patients are more likely to develop drug-induced parkinsonism [6], [65]. The latter can be explained by differences in proposed pathophysiology between the two conditions (see below). The incidence of acute dystonia was twice as high in men as in women in one study [6]. Clinical features of dystonia also seem to differ per age category, with younger patients showing more severe and generalized involvement of the trunk and extremities, while older individuals tend to show more restricted involvement of the neck, face, tongue, and upper extremities [42], [6]. It is difficult to know if some of these differences (particularly the gender differences) have to do with the use of higher doses of antipsychotic medications in men versus women with acute psychosis.

*Medication-Induced Movement Disorders*, ed. Joseph H. Friedman. Published by Cambridge University Press.
© Cambridge University Press 2015.

# Drugs inducing acute dystonia

## Dopamine receptor blocking agents

Dopamine receptor blocking drugs (DRBs) are used primarily as antipsychotic medications, but are also used as antiemetics and gastrointestinal promotility agents. This class of drug is the one most often associated with acute dystonic reactions. Acute dystonic reactions occur in about 1%–3% of patients receiving antipsychotic medication [6], [61], [5]. Whereas acute dystonia tends to occur more frequently with use of highly potent DRBs like haloperidol [65], newer atypical antipsychotics such as aripiprazole and olanzapine can also induce these side effects (see Tables 2.1 and 2.2). The frequency of acute dystonic reactions in patients using haloperidol was as high as 16% in the study by Swett [65], while others have reported an incidence of 7.3%, 2.3%, and 2% [64], [61], [5].

**Table 2.1** Overview of drug-induced acute dystonia cases

| Drug Category: Paper: | Drug: | Description: | Treatment: |
|---|---|---|---|
| **Antipsychotics** | | | |
| Singh et al. 2007 | Aripiprazole | Male, 10 y. Acute torticollis, after 3 days of treatment. | Benztropine |
| Shangadia et al. 2007 | Aripiprazole | Female, 19 y. Dystonia neck and jaw, 3 d after start (anecdotal). | Withdrawal, spontaneous recovery |
| Varkula and Dale 2008 | Aripiprazole | Male, 20 y. Torticollis and dysarthria, 30 h after start treatment. | Diphenhydramine |
| Saddichha et al. 2011 | Aripiprazole | Female, 33 y. Acute neck dystonia after 1 week drug use, in combination with fluoxetine. | Trihexyphenidyl |
| Chen and Liou 2013 | Aripiprazole | Female, 32 y. Acute dystonia, akathisia, and parkinsonism after 1 week treatment. | Biperiden, lorazepam. |
| Kastrup et al. 1994 | Clozapine | Male, 50 y. Acute torticollis and orolingual dystonia, week 6 of treatment and 2 days after discontinuation of diazepam. | Biperiden |
| Christodou-lou and Kalaitzi 2005 | Haloperidol | Female, 35 y. Laryngeal dystonia, 1 hour after drug intake. | Biperiden |
| Chakravarty 2005 | Haloperidol | Male, elderly. Laryngal dystonia after two doses of haloperidol and risperidone. | Withdrawal, spontaneous recovery |
| Schneider and Bhatia 2009 | Haloperidol | Male, 8 y. Dystonic spasms, oculogyric crises after several days. | Diphenhydramine |
| Alevizos et al. 2003 | Olanzapine | Male, 50 y. Torticollis, orolingual dystonia, 2 hours after single dose (history risperidone). | Biperiden, orphenadrine |
| Vena et al. 2005 | Olanzapine | Male, 21 y. Acute dystonia neck, torso, and face, 1 hour after drug ingestion. | Diphenhydramine, benzatropine, lorazepam |
| Robert et al. 2009 | Olanzapine | Female, 73 y. Acute camptocormia, after 1 week drug use. | Withdrawal, spontaneous recovery |

**Table 2.1** (cont.)

| Drug Category: | | | |
|---|---|---|---|
| **Paper:** | **Drug:** | **Description:** | **Treatment:** |
| Namdeorao et al. 2009 | Olanzapine | Female, 47 y. Acute blepharospasm and oromandibular dystonia), after 7 d of use. | Trihexyphenidyl, clonazepam |
| Linazasoro et al. 1991 | Sulpiride | Male, 15 y. Oculogyric crisis, retrocollis, opisthotonus, dystonia hand, 4 hours after single dose. | Biperiden |
| Dew 2004 | Ziprasidone | Female, 31 y. Torticollis and lingual dystonia, start after third dose. | Benztropine, Diphenhydramine |
| Yumru et al. 2006 | Ziprasidone | Male, 18 y. Torticollis and dystonic posture torso, 4 h after second dose. | Biperiden |
| Duggal 2007 | Ziprasidone | Male, 18 y. Laryngeal dystonia after 3 days treatment. | Benztropine |
| Mellacheruvu et al. 2007 | Ziprasidone | Male, 51 y. Laryngeal dystonia, 30 min after first dose.<br>Male, 21 y. Laryngeal dystonia, 20 min after first dose. | Diphenhydramine<br><br>Benztropine |
| Duggal 2008 | Ziprasidone | Male, 20 y. Acute Pisa syndrome with pharyngolaryngeal dystonia after dose increase. | Benztropine |
| Viana et al. 2009 | Ziprasidone | Female, 28 y. Oculogyric crisis after 7 months of drug use. Priorly same reaction to haloperidol. | Clonazepam |
| **Antidepressants** | | | |
| Finder et al. 1982 | Amitriptyline | Female, 30 y. Torticollis, after two doses. | Benztropine |
| Dominguez-Moran et al. 2001 | Fluoxetine | Female, 32 y. Paroxysmal hemidystonia, after 2 days of treatment. | Withdrawal, spontaneous recovery |
| Méndez Guerrero et al. 2013 | Mirtazapine | Female, 61 y. Pisa syndrome with laterocollis after single dose. | Withdrawal, spontaneous recovery |
| Arnone et al. 2002 | Paroxetine | Male, 67 y. Acute torticollis, oculogyric crisis and opisthotonus, 1 w use. | Procyclidine |
| **Antiepileptics** | | | |
| Kerrick et al. 1995 | Felbamate | Male, 13 y. Dystonia extremities, trunk, and neck, 3 hours after last dose. | Diphenhydramine |
| **Antiemetics** | | | |
| Madej 1985 | Domperidone | Female, 21 y. Oculogyric crisis, torticollis, dystonia upper limbs, 2 m after dose. | Thiopentone |
| Bonuccelli et al. 1991 | Domperidone | Female, 16 y. Acute orolingual dyskinesia and eye and head dystonia after 12 h treatment.<br>Female, 28 y. Acute orolingual dyskinesia during third day of treatment. | Withdrawal, spontaneous recovery<br>Withdrawal, spontaneous recovery |

**Table 2.1** (cont.)

| Drug Category: | | | |
| --- | --- | --- | --- |
| **Paper:** | **Drug:** | **Description:** | **Treatment:** |
| Venkate-swaran 1972 | Metoclopramide | Male, 25 y. Tongue, jaw, and lower limb dystonia, within 36 h of drug use. | Benztropine |
| Lu and Chu 1988 | Metoclopramide | Male, 65 y. Dystonia neck and face with myoclonus, 2 h after last intake. | Withdrawal, spontaneous recovery |
| Newton-John 1988 | Metoclopramide | Male, 16 y. Laryngeal and tongue dystonia, 30 m after last dose. | Benztropine |
| | | Male, 35 y. Laryngeal and tongue dystonia, trismus, start second day of drug use. | Benztropine |
| Schneider 2009 | Metoclopramide | Female, 24 y. Acute retrocollis and oromandibular dystonia. | Procyclidine |
| Silfeler 2012 | Metoclopramide | Males, 6, 8, and 15 y. Dysarthria, trismus, dystonic movement arms, 30 min after drug intake. | Biperiden |
| Patel 2011 | Ondansetron | Male, 4 y. Upper limb dystonia, trismus, and seizures, 30 m after drug administration. | Lorazepam |
| Schumock and Martinez 1991 | Prochlorperazine | Female, 23 y. Acute oculogyric crisis with opisthotonus. | Benztropine |
| Reecer 1993 | Prochlorperazine | Male, 18 y. Isolated tongue dystonia (patient with quadriplegia after trauma). | Diphenhydramine |
| **Stimulants** | | | |
| Panagiotis et al. 2012 | Donepezil | Female, 74 y. Acute Pisa syndrome, 3 hours after start medication. | Withdrawal, spontaneous recovery |
| Waugh 2013 | Methylphenidate | Male, 23 m. Facial dystonia, torticollis, 4 h after intake supra therapeutic dose. | Diphenhydramine |
| Dhikav and Anand 2013 | Rivastigmine | Female, 75 y. Neck and upper limb dystonia, 3 h after dose increase. | Diazepam |
| **Miscellaneous** | | | |
| Incecik 2011 | Albendazole (antihelminth) | Male, 9 y. Torticollis and buccolingual dystonia, 4 hours after intake. | Diazepam |
| Akindele and Odejide 1976 | Amodiaquine (antimalarial) | Male, 7 y. Tongue protrusion, after two days of treatment. | Benztropine |
| Micheli 1987 | Cinnarizine and Flunarizine (calcium blockers) | Male, 37 y. Acute torticollis after 3 days of medication use. Eleven older patients had parkinsonism. | Gradual decrease despite continuation |

**Table 2.1** (cont.)

| Drug Category: | | | |
|---|---|---|---|
| **Paper:** | **Drug:** | **Description:** | **Treatment:** |
| Howrie 1986 | Benztropine (AcH-antag) | Male, 20 m. Acute buccolingual, torticollic, and tortipelvic dystonia several hours after ingestion. | Spontaneous recovery |
| Hooker 1988 | Diazepam | Female, 25 y. Torticollis, 9 hours after ingestion drug. Female, 39 y. Buccolingual dystonia. | Diphenhydramine Diphenhydramine |
| Dubow 2008 | Foscarnet (antiviral) | Female, 55 y. Acute dystonic posturing of arms and face and anarthria, 30 min after single dose. | Diphenhydramine |
| Song 2005 | Lamivudine (antiviral) | Male, 24 y. Torticollis, lingual dystonia, dystonic posture, after 2 days of medication use. | Scopolamine |
| Castrioto 2008 | Midodrine (vasopressor) | Female, 57 y. Acute cranio-cervical dystonia after adding midodrine to perphenazine (typical AP) | Withdrawal, spontaneous recovery |
| Kapur 1999 | Ranitidine (H2-antagonist) | Male, 26 y. Opisthotonus and rigidity in all limbs, after second dose. | Benztropine |
| López-Alemany 1997 | Sumatriptan (5-HT agonist) | Female, 40 y. Oral dystonia and akathisia, 1 h after intake. | Withdrawal, spontaneous recovery |
| Burke 1985 | Tetrabenazine (DA depleter) | Female, 22 y. Recurrent oculogyric crises after dose increase. | Diphenhydramine |
| Uca 2014 | Varenicline (ACh-agonist) | Male, 25 y. Torticollis and tongue dystonia, after 7 days of daily use. | Biperiden |

Metoclopramide, an antiemetic, was shown to cause acute dystonic reactions in 0.5% (12 of 2557 patients receiving the drug for the first time), although the incidence in younger patients was higher (1.2%). In patients using prochlorperazine, 4 of 2811 (0.1%) developed acute dystonia [7]. Proposed pathophysiological mechanisms of acute dystonic reactions induced by DRBs are discussed below.

## Other medications reported to cause acute dystonic reactions

Many different drugs have been associated with acute dystonic reactions, including antiepileptics, antidepressants, antiviral agents, calcium blocking agents, and triptans (see Table 2.1). Although the pathogenesis is unknown, many of the reported drugs inducing acute dystonic reactions probably interact with dopaminergic and/or cholinergic systems and sigma receptors, as discussed below.

Some cases of acute dystonia after use of serotonin reuptake inhibitors (SSRI) have been described. SSRIs increase levels of serotonin, which is known to interact with dopaminergic systems. It has been suggested that acute dystonia may be caused by inhibition of dopamine activity secondary to serotonin increase; binding of SSRIs to sigma receptors might also play a role [4]. Although probably rare, dystonic reactions to triptans (serotonin agonists) have been described, possibly acting via a similar mechanism as SSRIs [38].

Acute dystonic reactions to dopamine-depleting drugs like tetrabenazine have been described, but are probably rare. Again, an imbalance between striatal dopaminergic and cholinergic systems, with a relative overactivity of the latter, has been suggested to explain this reaction [11].

**Table 2.2:** Prevalence and comparison studies of neuroleptic-induced acute dystonia

| Paper: | Drug: | Outcome: |
|---|---|---|
| Ayd and Baltimore 1961 | Phenothiazines | Of 3775 patients treated with neuroleptic from phenothiazine group, 1472 developed extrapyramidal reactions, of which 87 dystonia (2.3%). |
| Swett 1975 | Phenothiazines, butyrophenone or thioxanthene. | Of 1152 patients treated with one or more neuroleptics 116 developed acute dystonia (10,1%), torticollis (n= 35), facial dystonia (n=44), or other. Highest frequency with haloperidol (32/200, 16%) and long-acting injectable fluphenazine (11,7%). |
| Spina et al. 1993 | Typical antipsychotics | Of 646 patients treated with one or more neuroleptics 34 developed acute dystonia (5.3%). Patients on haloperidol had a higher frequency of acute dystonia (16/218, 7.3%) and patients without anticholinergic prophylaxis higher than patients with prophylaxis (8.5% vs. 2.8%). |
| Simpson and Lindenmayer 1997 | Risperidone vs. haloperidol | Eight-week trial with 523 patients (completed by 253) received risperidone (n=344, 0, 6, 10 or 16 mg/d) or haloperidol (n=83, 20 mg/d) after 1 w washout. Acute dystonia in 6/344 (1.7%) on risperidone and 2/83 (2.3%) on haloperidol. |
| Arvanitis and Miller 1998 | Quetiapine vs. haloperidol | Six-week trial comparing quetiapine (n=258, 75, 150, 300, 600 or 750 mg/d) with haloperidol (n=52, 12 mg/d) after 1 w washout. Acute dystonia is 2/258 (0.8%) on quetiapine and 1/52 (2%) on haloperidol (also 2% on placebo). |
| Chan et al. 2010 | Risperidone vs. olanzapine | Concomitant anticholinergics for acute dystonia or parkinsonism were used in 14/35 (40%) on risperidone and 4/35 (11%) on olanzapine. |

Drug-induced dystonia in a very young child after administration of methylphenidate, inhibiting the reuptake of dopamine, has been described. It was argued that a relatively high proportion of dopamine D2 receptors in young people could account for this increased sensitivity [74]. Cholinesterase-inhibitors occasionally cause dystonic reactions, probably via changing the dopamine-acetylcholine balance via enhancement of acetylcholine [50], [19].

Cinnarizine and flunarizine, both calcium blockers, have been shown to induce acute dystonic reactions as well. Both drugs are derivatives of piperazine, like many antipsychotics and antidepressant drugs, thus likely explaining their extrapyramidal side effects (which can include drug-induced parkinsonism) via dopamine receptor-blocking activity [47]. Related to this, several patients with untreated hyperparathyroidism and hypocalcemia have been reported with severe acute dystonia after administration of low dose neuroleptics [42]. Calcium signaling is important for dopamine synthesis, so impaired dopamine synthesis due to low calcium could also play a role [47].

Antihistaminergic drugs have occasionally been associated with acute dystonic reactions. With most antihistaminergic drugs also having anticholinergic properties, it has been postulated that a compensatory increase in cholinergic activity following blockade may be responsible for the dystonic reaction [32], [20].

The same mechanism of proposed compensatory cholinergic excess might play a role in acute dystonic reactions after administration of anticholinergics [28], and might partly explain why tricyclic antidepressants have been associated with acute dystonic reactions as well [24].

Some other medications not mentioned above have been associated with acute dystonia, including antiviral medications [22], [63], antihelminths [29], antimalarial medication [1], and benzodiazepines [27].

# Pathophysiology

## Dopamine and acetylcholine

The exact pathogenesis of acute medication-induced dystonia is not entirely understood, but seems to involve a combination of presynaptic dopaminergic mechanisms, changes of sensitivity of dopamine receptors, and cholinergic influences. Animal studies have shown that several species of primates exposed to the acute administration of a variety of neuroleptic drugs developed a clinical syndrome indistinguishable from that seen in humans experiencing acute dystonic reactions. While a range of antipsychotics could evoke these symptoms, a neuroleptic with exceptionally high intrinsic anticholinergic activity, thioridazine, was ineffective [41]. This observation is in accordance with other findings regarding the role of the cholinergic system in acute dystonic reactions. Anticholinergic drugs are an effective treatment of medication-induced acute dystonia in humans, and Marsden and Jenner showed that anticholinergic drugs could also abolish acute dystonic reactions in other primates. It was additionally shown that cholinergic enhancement (by administration of a cholinesterase inhibitor) intensified the dystonic symptoms induced by DRBs [41]. Further exploration of underlying mechanisms showed that disruption of both presynaptic storage and synthesis of catecholamines (probably dopamine, as neuroleptics with little noradrenaline antagonist action like haloperidol are very potent at producing acute dystonia) prevented neuroleptic-induced dystonia. It was concluded that acute dystonic reactions could be produced by a compensatory effect of increased dopamine synthesis and release resulting from postsynaptic dopamine receptor blockade [41], [35].

Involvement of the postsynaptic receptors themselves is a further/additional possibility. Inhibition of apomorphine-induced stereotypy by neuroleptics was investigated in rats via assessment of dopamine levels and markers of dopamine turnover (homovanillic acid, HVA, and dihydroxyphenylacetic acid, DOPAC). The drug butaperazine, which was previously shown to induce acute dystonic reactions after administration of a single dose in 8 of 13 schizophrenic patients, caused elevation of striatal and mesolimbic HVA and DOPAC concentrations with no change in dopamine levels, indicating an increased turnover and release of dopamine. Although these changes were a maximum of 12 hours after administration of the drug, they were still evident after 24 hours.

Apomorphine-induced stereotypies were reduced to 50% of their maximum 12 hours after administration of butaperazine and returned to slightly above baseline values (100%) by 24 hours. These data support the hypothesis that a combination of persisting compensatory dopamine release and slightly supersensitive dopamine receptors (as judged by exaggerated apomorphine-induced stereotypies) is responsible for acute dystonic reactions [35], [41].

# Dopamine receptor subtypes and idiosyncrasy

It remains unknown why only a small number of susceptible individuals experience acute dystonic reactions. This may represent an idiosyncratic reaction of the minority, which might be associated with genetic factors. Carriage of genetic alterations associated with autosomal recessive primary dystonia has been suggested as relevant, although the relative low incidence of gene carriage cannot account for the incidence of acute dystonic reactions in about 2% receiving antipsychotic medications [41].

Alternatively, any person might have the capacity to develop acute dystonia if given a big enough dose of DRB but, in usual clinical practice, only a small proportion achieve high enough concentrations of the drug to cause the problem [41]. Some studies have shown that patients exhibiting acute dystonic reactions, when compared to patients without this phenomenon, had similar plasma levels but higher concentrations of DRBs in erythrocytes. It was suggested that this cell-bound concentration may provide a better indication of cerebral drug levels [25].

Early studies in 1-methyl-4-phenyl-1,2,3,6- tetrahydropyridine (MPTP)-induced parkinsonian monkeys suggested that dopamine D1 receptors were associated predominantly with the dyskinetic effect of levodopa, while the D2 receptor subtype is responsible for its antiparkinsonian effect [10]. Further experiments showed that both receptor subtypes are involved, while it was suggested that interactions with other neurotransmitter systems play a role as well [26].

Whether differential involvement of D1 and D2 dopamine receptors is implicated in medication-induced acute dystonia is not known. D2-receptor occupancy in patients with schizophrenia using neuroleptics has been linked to extrapyramidal side effects, including acute dystonia. In a double blind study, Raclopride-PET was performed after two weeks of treatment in 22 patients with first-episode schizophrenia who were randomly assigned to receive haloperidol 1 or 2.5 mg/day. The dose was increased to 5 mg/day in patients without a clinical response, who were called non-responders. The degree of D2-receptor occupancy predicted clinical outcome and extrapyramidal side effects; D2-receptor occupancy exceeding 65% predicted clinical improvement, and occupancy exceeding 78% predicted occurrence of extrapyramidal side effects. Acute dystonia occurred in one of the nonresponders while other extrapyramidal symptoms occurred in six, after dose increase [31]. These data suggest that drug-induced extrapyramidal side effects might be dose-dependent within an individual, so possibly in combination with individual susceptibility.

## Cholinergic excess

The basal ganglia play an important role in motor, cognitive, and affective behavioral functions, through selection of an appropriate response in a particular context and, in parallel, the suppression of inappropriate responses [53]. The basal ganglia receive input from the whole cortex and project it, via the thalamus, back to the cortex, mainly the frontal lobe. Striatal output is modulated via the so-called direct and indirect pathways of the basal ganglia circuits, involved in response initiation and inhibition, respectively. Acetylcholine, via its reciprocal interactions with dopamine, has an important role in the differential modulation of striatal output. Dopaminergic enhancement stimulates the direct pathway via D1 receptors and inhibits the indirect pathway via D2 receptors, while acetylcholine mainly activates the indirect pathway. The concept of this functional antagonism between acetylcholine and dopamine in the striatum has led to the concept that an imbalance between dopaminergic and cholinergic influences in the striatum is involved in movement disorders like Parkinson's disease, but probably also in dystonia [8]. Anticholinergic medications are helpful in all types of dystonia, which is thought to reflect a relative hypercholinergic state of the striatum in dystonia patients [2], [8], [30]. Whether patients with acute drug-induced dystonia have a cholinergic excess is not known directly, although treatment with anticholinergics is remarkably effective in this condition as well, with improvement of symptoms within minutes after intravenous administration [21].

## Neuroanatomical correlates and other receptors

It is interesting to hypothesize why involvement of cranial and cervical structures is so often seen in acute drug-induced dystonic reactions (see Table 2.1). Another related question is why young patients seem to show the most severe and generalized dystonic reactions, while in older patients involvement seems more restricted to the cranial and cervical regions [6]. Possibly, age-related differences in dopamine receptors play a role. It had been shown that D2 dopamine receptor density declines with age, in striatal as well as in extrastriatal areas [73]. Like the cortex, the basal ganglia exhibit a somatotopic organization; for example, the putamen is characterized by a dorsoventral topography of somatotopic representations with leg dorsal, arm in the center, and face ventral [56]. Hypothetically, anatomical differences in age-related receptor density decline might explain these age differences, with relatively preserved ventral D2 receptor density in elderly people, and subsequent higher sensitivity to dopaminergic blockade or facilitation.

Sigma receptors might also play a role in the pathophysiology of acute dystonia, being especially present in brainstem nuclei controlling the muscles most often afflicted in neuroleptic-induced dystonia. Higher affinity of dopamine antagonists (neuroleptics and antiemetics) to sigma receptors in rats was correlated with a higher reported tendency of the drugs to produce acute dystonic reactions in humans [43]. Although the exact structure and nature of the sigma receptor are still being elucidated, it is known to modulate calcium signaling and neurotransmitter release, including acetylcholine [68]. Apart from the cranial nerve nuclei that subserve eye, lingual, facial, and masticatory movements, the red nucleus and cerebellum also contain high levels of sigma receptors. Animal studies have demonstrated the importance of the rubrocerebellar pathway, suggesting that sigma receptors might be involved in the central regulation of muscle tone and coordination [36]. The red nucleus has been associated with dystonic reactions in rats [43], and changes in its structure have been described in primary dystonia in humans as well [67]. The rubrospinal tract in humans mainly serves motor control of cranial, cervical, and upper extremity musculature and the red nucleus provides a junction where output from the basal ganglia can interact with output of the cerebellum for movement control of the head and face [52]. Alteration of sigma receptor–related activity at the level of the red nucleus or indirectly via the striatum might play a role in medication-induced dystonic reactions in humans.

# Treatment

Treatment of acute dystonic reactions relies on recognition of the phenomenon, withdrawal or dosage lowering of the causative drug, and administration of anticholinergic drugs. Intravenous anticholinergics such as benztropine, biperiden, or trihexyphenidyl are highly effective within minutes, although most patients are additionally treated with oral anticholinergics for some weeks to prevent recurrence [21]. Benzodiazepines may also be helpful, but are not as effective as anticholinergics [12]. It has been shown that prophylactic anticholinergic therapy lowers the incidence of acute dystonia in patients using typical neuroleptics [64]. However, the prophylactic administration of anticholinergic drugs to patients using antipsychotics is controversial and currently not recommended, because of the relatively low incidence of acute dystonic reactions in those receiving atypical neuroleptics and unwanted side effects from the anticholinergic medication itself.

# Conclusions

Drug-induced acute dystonia occurs most commonly after initiation of dopamine receptor blocking agents, but associations with several other medications have been described. Although the exact pathophysiology is unknown, interaction between postsynaptic dopamine receptor super-sensitivity and increased dopamine turnover and release provoked by the acute administration dopamine receptor blockers seems to play a role. The dramatic therapeutic effect of anticholinergics suggests an important role for acetylcholine as well, while the role of the less well described sigma receptors in striatal and extrastriatal areas remains to be elucidated.

# References

1. Akindele, M.O. and Odejide, A.O., 1976. Amodiaquine-induced involuntary movements. *BMJ (Clinical Research Ed.)*, 2(6029), pp. 214–215.

2. Albanese, A. and Lalli, S., 2012. Update on dystonia. *Current Opinion in Neurology*, 25(4), pp. 483–490.

3. Alevizos, B., Christodoulou, G. and Papageorgiou, C., 2003. Acute dystonia caused by low dosage of olanzapine. *Journal of Neuropsychiatry Clinical Neuroscience*, pp. 1–7.

4. Arnone, D., Hansen, L. and Kerr, J.S., 2002. Acute dystonic reaction in an elderly patient with mood disorder after titration of paroxetine: possible mechanisms and implications for clinical care. *Journal of Psychopharmacology*, 16(4), pp. 395–397.

5. Arvanitis, L.A. and Miller, B.G., 1997. Multiple fixed doses of "Seroquel" (quetiapine) in patients with acute exacerbation of schizophrenia: a comparison with haloperidol and placebo. The Seroquel Trial 13 Study Group. *Biological Psychiatry*, 42(4), pp. 233–246.

6. Ayd, F.J., 1961. A survey of drug-induced extrapyramidal reactions. *JAMA: The Journal of the American Medical Association*, 175, pp. 1054–1060.

7. Bateman, D.N. et al., 1989. Extrapyramidal reactions to metoclopramide and prochlorperazine. *The Quarterly Journal of Medicine*, 71(264), pp. 307–311.

8. Benarroch, E.E., 2012. Effects of acetylcholine in the striatum. Recent insights and therapeutic implications. *Neurology*, 79(3), pp. 274–281.

9. Bonuccelli, U. et al., 1991. Domperidone-induced acute dystonia and polycystic ovary syndrome. *Movement Disorders*, 6(1), pp. 79–81.

10. Boyce, S. et al., 1990. Differential effects of D1 and D2 agonists in MPTP-treated primates: functional implications for Parkinson's disease. *Neurology*, 40(6), pp. 927–933.

11. Burke, R.E. et al., 1985. Tetrabenazine induces acute dystonic reactions. *Annals of Neurology*, 17(2), pp. 200–202.

12. Burkhard, P.R., 2014. Acute and subacute drug-induced movement disorders. *Parkinsonism and Related Disorders*, 20 Suppl 1, pp. S 108–12.

13. Castrioto, A. et al., 2008. Acute dystonia induced by the combination of midodrine and perphenazine. *Journal of Neurology*, 255(5), pp. 767–768.

14. Chakravarty, A., 2005. Neuroleptic-induced acute laryngeal dystonia causing stridor: A lesson to remember. *Movement Disorders*, 20(8), pp. 1082–1082.

15. Chan, H. et al., 2010. A randomised controlled study of risperidone and olanzapine for schizophrenic patients with neuroleptic-induced acute dystonia or parkinsonism. *Journal of Psychopharmacology*, 24(1), pp. 91–98.

16. Chen, M.-H. and Liou, Y.-J., 2013. Aripiprazole-associated acute dystonia, akathisia and Parkinsonism in a patient with bipolar I disorder. *Journal of Psychopharmacology*, pp. 1–2.

17. Christodoulou, G., 2005. Antipsychotic drug-induced acute laryngeal dystonia: two case reports and a mini review. *Journal of Psychopharmacology*, 19(3), pp. 307–311.

18. Dew, R.E. and Hughes, D., 2004. Acute dystonic reaction with moderate-dose ziprasidone. *Journal of Clinical Psychopharmacotherapy*, 24(5), pp. 563–564.

19. Dhikav, V. and Anand, K.S., 2013. Acute dystonic reaction with rivastigmine. *International Psychogeriatrics*, **25**(8), pp. 1385–1386.

20. Donaldson, I. et al., 2011. *Marsden's Book of Movement Disorders*, Oxford University Press.

21. Dressler, D. and Benecke, R., 2005. Diagnosis and management of acute movement disorders. *Journal of Neurology*, **252**(11), pp. 1299–1306.

22. Dubow, J.S. et al., 2008. Acute dystonic reaction associated with foscarnet administration. *American Journal of Therapeutics*, **15**(2), pp. 184–186.

23. Duggal, H.S., 2008. Acute Pisa syndrome and pharnygolaryngeal dystonia due to ziprasidone. *The Journal of Neuropsychiatry and Clinical Neurosciences*, **20**(1), pp. 108–109.

24. Finder, E., Lin, K.M. and Ananth, J., 1982. Dystonic reaction to amitriptyline. *The American Journal of Psychiatry*, **139**(9), p. 1220.

25. Garver, D.L. et al., 1976. Pharmacokinetics of red blood cell phenothiazine and clinical effects. Acute dystonic reactions. *Archives of General Psychiatry*, **33**(7), pp. 862–866.

26. Grondin, R. et al., 1999. D1 receptor blockade improves L-dopa-induced dyskinesia but worsens parkinsonism in MPTP monkeys. *Neurology*, **52**(4), pp. 771–776.

27. Hooker, E.A. and Danzl, D.F., 1988. Acute dystonic reaction due to diazepam. *The Journal of Emergency Medicine*, **6**(6), pp. 491–493.

28. Howrie, D.L., Rowley, A.H. and Krenzelok, E.P., 1986. Benztropine-induced acute dystonic reaction. *Annals of Emergency Medicine*, **15**(5), pp. 594–596.

29. Incecik, F. et al., 2011. Albendazole-induced dystonic reaction: a case report. *The Turkish Journal of Pediatrics*, **53**(6), pp. 709–710.

30. Jankovic, J., 2013. Medical treatment of dystonia. *Movement Disorders*, **28**(7), pp. 1001–1012.

31. Kapur, S. et al., 2000. Relationship between dopamine D(2) occupancy, clinical response, and side effects: a double-blind PET study of first-episode schizophrenia. *The American Journal of Psychiatry*, **157**(4), pp. 514–520.

32. Kapur, V., Barber, K.R. and Peddireddy, R., 1999. Ranitidine-induced acute dystonia. *The American Journal of Emergency Medicine*, **17**(3), pp. 258–260.

33. Kastrup, O., Gastpar, M. and Schwarz, M., 1994. Acute dystonia due to clozapine. *Journal of Neurology, Neurosurgery and Psychiatry*, **57**(1), pp. 119–119.

34. Kerrick, J.M. et al., 1995. Involuntary movement disorders associated with felbamate. *Neurology*, **45**(1), pp. 185–187.

35. Kolbe, H. et al., 1981. Neuroleptic-induced acute dystonic reactions may be due to enhanced dopamine release on to supersensitive postsynaptic receptors. *Neurology*, **31**(4), pp. 434–434.

36. Leitner, M.L. et al., 1994. Regional variation in the ratio of sigma 1 to sigma 2 binding in rat brain. *European Journal of Pharmacology*, **259**(1), pp. 65–69.

37. Linazasoro, G., Martí Massó, J.F. and Olasagasti, B., 1991. Acute dystonia induced by sulpiride. *Clinical Neuropharmacology*, **14**(5), pp. 463–2.

38. López-Alemany, M., Ferrer-Tuset, C. and Bernácer-Alpera, B., 1997. Akathisia and acute dystonia induced by sumatriptan. *Journal of Neurology*, **244**(2), pp. 131–132.

39. Lu, C.S. and Chu, N.S., 1988. Acute dystonic reaction with asterixis and myoclonus following metoclopramide therapy. *Journal of Neurology, Neurosurgery and Psychiatry*, **51**(7), pp. 1002–1003.

40. Madej, T.H., 1985. Domperidone – an acute dystonic reaction. *Anaesthesia*.

41. Marsden, C.D. and Jenner, P., 1980. The pathophysiology of extrapyramidal side-effects of neuroleptic drugs. *Psychological Medicine*, **10**(1), pp. 55–72.

42. Marsden, C.D., Tarsy, D. and Baldessarini, R.J., 1975. Spontaneous and drug induced movement disorders in psychotic patients. In *Psychiatric Aspects of Neurologic Disease*. New York: Grune & Stratton, pp. 219–266.

43. Matsumoto, R.R. and Pouw, B., 2000. Correlation between neuroleptic binding to sigma(1) and sigma(2) receptors and acute dystonic reactions. *European Journal of Pharmacology*, **401**(2), pp. 155–160.

44. Mellacheruvu, S., Norton, J.W. and Schweinfurth, J., 2007. Atypical antipsychotic drug-induced acute laryngeal dystonia: 2 case reports. *Journal of Clinical Psychopharmacotherapy*, **27**(2), pp. 206–207.

45. Mendhekar, D. and War, L., 2014. Olanzapine induced acute Meige's syndrome. *Journal of Neuropsychiatry Clinical Neuroscience*, pp. 1–1.

46. Méndez Guerrero, A. et al., 2013. Acute Pisa syndrome after administration of a single dose of mirtazapine. *Clinical Neuropharmacology*, **36**(4), pp. 133–134.

47. Micheli, F. et al., 1987. Flunarizine- and cinnarizine-induced extrapyramidal reactions. *Neurology*, **37**(5), pp. 881–881.

48. Dominguez-Moran et al., 2001. Acute paroxysmal dystonia induced by fluoxetine. *Movement Disorders*, **16**(4), pp. 767–769.

49. Newton-John, H., 1988. Acute upper airway obstruction due to supraglottic dystonia induced by a neuroleptic. *BMJ (Clinical Research Ed.)*, **297**(6654), pp. 964–965.

50. Panagiotis, I. et al., 2012. Acute Pisa syndrome after administration of a single dose of donepezil. *The Journal of Neuropsychiatry and Clinical Neurosciences*, **24** (3), p. E26.

51. Patel, A. et al., 2011. Ondansetron-induced dystonia, hypoglycemia, and seizures in a child. *Annals of Pharmacotherapy*, **45** (1), p. e7.

52. Pong, M., Horn, K.M. and Gibson, A.R., 2008. Pathways for control of face and neck musculature by the basal ganglia and cerebellum. *Brain Research Reviews*, **58**(2), pp. 249–264.

53. Redgrave, P., Prescott, T.J. and Gurney, K., 1999. The basal ganglia: a vertebrate solution to the selection problem? *Neuroscience*, **89**(4), pp. 1009–1023.

54. Reecer, M.V., Clinchot, D.M. and Tipton, D.B., 1993. Drug-induced dystonia in a patient with C4 quadriplegia. Case report. *American Journal of Physical Medicine and Rehabilitation / Association of Academic Physiatrists*, **72**(2), pp. 97–98.

55. Robert, F. et al., 2010. Acute camptocormia induced by olanzapine: a case report. *Journal of Medical Case Reports*, **4**(1), p. 192.

56. Romanelli, P. et al., 2005. Somatotopy in the basal ganglia: experimental and clinical evidence for segregated sensorimotor channels. *Brain Research Reviews*, **48**(1), pp. 112–128.

57. Saddichha, S. et al., 2013. Aripiprazole associated with acute dystonia, akathisia, and parkinsonism in a single patient. *The Journal of Clinical Pharmacology*, **52**(9), pp. 1448–1449.

58. Schneider, S.A. et al., 2009. Recurrent acute dystonic reaction and oculogyric crisis despite withdrawal of dopamine receptor blocking drugs. *Movement Disorders*, **24**(8), pp. 1226–1229.

59. Schumock, G.T. and Martinez, E., 1991. Acute oculogyric crisis after administration of prochlorperazine. *Southern Medical Journal*, **84**(3), pp. 407–408.

60. Silfeler, I. et al., 2012. Development of acute dystonia in three brothers due to metoclopramide. *Journal of Research in Medical Sciences: The Official Journal of Isfahan University of Medical Sciences*, **17**(3), pp. 308–309.

61. Simpson, G.M. and Lindenmayer, J.P., 1997. Extrapyramidal symptoms in patients treated with risperidone. *Journal of Clinical Psychopharmacotherapy*, **17**(3), pp. 194–201.

62. Singh, M.K., DelBello, M.P. and Adler, C.M., 2007. Acute dystonia associated with aripiprazole in a child. *Journal of the American Academy of Child and Adolescent Psychiatry*, **46**(3), pp. 306–307.

63. Song, X., Hu, Z. and Zhang, H., 2005. Acute dystonia induced by lamivudine. *Clinical Neuropharmacology*, **28**(4), pp. 193–194.

64. Spina, E., Sturiale, V., Valvo, S., Ancione, M., Di Rosa, A.E., Meduri, M. and Caputi, A.P., 1993. Prevalence of acute dystonic reactions associated with neuroleptic treatment with and without anticholinergic prophylaxis. *International Clinical Psychopharmacology*, **8**(1), pp. 21–24.

65. Swett, C., 1975. Drug-induced dystonia. *The American Journal of Psychiatry*, **132**(5), pp. 532–534.

66. Uca, A.U., Kozak, H.H. and Uguz, F., 2014. Varenicline-induced acute dystonic reaction: a case report. *General Hospital Psychiatry*, **36**(3), pp. 361.e1–2.

67. van der Meer, J.N. et al., 2012. White matter abnormalities in gene-positive myoclonus-dystonia. *Movement Disorders*, **27**(13), pp. 1666–1672.

68. van Waarde, A. et al., 2011. The cholinergic system, sigma-1 receptors and cognition. *Behavioural Brain Research*, **221**(2), pp. 543–554.

69. Varkula, M. and Dale, R., 2008. Acute dystonic reaction after initiating aripiprazole monotherapy in a 20-year-old man. *Journal of Clinical Psychopharmacotherapy*, **28**(2), pp. 1–21.

70. Vena, J., Dufel, S. and Paige, T., 2006. Acute olanzapine-induced akathisia and dystonia in a patient discontinued from fluoxetine. *The Journal of Emergency Medicine*, **30**(3), pp. 311–317.

71. Venkateswaran, P.S. and Otto, A.G., 1972. Acute dystonia due to metoclopramide. *British Medical Journal*, **4**(5833), pp. 178–179.

72. Viana, B. de M. et al., 2009. Ziprasidone-related oculogyric crisis in an adult. *Clinical Neurology and Neurosurgery*, **111**(10), pp. 883–885.

73. Wang, G.J. et al., 1996. Age associated decrements in dopamine D2 receptors in thalamus and in temporal insula of human subjects. *Life Sciences*, **59**(1), pp. PL31–5.

74. Waugh, J.L., 2013. Acute dyskinetic reaction in a healthy toddler following methylphenidate ingestion. *Pediatric Neurology*, **49**(1), pp. 58–60.

75. Yumru, M. et al., 2006. Acute dystonia after initial doses of ziprasidone: A case report. *Progress in Neuro-Psychopharmacology and Biological Psychiatry*, **30**(4), pp. 745–747.

# Chapter 3

# Neuroleptic malignant syndrome

Atbin Djamashidian and Sean S. O'Sullivan

## Clinical vignette

A 21-year-old man with no previous psychiatric history was admitted to hospital with a two-month history of disturbed sleep and behavioral changes. He had developed paranoid delusions regarding family members and was becoming increasingly aggressive toward them. He was agitated and paranoid, and described auditory persecutory hallucinations. He was given 5mg of haloperidol and 2mg of lorazepam intramuscularly, and 2mg of haloperidol intravenously every four hours for three doses. Within 12 hours he developed a fever of 40.0°C, tremors, and tachycardia. He was started on broad-spectrum intravenous antibiotics for a presumed community-acquired pneumonia after a portable chest radiograph suggested possible lobar consolidation, and a full blood count showed a leucocytosis of 21,000/mm$^3$. By 24 hours after admission, he had become unresponsive, hypotensive, and rigid. Laboratory tests demonstrated a metabolic acidosis and a raised serum creatinine kinase (CK) level (36,000 IU). Cerebrospinal fluid (CSF) analyses were normal. Blood and CSF bacterial cultures were subsequently negative. Haloperidol was discontinued and dantrolene was administered intravenously. His recovery was complicated by acute renal failure requiring dialysis. He gradually became more responsive over the following week, but took two months to return to his premorbid baseline.

## Background

Neuroleptic malignant syndrome (NMS) is an idiosyncratic adverse reaction with potentially fatal outcome related to neuroleptic and other medications. Although the incidence of NMS is low, it is associated with a 5%–20% mortality rate and therefore a high index of suspicion is necessary (1).

Neuroleptic drugs were introduced in 1954 and probable cases of NMS were described in English in 1959 (2). However, these cases were not formally diagnosed as NMS. In 1960 Delay, in France, called these drug-related side effects 'syndrome malin des neuroleptiques' (3). For many years it was thought that this syndrome was extremely rare, although cases had been reported in Japan, France, and the UK (4). It was brought to broader attention by a review article by Caroff in 1980, which reviewed around 60 cases and concluded that the condition was underrecognized and could be fatal in around 20% of patients(5). A possible reason why NMS was not noticed earlier in the US may be that reports were published in different languages (4). By 1986 around 300 cases had been reported (4). Previously NMS was sometimes misdiagnosed as malignant catatonia or undertreated psychosis, resulting in further neuroleptic treatment and a delay in recognizing that this syndrome was iatrogenic (6).

## Neuroleptic medications

Neuroleptic medications, often referred to as neuroleptics, are a family of drugs broadly unified by their antagonistic actions on dopamine receptors. Neuroleptics also bind to numerous neurotransmitter receptors other than dopamine, including norepinephrine, epinephrine, acetylcholine, serotonin, and histamine. While the main therapeutic and extrapyramidal side effects of neuroleptics are thought to be attributable to the antagonism of dopamine at D2 receptors, their actions at the other neuroreceptors may be associated with various other side effects (7).

While this review will largely consider the neuroleptics used for the treatment of psychosis, which is their most commonly prescribed indication, it is

*Medication-Induced Movement Disorders*, ed. Joseph H. Friedman. Published by Cambridge University Press.
© Cambridge University Press 2015.

important to acknowledge that these drugs are not used exclusively for psychiatric symptoms. Neuroleptics are also frequently used for other indications such as nausea, vertigo, tic disorders, chorea, depression, or as "sleeping tablets". In the US, direct TV marketing to patients of aripiprazole for the treatment of depression has increased its sales. In some countries these medications may be dispensed without a prescription, and it is not uncommon for patients to be taking these medications chronically without being fully aware of the original indication for their use. Therefore, it is important to ask patients about all the tablets they are using, rather than specifically asking if they are on any medications for emotional problems. Several of the antipsychotic drugs (including haloperidol, fluphenazine, and risperidone) are available in long-acting injectable preparations for intramuscular administration. These depot injections must be specifically asked about when neuroleptic malignant syndrome is suspected, as they may not be remembered or volunteered by patients or their caregivers.

First-generation antipsychotic drugs are usually classified into three groups: phenothiazines, butyrophenones (e.g., haloperidol), and others (e.g., thiothixene, molindone, and loxapine), based on their structure. These all exhibit high affinity for D2 receptors, and all may be associated with extrapyramidal syndromes (EPS), including parkinsonism, dystonia, akathisia, and tardive dyskinesia. Second-generation antipsychotic drugs are characterized by generally lower affinities for D2 receptors and therefore with less EPS compared to first-generation antipsychotics (7). Second-generation neuroleptics such as olanzapine, clozapine, and ziprasidone have relatively greater affinities for serotonin (5 hydroxytryptamine) 5-HT2A receptors in particular, but also for noradrenergic receptors ($\alpha$ 1 and $\alpha$ 2), muscarinic acetylcholine receptors, histamine, and other dopamine (DA) subtype receptors. Aripiprazole is a second-generation neuroleptic which acts as a partial agonist at D2 and 5-HT1A receptors as well as an antagonist at the 5-HT2A and D2 receptors (7).

For a clinician treating a potential side effect of an antipsychotic medication, it is important to note the variability of duration of effect. The average plasma half-life of neuroleptics as a family is approximately 20 to 24 hours, ranging from 4–10 hours for shorter-acting drugs like ziprasidone and quetiapine, to up to 94 hours for others such as aripiprazole and its metabolites. Injectable neuroleptics like haloperidol and

fluphenazine decanoate have half-lives of approximately 3 weeks (7). Regardless of their serum half-lives, these drugs are all remarkably lipophilic and remain in the brain for very long periods of time, far surpassing their serum levels.

## Epidemiology

NMS is classically associated with the use of high-potency antipsychotics, such as butyrophenones and phenothiazines. Earlier case series in the era of first-generation neuroleptics described haloperidol and fluphenazine as being the most frequently-implicated drugs (8), with a presumed lower risk associated with newer second-generation neuroleptics. Convincing data of the lower risk is not available. The incidence of NMS in the 1980s was estimated between 0.2% and 1% (9). One prospective study over 6 months including 495 antipsychotic treated patients reported only one case of NMS (10), whereas others found a higher incidence up to 0.9 per cent (11). However, these incidence rates vary depending on the diagnostic criteria used or the survey techniques (4). Recent reports estimated the incidence much lower, between 0.07% and 0.15% (12). However, in a psychiatric hospital in the Northeast of the US only six out of 58,800 patients had been discharged with a diagnosis of NMS (0.001%) and none of the patients were diagnosed with NMS after 2010 (personal communication JH Friedman).

Increased physicians' vigilance, lower doses, and the use of atypical neuroleptics are likely responsible for the reduction in incidence of NMS (6).

## Risk factors

Most reports have been described in patients between 20 and 50 years, although it can affect all ages (13). Further, it is possible that clinicians fail to diagnose the condition in the elderly (14). The elderly are unlikely to be neuroleptically naïve if they have a primary psychotic disorder. New use of neuroleptics in the elderly is typically for dementia-related problems at very lose doses.

Some studies reported that men are affected more frequently, others reported the opposite, and some studies found no gender differences (4). Further, some speculated that postpartum women are more susceptible for developing NMS (15). It is unlikely that environmental factors are important in triggering NMS, as it has been reported worldwide in countries with hot and cool climates (4). Organic brain disease and affective disorders (16, 17) have been proposed as risk factors for NMS, although several cases with no neurological or psychiatric history have also been reported (18).

Around 17% of patients who developed NMS suffered from similar symptoms during earlier exposure to neuroleptic drugs (19). Once recovered, around 30% will develop NMS again when reexposed to the same neuroleptics (16, 19). All neuroleptic medications can cause NMS, although the incidence may vary with the drug. For example, clozapine is thought to have a tenfold lower potential to cause NMS compared to haloperidol (20). Case reports of NMS have also been reported with various nonneuroleptic drugs (see Table 3.1) and some authors have suggested calling these side effects "neuroleptic malignant-like disorders" as no exposure to neuroleptics occurred (21).

There are case reports of patients who developed NMS after a single low dose of haloperidol (22). However, it is generally accepted that higher doses, particularly of high-potency typical neuroleptics (23), rapid increase of dose or rate, and the use of depot preparations have been strongly associated with NMS. Further, dehydration, psychomotor agitation, exhaustion, and concurrent use of other psychotropic drugs have been suggested as risk factors (24). Alcohol abuse was diagnosed in 8% of patients with NMS in one study (25). These patients are considered at particular risk because of malnutrition, dehydration, and possibly an alcohol-induced sensitization of muscles to neuroleptics (24). A history of cocaine abuse was suggested as a risk factor for subsequent NMS development in patients later treated with neuroleptics (26). Caution is also required in patients with idiopathic or drug-induced catatonia, as they are thought particularly vulnerable (27). Previously-elevated serum creatinine kinase (CK) levels in patients treated for non-NMS psychotic episodes were shown to be a risk factor for future NMS in one case-control study (28). Switching from one neuroleptic to another (29), or discontinuation of neuroleptics (30), has also been reported to trigger NMS.

Families with NMS have been reported, suggesting that there are genetic risk factors (31). In particular, polymorphisms in the dopamine D2 receptor gene, the serotonin receptor, and the cytochrome P450 2D6 gene have been investigated as susceptibility factors for developing NMS (32), although the

**Table 3.1** Differential diagnosis of neuroleptic malignant syndrome. Table adapted from (56).

➤ Infectious
- Encephalitis or meningitis
- Brain abscess
- Rabies
- Sepsis
- Botulism
- Tetanus
- Any systemic infection causing secondary worsening of preexisting parkinsonism, especially in elderly

➤ Psychiatric
- Idiopathic malignant catatonia
- Delirium
- Severe depression
- Catatonia schizophrenia

➤ Neurological
- Parkinson's disease–dopaminergic medication withdrawal
- Nonconvulsive status epilepticus
- Structural lesions involving the midbrain
- Severe acute dystonic reactions

➤ Toxic or pharmacological
- Heat stroke
- Allergic drug reactions
- Heavy metal poisoning (e.g., lead, arsenic)
- Lithium, metoclopramide, carbamazepine, lamotrigine, venlafaxine, domperidone, amoxapine, baclofen, tetrabenazine, promethazine
- Salicylate poisoning
- Malignant hyperthermia
- Serotonin syndrome (monoamine oxidase inhibitors, triptans)
- Withdrawal from dopamine agonists
- Alcohol withdrawal

➤ Substance abuse
- Cocaine, amphetamines, ecstasy, and hallucinogen intoxication (e.g., phencyclidine)

➤ Endocrine/metabolic
- Pheochromocytoma
- Thyrotoxicosis
- Hypocalcemia
- Hypomagnesemia

➤ Miscellaneous
- Systemic lupus erythematosus
- Acute intermittent porphyria

data remains conflicting. Polymorphisms in the 5HT1A and 5HT2A receptor genes do not determine susceptibility to NMS (33). The TaqIA polymorphism of the D2 receptor gene has been identified as a risk factor in some (34) but not all studies (35).

## Diagnostic criteria and clinical features

NMS is a potentially fatal reaction to neuroleptic medication but has been reported in other drugs not mainly targeting the dopamine receptors. The clinical presentation of NMS is generally similar regardless of whether a first-generation or second-generation antipsychotic is implicated, although one study reported that rigidity may be a less prominent feature in clozapine-induced NMS (36). The diagnosis is clinical and no valid biomarker exists (37). Therefore a thorough clinical and laboratory assessment is required to exclude other potential causes of hyperthermia. Onset is usually over hours, although more rapid progressive forms exist. Changes in either mental status or rigidity were the initial manifestations of NMS in 82% of cases with a single presenting sign and were significantly more likely to be observed before hyperthermia and autonomic dysfunction (38, 39). Caroff and Mann reported that NMS began within one month of neuroleptic medication initiation in almost all cases, with 66% developing symptoms within 1 week (19).

There are no universally accepted diagnostic criteria for NMS (37). There has been a general recognition that the core clinical characteristics include a tetrad of fever, extrapyramidal symptoms, altered mentation, and autonomic instability (17). Mental status changes range from confusion to coma. To make a firm diagnosis of NMS the fever should be above 38°C (100.0°F) and severe rigidity or tremor should be present. Based on their study, Addonizio and colleagues proposed that three out of seven minor criteria are supportive for the diagnosis: heart rate above 100 beats per minute (96% of their cases), diaphoresis, peripheral white count above 10,800 cells/mm$^3$, elevated creatine phosphokinase, hypertension, confusion, and incontinence (17). In 2011 a multispecialist team containing psychiatrists, neurologists, anaesthesiologists, and emergency medicine specialists proposed the following definition:

Exposure to dopamine antagonist or withdrawal of dopamine agonists within the last 72 hours, hyperthermia (>38°C, 100.4°F) measured orally on two occasions, rigidity, mental status alteration (reduced or fluctuating level of consciousness), at least four times the upper limit of normal creatine kinase levels, evidence of sympathetic nervous system lability (defined as 2 of the following: blood pressure elevation or fluctuation, diaphoresis, and urinary incontinence), hypermetabolism (defined as heart rate increase >25% and respiratory increase by >50%), and a negative workup of infectious, toxic, metabolic, or other neurological causes (37). These criteria were recently validated with respect to the DSM-IV-TR criteria as the diagnostic reference standard, where a cutoff score of 64 (maximum, 100) was associated with a sensitivity of 83.2% and a specificity of 94.6% (40).

Apart from rigidity, tremor, freezing of gait, sialorrhea, hypomimia, bradykinesia, blepharospasm, chorea, and oculogyric crisis have been reported (4, 41).

All criteria are problematic because they are linked. Fever produces tachycardia, tachypnea, and diaphoresis, regardless of the cause. Fever also produces mental status changes in the elderly, and may dramatically worsen parkinsonism induced by a neuroleptic. In one review of patients thought to have NMS, half had infectious etiologies (42).

## Pathophysiology

The pathophysiology of NMS is still poorly understood. However, the rapid reduction in dopamine receptor D2 activity is considered to play a main role (43), although reports of NMS developing after several months of exposure make this explanation less than universal. The importance of an acute reduction in dopamine activity as the major mechanism driving NMS is suggested by the following: The neuroleptics causing NMS all block dopamine receptors, and the closely related parkinsonism-hyperpyrexia syndrome is caused by an abrupt reduction of dopamine replacement therapies; the likelihood of developing NMS is correlated with the relative dopamine-blocking potency of the neuroleptics implicated (44); NMS is thought to respond to dopamine replacement therapy; and studies on the cerebrospinal fluid of patients with NMS reveal reductions in homovanillic acid, dopamine's main metabolite (45). An NMS-like syndrome ascribed to reserpine (46), as well as a similar syndrome in people with Parkinson's disease who stop their medication, also support this theory.

One proposed model of NMS pathogenesis suggests profound sympatho-adrenergic dysfunction caused by dopamine antagonists interrupting the normally present tonic inhibitory modulation of sympathetic nervous system function (38). It has been suggested that D2 receptor antagonism could remove tonic inhibition from the sympathetic nervous system leading to sympatho-adrenal hyperactivity and thus causing tachycardia, thermo-dysregulation, labile blood pressure, urinary symptoms, and pallor (38). The sympathetic nervous system is regulated by the lateral and posterior hypothalamus, and most dorsal hypothalamic spinal projection neurons are dopaminergic and appear to be involved in autonomic functions (47). An injection of dopamine or the dopamine agonist apomorphine into the preoptic-anterior hypothalamus causes a reduction in core temperature (48). Therefore, the blockade of these hypothalamic dopamine sites with neuroleptic drugs has been implicated in causing the NMS hyperthermia (49). However, NMS can be caused by a variety of different drugs with different modes of action (e.g., lithium, SSRIs, carbamazepine); and therefore reduction in D2 receptor availability cannot account for all these cases. Similarly, the low incidence of NMS compared to drug-induced parkinsonism as a complication of dopaminergic receptor blockade suggests that other mechanisms may be implicated in NMS. Furthermore, the sympathetic changes are linked to each other.

The possibility of a direct toxic effect on skeletal muscle caused by neuroleptics has been investigated following reports of in vitro chlorpromazine inducing muscle contractures (50). However, subsequent studies did not demonstrate an increased sensitivity to neuroleptic drugs when comparing muscle from NMS patients and from normal patients (51). While these negative findings may apparently refute a susceptibility to a direct neuroleptic-induced muscle injury in NMS patients, it is worth acknowledging that they do not account for in vivo circumstances which are known to increase the risk of NMS, such as exhaustion, psychomotor agitation, or dehydration (24).

The possibility of an underlying pharmacogenetic defect in skeletal muscle as a cause of NMS has also been investigated, largely because of its clinical overlap with malignant hyperthermia (MH)—a syndrome caused by inhalational anesthetics and succinylcholine. Both conditions are characterized by hyperthermia, rigidity, an increased creatine kinase level, and a similar mortality rate (24). However, conflicting results have been reported regarding the prevalence of malignant hyperthermia susceptibility among NMS patients (24).

Other potential mechanisms that have been invoked to explain NMS include abnormalities of N-methyl-D-aspartate (NMDA) glutamate receptors (52), excessive glutamatergic transmission secondary to dopaminergic blockade, or reduced gamma-aminobutyric acid (GABA) activity (45). More recently, an immunologic mechanism for NMS development was hypothesized, following reports of the temporal evolution of a variety of acute phase reactants in an instance of neuroleptic malignant syndrome (53). Large studies are required to further investigate these hypothesized pathways in the development of NMS.

## Laboratory tests

Fever and rigidity contribute to muscle injury and necrosis, causing increased serum CK levels, aldolase, lactic dehydrogenase, and transaminase levels. Muscle necrosis can rapidly turn into rhabdomyolysis with electrolyte derangement. CK levels have been shown to correlate with the prognosis of NMS (25) and usually normalize when patients recover (54). Monitoring of serum CK levels is important to indicate the severity of rhabdomyolysis and the associated risk of developing myoglobinuric renal failure. Leucocytosis, ranging from a slight elevation between 10,000 and 40,000/mm$^3$, with or without shift, may be seen (16, 24). Abnormally low serum iron concentrations (more than two standard deviations lower than the normal range) have been found to be a sensitive but not specific marker for NMS (55). Cerebrospinal fluid (CSF) examination is normal in 95% of patients (19), although some have reported a reduction in the dopamine metabolite homovanillic acid (56). However, these reports need to be interpreted with care, as patients with schizophrenia also have lower homovanillic acid levels (HVA) (57), and multiple other factors may alter HVA. Magnetic resonance imaging (MRI) and computed tomography (CT) are usually unremarkable, although cases of basal ganglia and cerebellar damage, likely due to hyperthermia, have been reported (58). Electroencephalography (EEG) may show abnormal slowing due to the metabolic encephalopathy (24).

## Differential diagnosis

Neuroleptic malignant syndrome is a diagnosis of exclusion; therefore it is of paramount importance to exclude structural lesions and infectious diseases such as viral encephalitis, sepsis, and brain abscess (56) (Table 3.2). It is important to acknowledge that the majority of patients using neuroleptics who develop fever and rigidity will not have NMS.

Parkinsonism-hyperpyrexia syndrome is clinically identical to NMS except that it occurs in patients with preexisting treated parkinsonism. This syndrome develops following a rapid reduction of dopamine replacement therapies, and was initially described in patients with Parkinson's disease taking a "drug holiday" (59). Rigidity, stiffness, and tremor usually occur between 18 hours and 7 days, and within 72 to 96 hours patients develop high fever and reduced consciousness ranging from confusion to coma. Later on patients develop autonomic dysfunction with tachycardia, labile blood pressure, and diaphoresis. Elevated CK levels and leukocytosis may occur. A poorer outcome has been observed in older patients and those who have more severe premorbid parkinsonism (60). Physician-endorsed "drug holidays" are no longer clinically encountered, but parkinsonism-hyperpyrexia syndrome may still be seen in the setting of poor patient compliance, and when patients become acutely unable to take their medications as occurs with gastrointestinal and other surgeries. Although parkinsonism-hyperpyrexia syndrome is most commonly seen in patients with idiopathic Parkinson's disease, it has been also observed in patients with atypical parkinsonism such as progressive supranuclear palsy, multiple system atrophy, and vascular parkinsonism (60).

The treatment of parkinsonism-hyperpyrexia syndrome is similar to NMS (see below). Dopaminergic medication which has been stopped should be restarted immediately. In patients who cannot swallow medication, administration via a nasogastric tube is necessary or the transdermal dopamine agonist rotigotine (8–16mg) can be applied. Patients may require intensive care and supportive treatment including fluid replacement, antipyretic medication, and cooling blankets (60). One randomized-controlled trial found that pulse methylprednisolone therapy reduced the illness duration and improved symptoms of 20 Parkinson's disease patients with parkinsonism-hyperpyrexia syndrome (61).

## Malignant catatonia

While malignant catatonia shares features including fever, hyperthermia, rigidity, elevated creatinine kinase, and white blood count with NMS, clinical and laboratory features may offer clues to distinguish these conditions. Malignant catatonia may have a prodrome that is characterized by excessive and purposeless motor activity in both the upper and lower limbs (hyperkinesis), restlessness, stereotypy, impulsivity, frenzy, and combativeness (62), and this extreme psychotic excitement helps differentiate this disorder from NMS (63). In general, laboratory abnormalities are more often seen in NMS than catatonia, with some authors suggesting a reduced serum iron level as being most useful in pointing to an NMS diagnosis (64).

There are four other recognized drug-induced hyperthermia syndromes: serotonin syndrome, anticholinergic syndrome, sympathomimetic syndrome mainly caused by illicit drugs, and malignant hyperthermia.

## Serotonin syndrome

Serotonin syndrome (SS) usually occurs during serotonin agonist polypharmacotherapy(65). Like NMS, serotonin syndrome is a diagnosis of exclusion. Clinical features of SS include mood changes and a clouded sensorium; autonomic symptoms such as tachycardia, diaphoresis, labile blood pressure, and nausea; and neurological symptoms including tremor, myoclonus, brisk reflexes, rigidity, and ataxia (65). Despite this overlap, a few clinical differences may help in differentiating NMS from SS (see Table 3.2).

## Malignant hyperthermia

MH is a rare autosomal dominant disorder of the skeletal muscle usually caused by a mutation of the RYR-1 channel gene. MH is characterized by extreme hypermetabolic crisis after inhalation of, e.g., halothane; exposure to succinylcholine, which is a depolarizing neuromuscular blocking agent; or as a result of severe exercise or heat. The mortality rate is about 10% and symptoms emerge usually within minutes to hours. The initial symptoms include autonomic dysfunction with tachycardia and tachypnea followed by severe hyperthermia, rigidity, and metabolic acidosis, potentially leading to multiple organ failure. The therapy has been well established and consists of supportive care, dantrolene, and hyperventilation of 100% oxygen (66) (see Table 3.2).

**Table 3.2** Differential diagnosis between neuroleptic malignant syndrome, serotonin syndrome, and malignant hyperthermia adapted from (67). NMS=neuroleptic malignant syndrome, SS=serotonin syndrome, MH=malignant hyperthermia, CK=creatinine kinase, ECT=electroconvulsion therapy. **=causative agents should be withdrawn prior to therapy.

| | NMS | SS | MH |
|---|---|---|---|
| Onset | Subacute (days) | Subacute (days) | Acute (usually within hours, but occasionally longer) |
| Age | Adults | All ages | Children, young adults |
| Risk factors | Idiosyncratic | Dose related | Genetic |
| Resolution | Gradual within 14 days | Usually within <24h | May take several weeks up to 2 months |
| Fever | ++ | ++ | +++ |
| Confusion | +++ | +++ | + |
| Dysautonomia | +++ | +++ | +++ |
| Motor features | Tremor, rigidity | Myoclonus, brisk reflexes, stereotypies | |
| Elevated CK | +++ (>90%) | + (<20%) | +++ |
| Leucocytosis | +++ (<90%) | + (<15%) | ++ (case reports) |
| Diaphoresis | ++ | ++ | +++ |
| Metabolic acidosis | + | + | ++ |
| Therapy** | bromocriptine benzodiazepines dantrolene amantadine ECT | methysergide cyproheptadine | dantrolene azumolene |

## Anticholinergic syndrome

A variety of different drugs can cause anticholinergic syndrome, including tricyclic antidepressants, antihistamines, and belladonna alkaloids. Children are at higher risk of developing this syndrome as they have a lower sweat rate. Anticholinergic syndrome is caused by blockage of both central and peripheral muscarinic acetylcholine receptors. Symptoms caused by central blockage of the muscarinic receptor include confusion, agitation, myoclonus, tremor, and hallucinations, and can ultimately lead to coma and convulsions. Rigidity is, however, absent. In contrast to the other drug-induced hyperthermias, patients also suffer from peripheral symptoms such as dry mouth, mydriasis, blurred vision, urinary retention, and tachycardia (66).

## Sympathomimetic syndrome

This syndrome is mainly caused by illicit drugs such as cocaine and ecstasy but also nonselective monoamino-oxidase inhibitors. Symptoms include anxiety, panic attacks, and confusion. The exact mechanism by which these drugs cause hyperthermia is unknown but it is believed that alteration of the serotonin, dopamine, and norepinephrine levels cause dysfunction of central thermoregulation. Therapy includes withdrawal of the causative agent, supportive care, and vigorous cooling of the core temperature. Benzodiazepines or anticonvulsive therapy may be used, and some have suggested cautiously administered dantrolene (66).

## Complications

Complications are usually the consequence of dehydration, electrolyte derangement, fever, rigidity, and immobility (43). Hyperkalemia and hyperphosphatemia, due to potassium and phosphate release by the necrotic myocytes into the blood stream, can cause hypocalcemia, which in turn can lead to arrhythmias and myocardial infarction (54). In such cases continuous cardiac monitoring may be required. Seizures can occur as a consequence of hyperpyrexia and electrolyte derangement (54). Aspiration pneumonia because of swallowing problems combined with altered mentation, and respiratory failure due to chest wall rigidity may require intubation (43).

After cardiac arrhythmias and hypotension, which occur early, acute tubular necrosis due to myoglobinuria is the most common serious longer duration problem (68) and occurs in about 67% of patients in whom urine was tested (69). The risk of this complication may be reduced by early action to increase hydration, and by closely monitoring CK and myoglobin levels. Deep venous thrombosis and pulmonary embolism due to dehydration and immobility (43) and disseminated intravascular coagulation (70) have been reported.

## Treatment

No prospective randomized treatment trials have been published and no medication has been approved to treat NMS (71). Therefore, treatment of NMS centers on early diagnosis, withdrawal of neuroleptic medications, and initiation of supportive therapies. Neuroleptics cannot be removed by dialysis, and blood concentrations decline slowly.

## Supportive therapy

The most urgent aim is to discontinue the causative agent and to treat hyperthermia. Cooling blankets or sometimes ice packs in the axilla, or more extreme methods such as ice water gastric lavage (54) or endovascular cooling (72) may be required. Withdrawal of neuroleptics or the causative agent will usually lead to improvement within two weeks unless depot preparations have been administered (65). Electrolytes, CK levels, and renal function should be monitored once or twice daily and ECG monitoring may be required. Symptomatic treatment includes rehydration and supportive treatment, which can even require mechanical ventilation or pacemaker implantation, with case reports of recurrent cardiac arrest described in NMS. If CK levels are highly raised, vigorous administration of intravenous fluids in combination with urine alkalinization may prevent renal failure and subsequently rhabdomyolysis (54). Clonidine has been used successfully to manage autonomic dysfunction, including blood pressure lability, in small case series of NMS (73). Low-molecular heparin should be administered to prevent deep venous thrombosis. In cases where CK is markedly elevated and rigidity is severe, paralysis

should be induced until agents to reverse the NMS can take effect. Pyrexia and breathing will be easier to manage, and the risk of renal failure will be reduced.

## Pharmacological therapy

For a schematic flow chart see Figure 3.1. Benzodiazepine may be helpful to improve catatonic symptoms such as mutism and immobility (71) and may help to improve agitation. However, this is based only on case series, as a clinical trial did not show any benefit of benzodiazepine (74).

The use of dopamine agonists has been positively correlated with faster recovery and halved mortality (56). However, the correct diagnosis of NMS is critical, as bromocriptine, for example, can cause worsening of serotonin syndrome (71). While bromocriptine has historically been used most often and is considered the drug of choice (75), other dopaminergic agents are equally effective. Some suggest the use of amantadine as it may also reverse parkinsonism in these patients (56); however, so should dopamine agonists.

In parkinsonism-hyperpyrexia syndrome L-dopa or dopamine agonist therapy should be restarted as soon as possible (76). CK levels are usually lower and hospitalization days are shorter compared to patients with NMS (76).

Dantrolene inhibits calcium release from the sarcoplasmic reticulum, decreasing available calcium for ongoing muscle contracture. This muscle relaxant, alone or in combination with benzodiazepines and dopamine agonists, can be beneficial for patients with extreme hyperthermia and hypermetabolism (56). Coadministration with calcium channel blockers should be avoided because of cardiovascular collapse (56). While the use of dantrolene is considered a treatment of first choice in many current pharmacologic and psychiatric textbooks, it is important to acknowledge that its use is largely based on small case series and a robust evidence base is lacking. In particular, a retrospective review of 271 case reports found that dantrolene is associated with a prolongation of clinical recovery when used in combination therapy, and was associated with a higher overall mortality when used as monotherapy in NMS (77).

In patients with severe NMS, with fever above 40.0°C, severe rigidity, catatonia or coma, and a heart rate above 120 beats per minute, and who are pharmacoresistant, case reports have suggested that six to ten treatments with electroconvulsive therapy

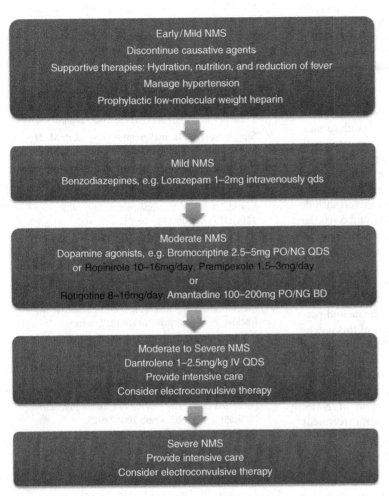

**Figure 3.1:** Flow chart of treatment options in patients with neuroleptic malignant syndrome (NMS). PO=per os, NG=nasogastric tube, bd=bis in die (twice per day), qds=quaque die (four times per day), IV=intravenously.

Early/Mild NMS
Discontinue causative agents
Supportive therapies: Hydration, nutrition, and reduction of fever
Manage hypertension
Prophylactic low-molecular weight heparin

Mild NMS
Benzodiazepines, e.g. Lorazepam 1–2mg intravenously qds

Moderate NMS
Dopamine agonists, e.g. Bromocriptine 2.5–5mg PO/NG QDS
or Ropinirole 10–16mg/day, Pramipexole 1.5–3mg/day
or
Rotigotine 8–16mg/day, Amantadine 100–200mg PO/NG BD

Moderate to Severe NMS
Dantrolene 1–2.5mg/kg IV QDS
Provide intensive care
Consider electroconvulsive therapy

Severe NMS
Provide intensive care
Consider electroconvulsive therapy

(ECT) may be useful (56, 78). However, there are no prospective, randomized, controlled data supporting its efficacy. In a retrospective review of ECT, Trollor and colleagues concluded it is the preferred treatment in severe NMS, cases where the underlying psychiatric diagnosis is psychotic depression or catatonia, and in cases where lethal catatonia cannot be ruled out. However, they note that ECT has been associated with cardiovascular complications, which occurred in 4 of 55 patients, including two patients with ventricular fibrillation and cardiac arrest with permanent anoxic brain injury (78).

Most patients require continuation of neuroleptic treatment and no accepted guidelines have been published for further treatment. Rechallenge with neuroleptics of the same milligram potency as the original stimulus in six patients resulted in recurrent NMS in five of the six patients, with two deaths. Rechallenge with less potent antipsychotics, such as thioridazine, was safe in nine of 10 cases (44). Generally, it is recommended to wait for 2 weeks after symptoms have resolved and then, if possible, to switch to a low dose of a low potency neuroleptic such as chlorpromazine or thioridazine (65), or a second-generation antipsychotic.

## Prognosis

The mortality rate was 76% in the 1960s but has dropped significantly over recent years and estimates now vary between 10% and 20% (54). Earlier recognition and treatment of NMS is the most likely factor contributing to the decline in mortality. Causes of death in NMS include cardiorespiratory arrest, acute renal failure, and disseminated intravascular coagulation. Most cases nowadays recover within two weeks (54). Patients receiving depot neuroleptic preparations generally have a prolonged duration of illness, and have a worse prognosis. Poor prognostic outcome has also been reported in patients with organic brain disease and those with extreme fever peaks and longer duration of hyperthermia (56). One study of 208 cases of NMS found that mortality was considerably lower for those with second-generation antipsychotic NMS (3.0%) compared with NMS following first-generation antipsychotic use (16.3%), and the former were more likely to have received supportive treatment (36). Persistent neurological complications described in NMS survivors include parkinsonism, dementia, dyskinesia (41), and cerebellar syndrome (79), as a result of parenchymal damage due to hyperpyrexia.

## Conclusions

While NMS is a relatively rare disorder, the frequent use of neuroleptic medications in medicine and psychiatry behooves clinicians to be aware of this potentially fatal syndrome. Hopefully, NMS will become less common due to the increasing use of second-generation antipsychotics, more conservative antipsychotic prescribing patterns, increased awareness of risk factors, and the earlier recognition of NMS. Prevention, early recognition, and prompt treatment remain of paramount importance.

## References

1. Robottom BJ, Weiner WJ, Factor SA. Movement disorders emergencies. Part 1: Hypokinetic disorders. *Archives of Neurology*. 2011;**68**(5):567–72. Epub 2011/05/11.

2. Preston J. Central nervous system reactions to small doses of tranquilizers; report of one death. *American Practitioner and Digest of Treatment*. 1959;**10**(4):627–30. Epub 1959/04/01.

3. Delay J, Pichot P, Lemperiere T, Ellisalde B, Peigne F. Un neuroleptique majeur non phenothiazine et non reserpinique l'haloperidol dans le traitment des psychoses. *Ann Med Psychol*. 1960;**118**:145–152.

4. Mann SC, Caroff S, Lazerus A, Keck PE. *Neuroleptic malignant syndrome and related conditions*. American Psychiatric Pub. 2008.

5. Caroff SN. The neuroleptic malignant syndrome. *The Journal of Clinical Psychiatry*. 1980;**41**(3):79–83. Epub 1980/03/01.

6. Caroff SN, Mann SC, Sullivan K, Campbell B. Neuroleptic malignant syndrome in movement disorder emergencies: diagnosis and treatment. 2013:43–57.

7. Lieberman JA, Tasman A. Antipsychotic drugs. In: Lieberman JA, Tasman A, editors. *Handbook of Psychiatric Drugs*. Chichester, England: John Wiley & Sons; 2006.

8. Chaimowitz GA, Gomes U, Maze SS. Neuroleptic malignant syndrome. *CMAJ: Canadian Medical Association Journal = Journal de l'Association Medicale Canadienne*. 1988;**138**(1):51–3. Epub 1988/01/01.

9. Sing A. Neuroleptic malignant syndrome. *Br Med J (Clin Res Ed)*. 1983;**287**(6391):560–1. Epub 1983/08/20.

10. Friedman JH, Davis R, Wagner RL. Neuroleptic malignant syndrome. The results of a 6-month prospective study of incidence in a state psychiatric hospital. *Clinical Neuropharmacology*. 1988;**11**(4):373–7.Epub 1988/08/01.

11. Keck PE, Jr., Sebastianelli J, Pope HG, Jr., McElroy SL. Frequency and presentation of neuroleptic malignant syndrome in a state psychiatric hospital. *The Journal of Clinical Psychiatry*. 1989;**50**(9):352–5. Epub 1989/09/01.

12. Mehndiratta P, Spolter Y, Igboeli B, Sajatovic M, Buckley P. *Neuroleptic Malignant Syndrome. Neuromuscular Disorders in Clinical Practice*. New York: Springer, 2014:1487–500.

13. Croarkin PE, Emslie GJ, Mayes TL. Neuroleptic malignant syndrome associated with atypical antipsychotics in pediatric patients: a review of published cases. *The Journal of Clinical Psychiatry*. 2008;**69**(7):1157–65. Epub 2008/06/25.

14. Margetic B, Aukst-Margetic B. Neuroleptic malignant syndrome and its controversies. *Pharmacoepidemiology and Drug Safety*. 2010;**19**(5):429–35. Epub 2010/03/23.

15. Alexander PJ, Thomas RM, Das A. Is risk of neuroleptic malignant syndrome increased in the postpartum period? *The Journal of Clinical Psychiatry*. 1998;**59**(5):254–5. Epub 1998/06/19.

16. Rosebush P, Stewart T. A prospective analysis of 24 episodes of neuroleptic malignant syndrome. *The American Journal of Psychiatry*. 1989;**146**(6):717–25. Epub 1989/06/01.

17. Addonizio G, Susman VL, Roth SD. Neuroleptic malignant syndrome: review and analysis of 115 cases. *Biological Psychiatry*. 1987;**22**(8):1004–20. Epub 1987/08/01.

18. Friedman LS, Weinrauch LA, D'Elia JA. Metoclopramide-induced neuroleptic malignant syndrome. *Archives of Internal Medicine*. 1987;**147**(8):1495–7. Epub 1987/08/01.

19. Caroff SN, Mann SC. Neuroleptic malignant syndrome. *Psychopharmacology Bulletin*. 1988;**24**(1):25–9. Epub 1988/01/01.

20. Stubner S, Rustenbeck E, Grohmann R, Wagner G, Engel R, Neundorfer G, et al. Severe and uncommon

involuntary movement disorders due to psychotropic drugs. *Pharmacopsychiatry*. 2004;**37** Suppl 1: S54–64. Epub 2004/03/31.

21. Ohkoshi N, Satoh D, Nishi M, Shoji S. Neuroleptic malignant-like syndrome due to donepezil and maprotiline. *Neurology*. 2003;**60**(6):1050–1. Epub 2003/03/26.

22. Aisen PS, Lawlor BA. Neuroleptic malignant syndrome induced by low-dose haloperidol. *The American Journal of Psychiatry*. 1992;**149**(6):844. Epub 1992/06/01.

23. Tural U, Onder E. Clinical and pharmacologic risk factors for neuroleptic malignant syndrome and their association with death. *Psychiatry and Clinical Neurosciences*. 2010;**64**(1):79–87. Epub 2010/04/27.

24. Adnet P, Lestavel P, Krivosic-Horber R. Neuroleptic malignant syndrome. *British Journal of Anaesthesia*. 2000;**85**(1):129–35. Epub 2000/08/06.

25. Levenson JL. Neuroleptic malignant syndrome. *The American Journal of Psychiatry*. 1985;**142**(10):1137–45. Epub 1985/10/01.

26. Akpaffiong MJ, Ruiz P. Neuroleptic malignant syndrome: a complication of neuroleptics and cocaine abuse. *The Psychiatric Quarterly*. 1991;**62**(4):299–309. Epub 1991/01/01.

27. White DA, Robins AH. Catatonia: harbinger of the neuroleptic malignant syndrome. *The British Journal of Psychiatry: The Journal of Mental Science*. 1991;**158**:419–21. Epub 1991/03/01.

28. Hermesh H, Manor I, Shiloh R, Aizenberg D, Benjamini Y, Munitz H, et al. High serum creatinine kinase level: possible risk factor for neuroleptic malignant syndrome. *Journal of Clinical Psychopharmacology*. 2002;**22**(3):252–6. Epub 2002/05/15.

29. Reeves RR, Mack JE, Torres RA. Neuroleptic malignant syndrome during a change from haloperidol to risperidone. *The Annals of Pharmacotherapy*. 2001;**35**(6):698–701. Epub 2001/06/21.

30. Amore M, Zazzeri N. Neuroleptic malignant syndrome after neuroleptic discontinuation. *Progress in Neuropsychopharmacology and Biological Psychiatry*. 1995;**19**(8):1323–34. Epub 1995/12/01.

31. Otani K, Horiuchi M, Kondo T, Kaneko S, Fukushima Y. Is the predisposition to neuroleptic malignant syndrome genetically transmitted? *The British Journal of Psychiatry: The Journal of Mental Science*. 1991;**158**:850–3. Epub 1991/06/01.

32. Kawanishi C. Genetic predisposition to neuroleptic malignant syndrome: implications for antipsychotic therapy. *American Journal of Pharmacogenomics: Genomics-Related Research in Drug Development and Clinical Practice*. 2003;**3**(2):89–95. Epub 2003/05/17.

33. Kawanishi C, Hanihara T, Shimoda Y, Suzuki K, Sugiyama N, Onishi H, et al. Lack of association

34. Suzuki A, Kondo T, Otani K, Mihara K, Yasui-Furukori N, Sano A, et al. Association of the TaqIA polymorphism of the dopamine D(2) receptor gene with predisposition to neuroleptic malignant syndrome. *The American Journal of Psychiatry*. 2001;**158**(10):1714–6. Epub 2001/10/02.

35. Kishida I, Kawanishi C, Furuno T, Kato D, Ishigami T, Kosaka K. Association in Japanese patients between neuroleptic malignant syndrome and functional polymorphisms of the dopamine D(2) receptor gene. *Molecular Psychiatry*. 2004;**9**(3):293–8. Epub 2004/04/20.

36. Trollor JN, Chen X, Chitty K, Sachdev PS. Comparison of neuroleptic malignant syndrome induced by first- and second-generation antipsychotics. *The British Journal of Psychiatry: The Journal of Mental Science*. 2012;**201**(1):52–6. Epub 2012/05/26.

37. Guerra R, Caroff SN, Cohen A, Carroll B, De Roos F, Francis A, et al. An international consensus study of neuroleptic malignant syndrome diagnostic criteria using the Delphi method. *J Clin Psychiatry*. 2011; Sep;**72**(9):1222–8.

38. Gurrera RJ. Sympathoadrenal hyperactivity and the etiology of neuroleptic malignant syndrome. *The American Journal of Psychiatry*. 1999;**156**(2):169–80. Epub 1999/02/16.

39. Velamoor VR, Norman RM, Caroff SN, Mann SC, Sullivan KA, Antelo RE. Progression of symptoms in neuroleptic malignant syndrome. *The Journal of Nervous and Mental Disease*. 1994;**182**(3):168–73. Epub 1994/03/01.

40. Gurrera RJ, Velamoor V, Cernovsky ZZ. A Validation study of the International Consensus Diagnostic Criteria for Neuroleptic Malignant Syndrome. *Journal of Clinical Psychopharmacology*. 2013. Epub 2013/08/27.

41. Kurlan R, Hamill R, Shoulson I. Neuroleptic malignant syndrome. *Clinical Neuropharmacology*. 1984;**7**(2):109–20. Epub 1984/01/01.

42. Sewell DD, Jeste DV. Distinguishing neuroleptic malignant syndrome (NMS) from NMS-like acute medical illnesses: a study of 34 cases. *The Journal of Neuropsychiatry and Clinical Neurosciences*. 1992;**4**(3):265–9. Epub 1992/01/01.

43. Pelonero AL, Levenson JL, Pandurangi AK. Neuroleptic malignant syndrome: a review. *Psychiatr Serv*. 1998;**49**(9):1163–72. Epub 1998/09/15.

44. Shalev A, Hermesh H, Munitz H. Mortality from neuroleptic malignant syndrome. *The Journal of Clinical Psychiatry*. 1989;**50**(1):18–25. Epub 1989/01/01.

45. Nisijima K, Ishiguro T. Cerebrospinal fluid levels of monoamine metabolites and gamma-aminobutyric

acid in neuroleptic malignant syndrome. *Journal of Psychiatric Research*. 1995;**29**(3):233–44. Epub 1995/05/01.

46. Burke RE, Fahn S, Mayeux R, Weinberg H, Louis K, Willner JH. Neuroleptic malignant syndrome caused by dopamine-depleting drugs in a patient with Huntington disease. *Neurology*. 1981;**31**(8):1022–5. Epub 1981/08/01.

47. Cechetto DF, Saper CB. Neurochemical organization of the hypothalamic projection to the spinal cord in the rat. *The Journal of Comparative Neurology*. 1988;**272**(4):579–604. Epub 1988/06/22.

48. Cox B, Kerwin R, Lee TF. Dopamine receptors in the central thermoregulatory pathways of the rat. *The Journal of Physiology*. 1978;**282**:471–83. Epub 1978/09/01.

49. Henderson VW, Wooten GF. Neuroleptic malignant syndrome: a pathogenetic role for dopamine receptor blockade? *Neurology*. 1981;**31**(2):132–7. Epub 1981/02/01.

50. Kelkar VV, Doctor RB, Jindal MN. Chlorpromazine-induced contracture of frog rectus abdominis muscle. *Pharmacology*. 1974;**12**(1):32–8. Epub 1974/01/01.

51. Adnet PJ, Krivosic-Horber RM, Adamantidis MM, Haudecoeur G, Adnet-Bonte CA, Saulnier F, et al. The association between the neuroleptic malignant syndrome and malignant hyperthermia. *Acta Anaesthesiologica Scandinavica*. 1989;**33**(8):676–80. Epub 1989/11/01.

52. Weller M, Kornhuber J. A rationale for NMDA receptor antagonist therapy of the neuroleptic malignant syndrome. *Medical Hypotheses*. 1992;**38**(4):329–33. Epub 1992/08/01.

53. Anglin RE, Rosebush PI, Mazurek MF. Neuroleptic malignant syndrome: a neuroimmunologic hypothesis. *CMAJ: Canadian Medical Association Journal = Journal de l'Association Medicale Canadienne*. 2010;**182**(18): E834–8. Epub 2010/08/11.

54. Wijdicks E. Neuroleptic malignant syndrome. In: Aminoff MJ, Wilterdink JL, eds. UpToDate: wwwUptodatecom. 2013.

55. Lee JW. Serum iron in catatonia and neuroleptic malignant syndrome. *Biological Psychiatry*. 1998;**44**(6):499–507. Epub 1998/10/20.

56. Strawn JR, Keck PE, Jr., Caroff SN. Neuroleptic malignant syndrome. *The American Journal of Psychiatry*. 2007;**164**(6):870–6. Epub 2007/06/02.

57. Wieselgren IM, Lindstrom LH. CSF levels of HVA and 5-HIAA in drug-free schizophrenic patients and healthy controls: a prospective study focused on their predictive value for outcome in schizophrenia. *Psychiatry Research*. 1998;**81**(2):101–10. Epub 1998/12/19.

58. Lyons JL, Cohen AB. Selective cerebellar and basal ganglia injury in neuroleptic malignant syndrome.

*Journal of Neuroimaging: Official Journal of the American Society of Neuroimaging*. 2013;**23**(2):240–1. Epub 2011/03/23.

59. Sechi GP, Tanda F, Mutani R. Fatal hyperpyrexia after withdrawal of levodopa. *Neurology*. 1984;**34**(2):249–51. Epub 1984/02/01.

60. Newman EJ, Grosset DG, Kennedy PG. The parkinsonism-hyperpyrexia syndrome. *Neurocritical Care*. 2009;**10**(1):136–40. Epub 2008/08/21.

61. Sato Y, Asoh T, Metoki N, Satoh K. Efficacy of methylprednisolone pulse therapy on neuroleptic malignant syndrome in Parkinson's disease. *Journal of Neurology, Neurosurgery, and Psychiatry*. 2003;**74**(5):574–6. Epub 2003/04/18.

62. Chalasani P, Healy D, Morriss R. Presentation and frequency of catatonia in new admissions to two acute psychiatric admission units in India and Wales. *Psychological Medicine*. 2005;**35**(11):1667–75. Epub 2005/10/13.

63. Castillo E, Rubin RT, Holsboer-Trachsler E. Clinical differentiation between lethal catatonia and neuroleptic malignant syndrome. *The American Journal of Psychiatry*. 1989;**146**(3):324–8. Epub 1989/03/01.

64. Rosebush PI, Mazurek MF. Catatonia and its treatment. *Schizophrenia Bulletin*. 2010;**36**(2):239–42. Epub 2009/12/09.

65. Perry PJ, Wilborn CA. Serotonin syndrome vs neuroleptic malignant syndrome: a contrast of causes, diagnoses, and management. *Annals of Clinical Psychiatry: Official Journal of the American Academy of Clinical Psychiatrists*. 2012;**24**(2):155–62. Epub 2012/05/09.

66. Musselman ME, Saely S. Diagnosis and treatment of drug-induced hyperthermia. *American Journal of Health-System Pharmacy: AJHP: Official Journal of the American Society of Health-System Pharmacists*. 2013;**70**(1):34–42. Epub 2012/12/25.

67. Munhoz RP, Moscovich M, Araujo PD, Teive HA. Movement disorders emergencies: a review. *Arquivos de Neuro-Psiquiatria*. 2012;**70**(6):453–61. Epub 2012/06/16.

68. Huerta-Alardin AL, Varon J, Marik PE. Bench-to-bedside review: Rhabdomyolysis – an overview for clinicians. *Crit Care*. 2005;**9**(2):158–69. Epub 2005/03/19.

69. Caroff S, Mann SC, Stephan C, Lazarus A, Sullivan K, Macfadden W. Neuroleptic malignant syndrome: Diagnostic issues. *Psychiatric Annals*. 1991;**21**(3):130–47.

70. Lowy A, Wilson A, Sachdev P, Lindeman R. Disseminated intravascular coagulopathy and thrombocytopenia associated with clozapine-induced neuroleptic malignant syndrome. *Australian and New Zealand Journal of Medicine*. 1995;**25**(4):368. Epub 1995/08/01.

71.  Bienvenu OJ, Neufeld KJ, Needham DM. Treatment of four psychiatric emergencies in the intensive care unit. *Critical Care Medicine*. 2012;**40**(9):2662–70. Epub 2012/06/27.

72.  Diedler J, Mellado P, Veltkamp R. Endovascular cooling in a patient with neuroleptic malignant syndrome. *Journal of the Neurological Sciences*. 2008; **264** (1–2): 163–5. Epub 2007/08/21.

73.  Gregorakos L, Thomaides T, Stratouli S, Sakayanni E. The use of clonidine in the management of autonomic overactivity in neuroleptic malignant syndrome. *Clinical Autonomic Research: Official Journal of the Clinical Autonomic Research Society*. 2000;**10**(4):193–6. Epub 2000/10/12.

74.  Keck PE, Jr., Pope HG, Jr., Cohen BM, McElroy SL, Nierenberg AA. Risk factors for neuroleptic malignant syndrome. A case-control study. *Archives of General Psychiatry*. 1989;**46**(10):914–8. Epub 1989/10/01.

75.  Rosenberg MR, Green M. Neuroleptic malignant syndrome. Review of response to therapy. *Archives of Internal Medicine*. 1989;**149**(9):1927–31. Epub 1989/09/01.

76.  Serrano-Duenas M. Neuroleptic malignant syndrome-like, or–dopaminergic malignant syndrome–due to levodopa therapy withdrawal. Clinical features in 11 patients. *Parkinsonism and Related Disorders*. 2003;**9**(3):175–8. Epub 2003/02/08.

77.  Reulbach U, Dutsch C, Biermann T, Sperling W, Thuerauf N, Kornhuber J, et al. Managing an effective treatment for neuroleptic malignant syndrome. *Crit Care*. 2007;**11**(1): R4. Epub 2007/01/16.

78.  Trollor JN, Sachdev PS. Electroconvulsive treatment of neuroleptic malignant syndrome: a review and report of cases. *The Australian and New Zealand Journal of Psychiatry*. 1999;**33**(5):650–9. Epub 1999/11/02.

79.  Lee S, Merriam A, Kim TS, Liebling M, Dickson DW, Moore GR. Cerebellar degeneration in neuroleptic malignant syndrome: neuropathologic findings and review of the literature concerning heat-related nervous system injury. *Journal of Neurology, Neurosurgery, and Psychiatry*. 1989;**52**(3):387–91. Epub 1989/03/01.

**Chapter**

**4**

# Serotonin syndrome

Dimitrios A. Nacopoulos and Hubert H. Fernandez

## Introduction

*Serotonin syndrome*, a medical condition that gained prominent attention with the death of Libby Zion, the 18-year-old daughter of Sydney Zion (a lawyer and writer for *The New York Times*), remains a serious, yet preventable condition. This potentially life-threatening syndrome, which results from excess levels of serotonin (5-Hydroxytryptimine or 5-HT) in the brain, is an important condition for clinicians to recognize. The serotonin syndrome itself has several features—including the classic triad of mental status changes, autonomic hyperactivity, and neuromuscular abnormalities.[1] These symptoms may not all be present, and occur with varying degrees of severity, which contributes to the heterogeneity of its clinical presentation. The more severe end of the spectrum can result in toxicity that can be fatal. The challenge is not only for clinicians to recognize these symptoms (as the diagnosis remains clinical); but, in addition, because the condition is not an idiosyncratic drug reaction, to also understand the syndrome at its basic level to prevent inadvertent drug interactions.

This chapter will cover the serotonin syndrome in detail, assessing the background and epidemiology, pathophysiology, clinical manifestations, diagnosis with discussion of commonly used clinical criteria, treatment, and a discussion of prevention.

## History

First described in 1959[8] as a "fatal toxic encephalitis" in a patient with tuberculosis receiving meperidine, it was only in 1982 that the term "serotonin syndrome" was coined by Insel and colleagues.[9] Prior to this, studies beginning in the 1960s on the effects of L-tryptophan (a precursor to 5-HT) on the CNS

observed signs such as hyperreflexia, clonus, ataxia, drowsiness, nystagmus, and restlessness. Subsequent studies demonstrated the interaction between antidepressants that produced these symptoms.[5] Hodge, in 1964, described the reduction of the central nervous system effects of L-tryptophan after administering a decarboxylase inhibitor.[5]

In 1984, the condition became recognized from the news headline case of Libby Zion, who died in a New York City hospital after administration of pethidine (Demerol, an opioid analgesic) and phenelzine (a nonselective and irreversible monoamine oxidase inhibitor or MAOI).[10] She presented with fever and agitation, and several hours later, suffered a cardiac arrest and could not be resuscitated. Spearheaded by efforts from her journalist father, the case became famous for its implications in restriction of duty hours for graduate medical residency programs (particularly the Accreditation Council on Graduate Medical Education or ACGME); but it also brought awareness of the *serotonin syndrome* to the medical community. In 1991, Sternbach published his report on serotonin syndrome, including his suggested diagnostic criteria.

## Epidemiology

Although the syndrome has been reported in all age groups, due to the lack of specific laboratory tests to diagnose the condition, serotonin syndrome may be underrecognized in practice. With the increasing number of proserotonergic medications prescribed in the general population, the incidence of serotonin syndrome is believed to be following suit.[2] The serotonin syndrome has been reported in patients with a variety of neurological and psychiatric conditions, including depression, bipolar disorder, obsessive

*Medication-Induced Movement Disorders*, ed. Joseph H. Friedman. Published by Cambridge University Press.
© Cambridge University Press 2015.

compulsive disorder, Parkinson's disease, eating disorders, and others.[5] There have been no laborious epidemiological assessments to date. There have been postmarketing surveillance studies on some serotoninergic drugs, such as nefazodone, with an incidence of 0.4 cases per 1000 patient-months.[3] Complicating future studies is the realization that because the diagnosis is clinical, identification among clinicians can vary greatly and thus may be a challenge. A 1998 English survey among general practitioners revealed that 85 percent of those prescribing the antidepressant nefazodone were not aware of "serotonin syndrome" as a clinical diagnosis![3] In primary care settings, patients presenting with very mild symptoms such as diarrhea may not have an assessment of other clinical findings such as hyperreflexia. Moreover, many clinicians may confuse serotonin syndrome with other diagnoses, such as *neuroleptic malignant syndrome*.[5]

Toxicity reports on the use of selective serotonin-reuptake inhibitors (SSRIs) from the 2002 Toxic Exposure Surveillance System (TESS), assessing case descriptions in a variety of clinical settings, reported an incidence of exposures at 26,733 to SSRIs that caused significant toxicity in 7,349 people and resulted in 93 deaths.[4] A 2004 report from TESS reported nearly double the incidence of exposures to SSRIs at 48,204, resulting in significant toxicity in 8,187 patients and 103 deaths.[7] Furthermore, patients may have only mild symptoms on presentation, which often are dismissed by the practitioner rather than associated with drug therapy. In the cases reviewed and subsequent criteria proposed by Sternbach in 1991 (reviewed in the section Diagnosis), mild or early cases of the disorder may not have been recognized.[1,5] Among those overdosing on SSRIs, serotonin syndrome has been reported in approximately 15% of patients.[4]

## Medications implicated

Recognizing drugs that are known to be associated with serotonin syndrome is also important for practitioners, and its underrecognition further contributes to the lack of proper epidemiological studies at this time. The syndrome may present after a single administration of a therapeutic serotonergic drug,[6] an inadvertent combination of drugs with interaction, or after overdose or subsequent to recreational use of some drugs. Many drugs and combinations of drugs with proserotonergic effects have been implicated in serotonin syndrome. Many classes of medications have been associated with this condition, including MAOIs, SSRIs, tricyclic antidepressants (TCAs), opiates, analgesics, herbal products, cough medications, antibiotics, drugs of abuse, weight-loss supplements, antinausea medications, antimigraine medications, and anticonvulsant medications.[1,5]

Triptan medications (5-HT agonists) used in headache conditions such as migraines have been implicated recently, with the United States Food and Drug Administration (FDA) issuing a warning in 2006 against the use of triptans concomitantly with an SSRI or a selective serotonin/norepinephrine reuptake inhibitor (SNRI) in the development of serotonin syndrome.[15] Subsequently, these suspected cases were reviewed and it was discovered that the majority did not meet either Sternbach's criteria or Hunter's criteria (both criteria are reviewed later in the section Diagnosis). Thus, the American Headache Society in a position paper in 2010 declared that there was not sufficient data to support limiting the use of triptans with SSRIs or SNRIs.[16]

Severe forms of the syndrome may be seen particularly after the administration of MAOIs, which are irreversible or nonselective, particularly those inhibiting monoamine oxidase subtype A, and notably when coadministered with meperidine, dextromethorphan, SSRIs, or methylenedioxymethamphetamine (MDMA, or the drug of abuse "ecstasy").[1,4] MAO inhibitors are subdivided into their selectivity for blocking two subtypes—type A and type B. Nonselective MAO inhibitors (MAOIs) can block both subtypes, and selective inhibitors block either type A or type B. Drug interactions associated with MAO inhibitors are largely related to inhibition of MAO-A and are therefore less likely with selective MAO-B inhibitors. Concomitant use of antidepressant medications or other serotonergic agents can potentially increase the risk for serotonin syndrome.

Most serious reactions have occurred with uses of MAO-A or nonselective MAO-B inhibitors, rather than with selective MAO-B inhibitors.[27] However, the FDA has issued a warning on the packages of MAO-B inhibitors used in Parkinson's disease (selegiline and rasagiline)[28, 29] that indicates this theoretical risk. As of yet, this is not a black-box contraindication for use of serotonergic agents with MAO-B inhibitors. The risk of serotonin syndrome with MAO-B inhibitors increases as the dose escalates above what is typically prescribed. The Parkinson Study Group found that of

4,568 PD patients treated with an antidepressant and selegiline, only 11 (0.24%) reported symptoms consistent with serotonin syndrome.[30] Only two patients (0.04%) experienced serious symptoms, and no fatalities occurred. No cases of serotonin syndrome have been reported with the use of rasagiline, an MAO-B inhibitor.[29] Use of meperidine, tramadol, methadone, propoxyphene, dextromethorphan, St. John's wort, and other MAO inhibitors (selective or nonselective) concurrent with MAO-B inhibitors is contraindicated, however.[27]

The addition of drugs that inhibit cytochrome isoforms CYP2D6 and CYP3A4 to SSRI therapy has been implicated in the condition as well. Due to the long serum half-life of certain SSRIs such as fluoxetine, even after discontinuation of the drug for up to five weeks, serotonin syndrome may still occur. Withdrawal from any of the implicated medications may also result in the syndrome.[1,6,10] Some patients may present with mild clinical features and after assessment of medication history, the use of a serotonergic medication is discovered (i.e., SSRIs). As will be

discussed later in the Diagnosis section, less severe clinical features are sometimes difficult to associate with a diagnosis of mild serotonin syndrome, versus mild serotonergic adverse effect. In any case, discontinuation of the medication will lead to symptomatic improvement. Typically, mild serotonergic adverse effects encountered with therapeutic efficacy will not advance to severe toxicity and severe serotonin syndrome unless an additional medication is added that leads to interaction, or an increase in dose of the suspected agent occurs.[14]

# Pathophysiology

Serotonin is the product of decarboxylation and hydroxylation of L-tryptophan in presynaptic neurons in the central nervous system (CNS). It is stored in presynaptic vesicles where it remains until a signal mediates its release for response in neurotransmission. Once the axon is stimulated, there is release of serotonin in the synaptic space, with 5-HT binding to postsynaptic receptors. There is a feedback system where presynaptic 5-HT receptors inhibit exocytosis of vesicles, and a reuptake mechanism allows for 5-HT to return to the presynaptic space, where it again is stored in vesicles for the following neurotransmission cycle. Finally, the enzyme monoamine oxidase subtype A metabolizes serotonin in the presynaptic cytoplasm to become hydroxyindoleacetic acid, which is released from the neuronal cytoplasm.[1]

Early studies by Smith and Prockop on the CNS effects of L-tryptophan in humans demonstrated findings of euphoria, drowsiness, nystagmus, signs of hyperreflexia, clonus, and imbalance.[13] In animal models, treatments implicated in inducing the syndrome included L-tryptophan or SSRIs given with MAOIs in combination, and simulation of the 5-HT receptor directly with 5-HT agonists.[5] In the CNS, serotonin is produced primarily in the midline raphe nuclei in the brainstem. The rostral end regulates wakefulness, behavior, food intake, thermoregulation, migraine, emesis, and sexual behavior.[1] The peripheral effects of serotonin include regulation of vascular tone and gastrointestinal motility.[1] Feedback systems and reuptake mechanisms control the quantity and actions of serotonin in the CNS (see Box 4.1). There are seven serotonin receptor families (5-HT1 to 5-HT7), with further subgroups in each (e.g., $5\text{-HT}_{1A}$, $5\text{-HT}_{1B}$, etc.). No single receptor appears to be solely responsible in the serotonin syndrome; however, stimulation of postsynaptic $5\text{-HT}_{1A}$ and $5\text{-HT}_{1B}$ receptors has been more commonly associated.[7] The 5-$HT_{2A}$ receptor subtype has also been demonstrated to contribute to developing serotonin syndrome.[1]

Other neurotransmitters that may be involved include N-methyl-D-aspartate (NMDA) receptor antagonists and γ-aminobutyric acid (GABA), but their mechanism and role remain unclear. Furthermore, CNS noradrenergic hyperactivity may be involved, as demonstrated with the degree of CNS noradrenergic concentration correlating with clinical outcome as levels increase.[12]

## Clinical Manifestations

The serotonin syndrome encompasses a clinical spectrum. Patients may demonstrate very mild findings of tachycardia, with slight anxiety, and on physical exam shivering, diaphoresis, mydriasis, with neurologic exam significant for intermittent tremor or myoclonus, and increased deep-tendon reflexes. The classic triad clinical features—mental status changes, dysautonomia, and neuromuscular abnormalities—may not be simultaneously present. Symptoms will typically develop rapidly, within minutes to hours after intake of a suspected drug or agent.[7] Mild symptoms may present as a subacute or chronic presentation.[1]

Moderate symptoms may include tachycardia, hypertension, and hyperthermia, with temperatures reaching as high as 40°C in some cases. Clinical features in moderate toxicity seen commonly are mydriasis, hyperactive bowel sounds, and sweating, with normal skin color. Reflexes are further increased in moderate intoxication, and lower extremity reflexes may be significantly greater in particular, with clonus seen in patellar deep-tendon reflexes. Other clonus may manifest, including ocular clonus. Ocular clonus represents a spectrum of abnormal eye movements that range from fine or slight oscillations of gaze in different directions, either triggered by rapid eye movements or spontaneously, to more obvious movements such as "ping-pong gaze" with short cycle, and alternating lateral gaze.[14] Startle response and mild agitation or hypervigilance may be present on cognitive testing. A dystonic posture following startle, involving repetitive rotation of the head while the neck is moderately extended, may also be seen.[1]

Severe toxicity can result in marked hypertension and tachycardia, with autonomic instability resulting in shock. Clinically, patients may be agitated severely and encephalopathic. Neuromuscular abnormalities

including myoclonus and rigidity, greater in the lower extremities, are characteristic. In a review by Dunkley and colleagues, life-threatening cases demonstrated progressive rigidity (particularly truncal) in serotonin toxicity resulting ultimately in intubation secondary to respiratory compromise.[11] Hyperthermia may result, with severe and life-threatening cases exceeding 41.1°C. Muscle hyperactivity and hyperthermia can be so severe that significant abnormal laboratory findings can occur—including metabolic acidosis, elevated creatinine kinase (even rhabdomyolysis), elevated serum aminotransferase and creatinine, and disseminated intravascular coagulopathy.[1]

Neuromuscular abnormalities are the clinical findings that appear to be the most significant, as demonstrated in a study assessing 2222 consecutive cases of serotoninergic drug overdose.[11] Hyperreflexia, clonus, myoclonus, ocular clonus, and other neuromuscular signs are typically encountered. Additional signs observed included dysautonomia, GI symptoms such as diarrhea, and signs of hyperactive bowel sounds. Mental status with agitation and encephalopathy were associated, but hyperthermia (temperature greater than 38°C) was only encountered in severe toxicity.[1]

## Diagnosis

At this time, no laboratory tests can definitively confirm the diagnosis of the serotonin syndrome. Clinical features are important in correct recognition of the condition, through careful history taking and physical examination. As mentioned in sections above, there have been several medications and drug interactions implicated in the serotonin syndrome, and these should be a focus of the clinician in diagnosis. History taking should include a thorough inquiry of the patient's use of prescription medication, including over-the-counter drugs. Serotonergic effects from some drugs should be considered, such as medications like opioids, and some antibiotics, such as linezolid.[14] Drugs of abuse and other illicit substances should also be documented. Other agents such as dietary supplements should be investigated in the history. As mentioned above in earlier sections, addition of new proserotonergic medications should be evaluated, either as monotherapy, but more importantly as an additional agent that may lead to drug interaction. The temporal relation of administration of these serotonergic agents is important, with administration within 5 weeks of presentation helpful in suggesting a diagnosis of serotonin syndrome.[11]

In 1991, Harvey Sternbach provided proposed diagnostic criteria for serotonin syndrome, based on his review of the literature, with 38 cases from ten case reports and two case series. With his review, published in the American Journal of Psychiatry, he described the most common clinical features from these cases and proposed criteria based on the presence of three of the ten most common symptoms and signs in the setting of a coincident administration of or increase in a known serotonergic agent (see Box 4.2—Sternbach's criteria). He also proposed that other etiologies be ruled out and a neuroleptic agent started prior to onset of symptoms as an exclusionary criterion.[5,11]

Sternbach's criteria pose some problems in diagnosis, namely, the favoring of symptoms relating to altered mental status can lead to misdiagnosis.[11] For instance, when anticholinergic toxicity occurs, serotonin syndrome may be diagnosed instead, mostly related to the presence of altered mental status and other subtle signs. Conversely, Sternbach's criteria are somewhat more likely to diagnose moderate or severe toxicity, and may exclude what is recognized now as mild, early, or subacute instances of serotonin syndrome.[1]

---

**BOX 4.2 – Sternbach's Criteria[5]**

1. Recent addition or increase in a known serotonergic agent
2. Absence of other possible etiologies (infections, metabolic, substance abuse, or drug withdrawal) have been ruled out
3. Absence of recent addition or increased dose of a neuroleptic agent
4. Minimum of three of the following symptoms:

   a. Altered mental status (confusion, hypomania)
   b. Agitation
   c. Myoclonus
   d. Hyperreflexia
   e. Diaphoresis
   f. Shivering
   g. Tremor
   h. Diarrhea
   i. Ataxia or incoordination
   j. Fever or hyperthermia

---

With these limitations in mind, others made attempts to create a scale of severity, as the argument was made that serotonin toxicity represented a spectrum from mild adverse effects to toxic and life-threatening states. Hegerl and colleagues created a serotonin syndrome scale in patients treated with paroxetine, correlating drug concentration with serotonergic symptoms.[17] Another paper by Randomoski, assessing a four-year period after Sternbach's work in 1991, reviewed 24 subsequent cases. Cases of serotonin syndrome were divided into mild state of serotonin related adverse effects, serotonin syndrome, and serotonin toxic states.[18]

Simpler criteria were proposed by Dunkley and colleagues in 2003, with their work titled "Hunter Serotonin Toxicity Criteria", commonly referred to as Hunter's criteria (Box 4.3—Hunter's criteria), a retrospective analysis of prospectively collected data studying all patients (n=2222) admitted to a toxicology service following serotonergic overdose. A clinical toxicologist verified diagnosis. The researchers found that although many clinical features were associated with toxicity, only certain features were needed for accurate prediction of serotonin toxicity (in other words, serotonin syndrome) as diagnosed by a clinical toxicologist. These features included clonus (including induced, spontaneous, or ocular), agitation, diaphoresis, tremor, and hyperreflexia. Not included were patients with life-threatening toxicity (requiring endotracheal intubation and assisted ventilation), but it was determined that in such patients, hypertonicity and hyperthermia with temperature >38°C were universal.[11] Hunter's criteria were found to be more sensitive (84% vs. 75%) and specific (97% vs. 96%) than Sternbach's and simpler to apply. As stated earlier in the chapter, clonus appears to be the most important clinical feature in diagnosis.[11] In their work, Dunkley and colleagues included muscle rigidity as a clinical feature in diagnosis solely on the analysis of occurrence in cases of life-threatening serotonin toxicity reviewed in the literature, rather than in the patients studied in the original SSRI dataset.[11]

Hunter's criteria have been adapted by other clinicians as well, notably Boyer and colleagues in the New England Journal of Medicine paper published in 2005.[1] However, there are fair numbers of case reports, published more recently, which use the original Sternbach criteria in diagnosis.[11] There are no consensus criteria as yet, but the diagnostic accuracy proposed in Hunter's criteria seems to bear merit in

---

**BOX 4.3 – Hunter's Criteria[11]**

Hunter serotonin toxicity criteria: decision rules
  If present with a known serotonergic agent:

1. IF (spontaneous clonus = yes) THEN serotonin toxicity = YES
2. ELSE IF (inducible clonus = yes) AND [(agitation = yes) OR (diaphoresis = yes)] THEN serotonin toxicity = YES
3. ELSE IF (ocular clonus = yes) AND [(agitation = yes) OR (diaphoresis = yes) THEN serotonin toxicity = YES
4. ELSE IF (tremor = yes) AND (hyperreflexia = yes) THEN serotonin toxicity = YES
5. ELSE IF (hypertonic = yes) AND (temperature > 38°C) AND [(ocular clonus = yes) OR (inducible clonus = yes)] THEN serotonin toxicity = YES
6. ELSE serotonin toxicity = NO

---

practical use. Indeed, certain clinical features appear to be somewhat pathognomonic and should be noted, particularly clonus of all types in the setting of a medication history involving serotonergic agents.

## Differential diagnosis

The differential diagnosis for serotonin syndrome and toxicity includes similarly presenting neurologic conditions. These include anticholinergic toxicity, malignant hyperthermia, and neuroleptic malignant syndrome. Serotonin syndrome, as mentioned above, is diagnosed clinically, in the setting of a serotonergic agent either being initiated, an escalation in dose, or in addition to another known serotonergic agent. In the other conditions mentioned above, this is not a feature.

Anticholinergic poisoning or toxicity is another condition that may present as an agitated delirium, but also featured should be normal reflexes and other typical clinical features such as mydriasis (which can also be seen in serotonin syndrome), dry mucosa, hot, dry, erythematous skin findings, absent bowel sounds (opposed to hyperactive bowel sounds seen in serotonin syndrome), and urinary retention—all typical findings of anticholinergic effects systemically.[1] Absent features in anticholinergic toxicity, that are typically seen in serotonin syndrome, include neuromuscular abnormalities such as clonus or rigidity. Other clinical features include mild hypertension,

tachycardia, tachypnea, and hyperthermia that is mild (less than 38.8°C typically).

Hyperthermia and hypertonicity are features of malignant hyperthermia, which is also a potentially life-threatening disorder occurring after inhalational anesthetic exposure or skeletal muscle relaxants in susceptible individuals. A family history of similar reactions is helpful in diagnosis. These individuals inherit this trait in an autosomal dominant fashion, with mutation in the ryanodine receptor gene (RYR), involving $Ca^{2+}$ regulation involved in muscle contraction.[19] The condition leads to a sudden rise in intramuscular $Ca^{2+}$; and contracture of the myofibrils leads to increased heat production (with elevation in core body temperature as high as 46°C in some cases[1]), as well as lactic acid and carbon dioxide excess.[20] Other clinical features include increased end-tidal carbon dioxide, and metabolic acidosis. Skin findings are characteristic. The skin becomes mottled in appearance, with alternating areas of blue, cyanotic tissue, and other areas that appear bright red with flushing. Rigidity encountered in this condition is very severe, but the muscle stretch reflexes are decreased, which helps differentiate neuromuscular abnormalities seen in serotonin syndrome.[1] Treatment of this condition requires use of the drug dantrolene, which acts on skeletal muscle binding to the ryanodine receptor, leading to reduction in intracellular $Ca^{2+}$ concentration.[20]

Neuroleptic malignant syndrome (NMS) is the condition that perhaps is most often compared to serotonin syndrome, due to similarities in clinical presentation. However, NMS occurs as an idiosyncratic reaction to dopamine antagonists such as neuroleptic medications, rather than serotonergic agents encountered in serotonin syndrome. Moreover, the clinical triad classically described in NMS consists of hyperthermia, severe muscle rigidity, and dysautonomia.[21] Also associated symptoms include bradykinesia or akinesia, in contrast to the hyperactive state exhibited in serotonin syndrome.[1] Bowel sounds may be decreased or normal. NMS develops typically with a slower onset of symptoms than seen in serotonin syndrome. Both conditions are potentially fatal, although it is notable that estimates of incidence of NMS in patients treated with antipsychotic agents have decreased over the years, likely due to increased awareness, resulting in earlier treatment.[21] Therefore, it is essential that a complete medication history be obtained, as is the case in suspected serotonin toxicity.

As with serotonin toxicity, there can be delayed onset of symptoms. Approximately 16% of cases of NMS develop within 24 hours after initiation of antipsychotic treatment, 66% within the first week, and virtually all cases within 30 days.[22] Laboratory analysis may be helpful in diagnosis, with serum creatine kinase, aldolase, transaminases, and lactic acid demonstrating elevated levels. However, these laboratory abnormalities are not specific to the condition.[21] Pharmacologic treatment includes benzodiazepines, dopaminergic agents such as bromocriptine or amantadine, and dantrolene. Nonpharmacologic treatment includes supportive care and electroconvulsive therapy (ECT) in moderate to severe cases.[22]

## Treatment

Initial steps in management of the serotonin syndrome begin with recognition of the suspected offending serotonergic agent and removal of that agent immediately. Depending on the agent in question, with some drugs having properties of long elimination half-lives, most cases of serotonin syndrome can resolve after supportive therapy is started and the offending agent is removed within 24 hours. Supportive care should be administered, agitation can be controlled with measures including pharmacologic treatment with $5-HT_{2A}$ antagonists, autonomic fluctuations may require treatment, and hyperthermia should be monitored. In all instances, due to the unpredictability of the condition, clinicians should be prepared for the most severe cases.

As mentioned in previous sections, the serotonin syndrome encompasses a wide clinical spectrum, and thus treatments are typically targeted to the degree of severity encountered. In milder cases of serotonin syndrome with subtle clinical signs such as hyperreflexia or tremor, management consists of supportive care and removal of the offending agent, along with treatment of symptoms with benzodiazepines. Benzodiazepines are used in serotonin syndrome particularly to control agitation, but should be administered in most cases. Chemical sedation with benzodiazepines is preferred over physical restraints in that physical restraints may increase risk for lactic acidosis and worsen hyperthermia secondary to forced isometric muscular contraction.[1] In animal models, diazepam improved survival in animals with serotonin toxicity, dampening the hyperadrenergic aspect of the serotonin syndrome that leads to

complications, particularly hyperthermia.[23] In moderate cases of serotonin toxicity, patients may require closer monitoring for vital signs and cardiorespiratory status and an appropriate stay in the hospital may require intensive care monitoring.

In severe cases, hyperthermia (body temperature greater than 41.1°C) may be encountered, and this should be treated. Supportive measures such as cooling blankets,[5] or other methods that are more invasive, should be considered, such as sedation and paralysis with neuromuscular blocking agents as well as intubation for airway protection.[1] Neuromuscular blocking agents should be used with caution, particularly in the case of succinylcholine. Succinylcholine may increase the risk of arrhythmia from hyperkalemia associated with rhabdomyolysis and should be avoided. Vecuronium, a nondepolarizing agent, should be used instead when hyperthermia is present in severe cases, followed by orotracheal intubation and ventilation.[1] Antipyretics are typically not used in the serotonin syndrome, due to the mechanism of hyperthermia in serotonin syndrome being secondary to increased muscle activity rather than from central hypothalamic alterations.[1]

$5-HT_{2A}$ antagonists are pharmacologic agents that can be used to directly target the serotoninergic overdrive encountered in serotonin syndrome.[1,24] Cyproheptadine is a $5-HT_{2A}$ agent recommended for serotonin syndrome, typically started at a dose of 12mg and then 2mg every 2 hours as long as symptoms continue. Doses up to 32mg have been used during a 24-hour duration of symptoms; typically 8mg doses are given every six hours for maintenance therapy. The drug binds to a large percentage of serotonin receptors; however, no efficacy has been clearly established in clinical studies.[24] Administration of cyproheptadine is oral, but it can be crushed so that it can be given through a nasogastric tube if necessary.

In some instances, other medications can be given alongside cyproheptadine, namely atypical antipsychotic agents with 5-HT2A antagonistic activities, although their efficacy has not been clearly determined. Olanzapine can be given at a dose of 10mg, typically administered sublingually. In more severe cases, the older antipsychotic medication chlorpromazine at 50 to 100mg can be administered intramuscularly.[1]

Autonomic instability may develop and in some instances requires intervention with low dose sympathomimetic amines such as norepinephrine, phenylephrine, and epinephrine. Conversely, patients with hypertension and tachycardia as a response to serotonin toxicity may require short-acting treatment with nitroprusside and esmolol.[1] Propranolol, with 5-HT1A antagonistic actions, should not be used as it may worsen autonomic instability, and also the reduction in heart rate may make it difficult to monitor the patient clinically.[11] Unlike with NMS and malignant hyperthermia, treatments including dantrolene and bromocriptine, a dopamine agonist, should not be used in the serotonin syndrome, and may worsen the condition.[25] When measures are implemented to treat serotonin syndrome, the mortality associated with the condition is significantly reduced to levels below one percent (<1%) and recovery is typical.[4]

## Prevention

Prevention begins with identification of medications and agents that can cause serotonin syndrome, and prior to prescribing medications or over-the-counter agents, practitioners should study these comprehensive reviews and be cautious in these instances.[1,2,3,4] Drug-drug interactions, in particular, warrant attention, as more severe serotonin toxicity is usually the result of a combination therapy of proserotonergic agents rather than toxicity from monotherapy.[1,8] In today's world of medicine, often computer-generated prescriptions warn of these potential interactions or risks, and these should be carefully evaluated. Some warnings, such as those advised when prescribing an initial SSRI or MAOI as monotherapy in an otherwise medication naïve patient may be considered less likely to produce serotonin syndrome. Typically, interactions with SSRIs and MAOIs should be avoided so as to prevent possible serotonin toxicity.[14] For the practitioner, based on systematic reviews of case reports of severe serotonin toxicity, MAOIs appear to be the agent that should warrant the most caution. As there are not many available MAOIs in use, it is suggested that these medications be kept in mind most importantly when prescribing medications.[14]

Awareness of the reported toxicity is important when using unfamiliar agents. There are many lists available of agents that have been implicated in serotonin toxicity.[1] As mentioned in the earlier sections (as in the case of triptans), some medications have warnings listed under one agency, but under a different organization are deemed fairly safe. This confuses the practitioner as well as the patient, but in general,

because this condition is reversible, counseling when prescribing the medications or agents that can produce toxicity is an important step. When changing medications, washout periods should occur with antidepressants. At this time, there is no testing for susceptibility, but this may be a future area of interest.[26]

## Conclusion

Serotonin syndrome has become part of our national attention after an unfortunate case brought attention to a preventable and reversible serious illness. The understanding of this condition is relatively recent, but as more serotonergic medications are prescribed, clinicians must be aware of and vigilant about this condition. The agents that have been implicated have been reported in detail, and although limited evidence exists, the condition is fairly treatable and preventable. In the ever-changing world of medications, clinicians should be cautious when prescribing medications that may result in serotonin syndrome.

## References

1. Boyer EW, Shannon M. The serotonin syndrome. *N Engl J Med* 2005;**352**:1112–20.

2. Sporer KA. The serotonin syndrome. Implicated drugs, pathophysiology and management. *Drug Saf* 1995;**13**(2):94–104.

3. Mackay FJ, Dunn NR, Mann RD. Antidepressants and the serotonin syndrome in general practice. *Br J Gen Pract* 1999;**49**:871–4.

4. Isbister GK, Bowe SJ, Dawson A, Whyte IM. Relative toxicity of selective serotonin reuptake inhibitors (SSRIs) in overdose. *J Toxicol Clin Toxicol* 2004;**42**:277–85.

5. Sternbach H. The serotonin syndrome. *Am J Psychiatry* 1991;**148**:705–13.

6. Gill M, LoVecchio F, Selden B. Serotonin syndrome in a child after a single dose of fluvoxamine. *Ann Emerg Med* 1999;**33**:457–9.

7. Arora B, Kannikeswaran N. The serotonin syndrome – the need for physician's awareness. *Int J Emerg Med* 2010;**3**(4):373–77.

8. Gillman PK. Serotonin syndrome: history and risk. *Fundam Clin Pharmacol* 1998;**12**(5):482–91.

9. Insel TR, Roy BF, Cohen RM, Murphy DL. Possible development of the serotonin syndrome in man. *Am J Psychiatry* 1982;**139**(7):954–5.

10. Asch DA, Parker RM. The Libby Zion case: one step forward or two steps backward? *N Engl J Med* 1988;**318**:771–5.

11. Dunkley EJ, Isbister GK, Sibbritt D, Dawson AH, Whyte IM. The Hunter Serotonin Toxicity Criteria: simple and accurate diagnostic decision rules for serotonin toxicity. *QJM* 2003;**96**:635–42.

12. Nisijima K, Shioda K, Yoshino T, Takano K, Kato S. Memantine, an NMDA antagonist, prevents the development of hyperthermia in an animal model for serotonin syndrome. *Pharmacopsychiatry* 2004;**37**:57–62.

13. Smith B, Prockop DJ. Central-nervous-system effects of ingestion of L-tryptophan by normal subjects. *N Engl J Med* 1962;**267**:1338–1341.

14. Buckley NA, Dawson AH, Isbister GK. Serotonin syndrome. *BMJ* 2014;**348**:g1626.

15. Evans RW. The FDA alert on serotonin syndrome with combined use of SSRIs or SNRIs and triptans: an analysis of the 29 case reports. *MedGenMed* 2007;**9**(3):48.

16. Evans RW, Tepper SJ, Shapiro RE, Sun-Edelstein C, Tietjen GE. The FDA alert on serotonin syndrome with use of triptans combined with selective serotonin reuptake inhibitors or selective serotonin-norepinephrine reuptake inhibitors: American Headache Society position paper. *Headache* 2010 Jun:**50**(6);1089–99.

17. Hegerl U, Bottlender R, Gallinat J, Kuss HJ, Ackenheil M, Moller HJ. The serotonin syndrome scale: first results on validity. *Eur Arch Psychiatry Clin Neurosci* 1998;**248**:96–103.

18. Radomski JW, Dursun SM, Reveley MAKSP. An exploratory approach to the serotonin syndrome: an update of clinical phenomenology and revised diagnostic criteria. *Med Hypotheses* 1999;218–24.

19. MacLennan DH, Duff C, Zorzato F, Fujii J, Phillips M, Korneluk RG, Frodis W, Britt BA, Wortont RG. Ryanodine receptor gene is a candidate for

20. Rosenberg H, Davis M, James D, Pollock N, Stowell K. Malignant hyperthermia. *Orphanet J Rare Dis* 2007;**24**:2–21.

21. Strawn JR, Keck PE, Caroff SN. Neuroleptic malignant syndrome. *Am J Psychiatry* 2007;**164**(6):870–6.

22. Caroff SN, Mann SC. Neuroleptic malignant syndrome. *Psychopharmocol Bull* 1988;**24**:25–29.

23. Nisijima K, Yoshino T, Yui K, Katoh S. Potent serotonin (5-HT2A) receptor antagonists completely prevent the development of hyperthermia in an animal model of the 5-HT syndrome. *Brain Res* 2001;**890**:23–31.

24. Graudins A, Stearman A, Chan B. Treatment of the serotonin syndrome with cyproheptadine. *J Emerg Med* 1988;**16**:615–9.

25. Snider SR, Hutt C, Stein B, Fahn S. Increase in brain serotonin produced by bromocriptine. *Neurosci Lett* 1975;**1**:237–41.

26. Porcelli S, Drago A, Fabbri C, Gibiino S, Calati R, Serretti A. Pharmacogenetics of antidepressant response. *J Psychiatry Neurosci* 2011;**36**:87–113.

27. Wimbiscus M, Kostenko O, Malone D. MAO inhibitors: risks, benefits, and lore. *Cleve Clin J Med.* 2010 Dec;**77**(12):859–82.

28. *Selegiline [package insert].* Morgantown, WV: Mylan Pharmaceuticals; 2009.

29. *Azilect [package insert].* Kansas City, MO: Teva Neuroscience; 2009.

30. Richard IH, Kurlan R, Tanner C, et al. Serotonin syndrome and the combined use of deprenyl and an antidepressant in Parkinson's disease. *Neurology.* 1997;**48**:1070–7.

predisposition to malignant hyperthermia. *Nature* 1990;**343**:559–61.

# Neuroleptic parkinsonism

Joseph H. Friedman

It is my contention, based on personal experience and common sense, based partly on extrapolation, not evidence-based studies, that parkinsonism is the single most important medication-induced movement disorder. In older patients it leads to loss of gait, diminished mobility, and falls. In younger patients it worsens stigmatization, an already severe problem for people with psychotic disorders. And it is very common. Twenty percent of nursing home residents in the U.S. are on antipsychotic drugs.

Vignette: a 78-year-old woman with a 15-year history of Parkinson's disease had uncontrolled motor fluctuations, but was usually able to walk by herself with a walker. She had a number of somatic complaints, including nausea, that had been present for several decades, with no explanations found. Within a month of entering a nursing home, her daughter called to let me know that her mother had become so stiff and slow that she could no longer feed herself, assist with her care, or walk. The patient had been started on metoclopramide for her nausea. The medical staff thought that the metoclopramide had been very successful in stopping the nausea and that the timing of her nursing home placement had been surprisingly prescient, as she was in an appropriate facility to handle such a precipitous decline.

One month after stopping the metoclopramide, the patient returned almost to her baseline level of motor function.

## Introduction

While drug-induced parkinsonism is the best understood of the drug-induced movement disorders, it still holds a number of mysteries. It is generally thought that drugs that block dopamine D2 receptors or reduce dopamine transmission cause a syndrome that mimics the motor aspects of idiopathic PD (IPD) (1). However, there are medications, such as lithium and valproic acid, that produce parkinsonism without known effect on dopamine transmission (2,3). Another interesting and unanswered question is the explanation for the extremely wide spectrum of responses to dopamine blocking drugs. Some patients on small doses develop extreme parkinsonism while others on very high doses of similar potency drugs do not (personal observation). While this may be due to early unmasking of subclinical idiopathic PD, there is only mild support for this hypothesis (4). The second generation of antipsychotic drugs, also known as "atypical" neuroleptics, all share the property of dopamine D2 receptor blockade, yet two, quetiapine and clozapine, do not cause parkinsonism, while all the others do (5). An explanation for these observations is debated, with one major theory holding that the ratio of 5HT2-A serotonin receptor blockade to dopamine D2 receptor blockade is the important determinant (6), whereas the second hypothesis maintains that the amount of time the drug actually binds to the D2 receptor, the "fast-off" theory, is the explanation (7). And patients who develop parkinsonism on their neuroleptic often have it resolve without any treatment (1). The observation that "pseudoparkinsonism will often spontaneously remit six to eight weeks after first presenting" (8) is present in much of the early literature on neuroleptic extrapyramidal side effects (9). It has even been suggested that only 1% of NIP cases fail to return to normal after discontinuation of neuroleptic (10) and that these likely suffered from idiopathic PD; yet some patients develop parkinsonism that neither progresses nor regresses after years of being off the offending

*Medication-Induced Movement Disorders*, ed. Joseph H. Friedman. Published by Cambridge University Press.

drug (11). Furthermore, although MIP is frequently treated with anti-PD medications, their efficacy is not clear (12). These issues remain unresolved.

Far and away the most common MIP is neuroleptic-induced parkinsonism (NIP). While it is commonly believed by authorities in the field that the second generation of antipsychotic drugs (SGA), the "atypical" neuroleptics, are less likely to cause this problem than the first generation, this is not supported by data (13–15), although several SGA have been shown to be less likely to cause this than haloperidol (16). Yet no differences were found between haloperidol and risperidone effects in neuroleptic naïve patients (17). The discrepancy between experience and the evidence base may lie in confounding factors inherent in studies of antipsychotic drugs in psychiatric patients, due to the long duration of parkinsonism even after all neuroleptics have been discontinued.

## Clinical aspects of MIP

Parkinsonism is defined as an "akinetic-rigid" syndrome. It is a disorder that looks like IPD. Most published studies of NIP are from the early years of neuroleptics. Since most patients on antipsychotics are treated for primary psychotic disorders which tend to be life-long, these drugs usually cannot be discontinued. In addition, psychosis tends to be treated very soon after presentation, often before psychiatrists, or at least attending-level psychiatrists, see the patient, making contemporary studies of NIP difficult.

NIP typically develops over weeks (18) but may develop within days. Onset depends partly on the route of administration, the drug itself, and its dose. Extrapyramidal disorders tend to occur more quickly with injected preparations.

NIP is clinically indistinguishable from IPD in individual cases (4,19). While there are some differences, in general, between the motor syndrome of IPD and medication-induced parkinsonism (MIP), these are statistical in nature, applying to large groups, and cannot be applied to individuals to distinguish one condition from the other. Drug-induced parkinsonism is thought less likely to cause tremor than IPD (18,20,21), and is more likely to be symmetric. However, IPD may be without tremor and may be symmetric. In some reports, NIP was asymmetric in over half the cases (12,22).

No study has compared age and gender matched groups to determine if these statistical differences may be age- or gender-related, since idiopathic PD generally affects older people, and men more than women.

The most commonly employed criteria for the diagnosis of parkinsonism, or a Parkinson syndrome, referred to as "the UK Brain Bank Criteria" (23), require bradykinesia as the fundamental abnormality, plus rest tremor, rigidity, or postural instability. Idiopathic Parkinson's disease (IPD) is defined as a progressive Parkinson syndrome with unilateral onset, persistent asymmetry, rest tremor, L-Dopa responsiveness maintained for five years, the presence of L-Dopa dyskinesias, and the absence of features that would suggest an alternative diagnosis such as eye movement abnormalities, dementia, corticospinal tract abnormalities, etc. The standard assessment tool in psychiatric studies of parkinsonism is the Simpson Angus Scale (24), which is heavily weighted toward rigidity and does not include bradykinesia. Unlike most reports in the psychiatric literature, no minimum score on a Parkinson assessment tool is used to define IPD in neurological reports. Patients either meet the UK Brain Bank Criteria or not. The feature of facial masking, considered a reflection of akinesia, is not a cardinal feature.

Akinesia is technically different than bradykinesia, but is subsumed under the term for purposes of classification. Parkinson patients move more slowly than normal. It takes them longer to dress, bathe, and perform chores of all types, particularly those involving finger dexterity, like buttoning. On tasks involving rapidly performed repetitive movements they show reduced power (25), similar to myasthenics, but also reduced amplitude, and frequently suffer transient arrests of movements. Bradykinesia, the single required cardinal feature in the UK criteria, is usually the most debilitating problem in early IPD. Akinesia refers to the reduction in spontaneous movements that are typically part of the syndrome. Patients blink less than others, producing a "staring" expression, which may lead, paradoxically, to tearing, when the underlying problem is dry eyes. They smile less. They move less as well, so that they are somewhat like statues. In the waiting room they sit still, not commonly crossing their legs, rubbing their hair, crossing their arms, etc. They swallow less than others, which may lead to drooling. Rigidity is the resistance to passive movement. This can be difficult to assess since it requires relaxation of the limb, something many people have great difficulty achieving.

Patients may or may not appreciate their own rigidity, which they will describe as "stiff." While this rigidity is often characterized as "cogwheel" because it is often ratchety, like a cogwheel, it often is not. The presence or absence of cogwheeling should not be construed as having any impact on the diagnosis of parkinsonism. The rigidity differs from that seen with spasticity in that it is not rate-dependent, nor is it associated with any change in reflexes. Interestingly, bradykinesia and akinesia, while related, may often be quite dissociated, with a very akinetic patient demonstrating very little slowness, and vice versa.

The tremor of parkinsonism is quite stereotypic, occurring at rest. It may occur with posture holding as well but resolves with movement. Complicating interpretation of tremor is the high prevalence of essential tremor and the occurrence of tremors due to medications. Lithium, in particular, frequently causes sustention and action tremor, independent of parkinsonism, as does valproic acid. Parkinsonian tremor most commonly affects the fingers or hands, usually starting on one side. Although frequently labeled a "pill rolling" tremor, because the tremors in the fingers, particularly the thumb, make it appear as if the affected hand is rolling a pill, the tremor often does not look like this, and may affect the hand rather than the fingers. Sometimes a single finger may be involved, most commonly the thumb, but usually all of the fingers are involved. After fingers and hands, the next most commonly involved body parts having tremor are the jaw and feet. Tremor of the tongue is not uncommon. Head tremor may occur but is very uncommon, whereas foot tremor is far more common in parkinsonism than in essential tremor. Vocal tremor does not occur.

The posture of parkinsonism is stooped. Patients tend to be flexed. They adopt a posture similar to that of an aged person, with flexion of the hip, shoulders and neck. They lose "associated movements," namely armswing, when they walk. Their stride is reduced in length, and the heel strike becomes less angled. Walking slows. Balance may be impaired, but not usually unless the NIP is severe.

## Epidemiology

The reported prevalence of NIP varies enormously, with figures generally ranging from 5%–90% (26). The long-term schizophrenia project from Nithsdale, Scotland, has figures varying from 27% (27)

in 1992 to 35% (14) ten years later. These studies, while community based, involved small numbers of patients; however, the 20-year follow-up study from 2002 included only 136 patients. Two inpatient studies reported a prevalence of 40% in Holland (28) and 20% (29) in Curacao, both with under 200 patients. A study of 1559 patients in 6 psychiatric hospitals in Italy reported that 66% had parkinsonism, as defined by a threshold score on the Simpson Angus Scale (30). Yet a recent study involving over 1400 patients receiving intramuscular or oral olanzapine for over a year found that only 0.3% had parkinsonism (31). A door-to-door study in Spain found that the prevalence of MIP was equal to that of IPD (32).

## Clinical course and treatment

Known risk factors for the development of parkinsonism include the choice of drug, with the "high"-potency neuroleptics having the greatest risk, and the age and gender of the patient. Genetic influences are being explored as well (33). Older people were at greater risk than younger (whereas younger are at greater risk for acute dystonic reactions) and women at greater risk than men (18). The observation that women are at greater risk is counterintuitive as women are typically given lower doses than men, and men are about 30% more likely than women to develop IPD than women.

How quickly parkinsonism develops varies considerably. Even in early reports where the patients had not ever been exposed to neuroleptics the time to onset was quite variable. One author (34) noted onset in the great majority by three weeks. Another report (35) described the majority being affected within the first week. The largest study (18) had 90% of patients affected by day 72, with half the patients affected by 30 days. A common issue for contemporary neurologists is in diagnosing NIP in an upper middle aged or elderly person who has been on neuroleptics for decades. Oftentimes the history suggests that the patient tolerated the drugs without a problem until recently, when the parkinsonian effects developed. The question then is whether the patient has simply become more sensitive to the drug side effects, as elderly people are, or whether the sensitivity is entirely due to the development of IPD.

The natural course of MIP is also unknown. A 1954 report (36) stated that the syndrome resolves, untreated, within 2 months with patients staying on their medication. Marsden also reported that NIP often resolves (37). A 1971 study found that almost half still had tremor after remaining on trifluoperazine 3 years (38). A study of NIP in the elderly (4) associated it with a high death rate and found that most surviving patients became and remained incapacitated. They also (4) found that 2/3 had resolution within 7 weeks of stopping the drug but that 11% did not by 18 months. A report following a cohort of long-term patients in a state psychiatric hospital found that parkinsonism increased over the 10 years of observation (39), with all patients still taking neuroleptics.

How long patients remain parkinsonian when lithium and valproic acid are stopped is unknown (see chapter 12). In general, when neuroleptics are stopped, the syndrome resolves over weeks to months, but prolonged parkinsonism lasting 18 months is not rare (10).

Most reports indicate that NIP is not a risk factor for the later development of tardive dyskinesia (29,39,40), but this is not clear. There are reports that neuroleptic parkinsonism increases the risk of the later development of idiopathic Parkinson's disease (4,41). A report on NIP in patients seen at a geriatrics clinic in England (4) found that 25% were found to have IPD at 41 months after drug discontinuation. This latter observation seems intuitive, since PD patients are extremely sensitive to neuroleptic side effects.

## Treatment

The drug treatment of MIP rests on several small studies and observations primarily published in the 1970s and 1980s. Many of the recommendations then were based on the percentages of neuroleptic treated patients who "needed" treatment for parkinsonism. Effects were often based on observations that considered parkinsonism as mild, moderate, or severe in a global assessment, and some used the Simpson Angus Scale (SAS), which, as noted above, is flawed. As one authority at the time noted, "methods of assessment were in many cases crude, subjective reports of symptoms from patients and were often unreliable" (12,42). Hardie and Lees (12) noted that "the value of anticholinergic drugs has probably been overestimated." A study of 12 subjects treated in double blind fashion with two anticholinergics or placebo reported that "considerable parkinsonism persisted in most cases in spite of treatment," with four subjects having no response (9). A study of 35 subjects reported no

difference in parkinsonism due to fluphenazine, whether amantadine, orphenadrine, or placebo was used (42). Yet other reports described "excellent" response in 33 subjects, with an onset of improvement within 24 hours, (35) and "highly effective" (43) responses. A study of 32 schizophrenic inpatients found that amantadine and biperiden, an anticholinergic, were equally effective (44) for MIP.

Unfortunately, in addition to the expected side effects of anticholinergics, including dry mouth, constipation, reduced bladder function, blurred vision, and memory impairment, a small but significant percentage of schizophrenics may abuse these drugs (45).

In a double blind trial 14 patients completed an assessment comparing amantadine to benztropine for all identified EPS, including MIP. Improvements were noted in rigidity and limb tremor but not facial tremor (46).

L-Dopa has been used to treat NIP despite the obvious theoretical problem of increasing dopamine in the face of receptor blockade. Hardie and Lees reported (12) a good outcome in 16 patients treated with L-Dopa, out of 26 patients with NIP. Of note is that only two patients had complete resolution of parkinsonism despite anti-PD medications. They found that the drug was well tolerated but only mildly effective. It did not worsen psychiatric problems. Other reports (47–49) also involved small numbers, also with disappointing motor outcomes. In schizophrenics treated with quetiapine or clozapine, who were thought to have idiopathic PD, the addition of L-Dopa did not induce psychiatric decline (50).

There are a number of case reports and small series advocating the benefits of electroconvulsive therapy (ECT) in MIP (51), but in this situation the ECT should be seen as an added advantage for treating the underlying psychiatric problem. It should never be the sole treatment for the parkinsonism, since the parkinsonism will recur after days to weeks, and there is minimal evidence that maintenance ECT will continue to provide benefit.

Interestingly, clozapine has been demonstrated to have major efficacy in treating tremor in IPD (52), even in patients who had not responded to anticholinergics (53), so that switching to clozapine from an alternative antipsychotic may be quite useful, especially when tremor is a significant factor.

There are few data concerning management of NIP in children. A British pediatric advisory group recommended the same approach for treating NIP in children and adolescents that they believed applies to adults, as the literature on treating nonadults is meager (54). Their recommendations are to stop the offending drug, if possible; replace lithium and valproate, if part of the treatment; substitute clozapine if an antipsychotic is required; and treat remaining Parkinson features with amantadine or an anticholinergic.

## Recognition

Parkinsonism is a common but underrecognized disorder. Although few studies have assessed this, it is common experience for neurologists to see patients referred for an evaluation only when parkinsonism is advanced, or tremor occurs. In two studies in Rhode Island, one in a nursing home used to teach geriatric medicine to physicians, approximately 50% of patients were found to have significant features of parkinsonism which were not identified in the nursing home medical record, either by the physician or the staff at any level, including physical therapists (55). In many cases parkinsonism was due to medication side effects. A second study by the same group reviewed all neurological inpatient consultations performed in a teaching hospital. All patients had been seen by at least four nonneurologist physicians, and often by more. Again, in only about 50% of patients with significant parkinsonism was the parkinsonism recognized (56). Most of these patients did not suffer from IPD, but the parkinsonism caused or was contributory to impaired gait in all the nursing home residents, and led to falls and hospitalization for many of the acute medically hospitalized patients.

## Stigma

The effect of bodily appearance has been studied to a very limited degree in idiopathic PD, and not at all in patients with MIP or tardive dyskinesia. A study of stigma in IPD reported that observers found patients with IPD to be "cold, withdrawn, unintelligent, and moody," in addition to being perceived as relating poorly to the interviewer (57). A study of U.S. practitioners expected increased "neuroticism" with increased masking (58). Another study of attitudes of 284 physicians from the U.S. or Taiwan viewing videotapes of people, Caucasians and Taiwanese, with a masked facial expression from IPD found that the patients with the greater masking were more likely to be deemed depressed, less sociable, less socially

supportive, and less cognitively intact, based simply on their facial appearance (59). IPD patients themselves feel stigmatized by their illness, as well (60). While only limited inferences may be drawn from the stigma associated with IPD to MIP, it seems likely that if a masked facial expression in an old person is associated with a negative impression by medical doctors, then a masked facial expression in a young person is even more likely to produce a negative impression, especially in the patient's community.

## Diagnosing IPD in patients on drugs that may cause parkinsonism

The only universally accepted method for distinguishing IPD from medication-induced parkinsonism in life is to stop the offending agent and observe the patient for months to years for clinical change. MIP is more likely symmetric (26). Whether the common nonmotor problems so often seen in IPD are less common in MIP, as seems intuitively likely, such as REM sleep behavior disorder, impaired olfaction, constipation, rhinorrhea, and other autonomic symptoms, has not been established, and even if present, could only be interpreted as supportive but not diagnostic. In the case of medication-exacerbated IPD, the patient will likely improve as the effects of the medication wear off and then decline again as IPD progresses. Imaging techniques, particularly SPECT scanning of the dopamine transporter, offers an approach that likely can reliably distinguish the two disorders (19) but has not yet been adequately tested. Transcranial ultrasound (TCU) has been used to distinguish IPD from other tremor disorders but probably is not useful for distinguishing IPD from NIP since it appears to be abnormal in neuroleptic parkinsonism in the same way as it is in IPD.

SPECT scanning for dopamine deficiency uses a radioactively labeled compound that binds to the dopamine transporter, thus labeling cells which secrete dopamine. This provides a reliable measure of the number of dopamine transporters, and, indirectly, the number of dopamine secreting cells, since the transporter is limited to the synapses of these neurons. Since in IPD there is a loss of 50%–30% of the cells before clinical signs are evident, there is usually a large gradient between normal and IPD. Different ligands have been approved in different countries for SPECT imaging to help diagnose IPD. While scanning cannot yet reliably distinguish different diseases affecting the substantia nigra, it is believed to be able to reliably distinguish a normal substantia nigra, as would be seen in medication-induced parkinsonism. Studies by Tinazzi et al. (19) have shown a strong correlation between an abnormal SPECT scan and motor progression over two years, suggesting that an abnormal scan is diagnostic of a basal ganglia degenerative disorder. Olivares et al. (61) followed their subjects for only 6 months and reported extremely good reliability of the scan for predicting a course suggestive of IPD.

TCU produces an estimate for the area on slices through the SN. In IPD the SN is "hyperechogenic," meaning that the SN echo-determined volume is larger than that seen in an age-matched control population. This counterintuitive observation reflects a pathological process that is not a direct reflection of the number of dopamine secreting cells, and is hypothesized to represent abnormal iron accumulation. In a 2009 review of 35 studies of 1534 patients with IPD who underwent TCU, 87% were abnormal, whereas 12% of the controls were, and 13% were inconclusive. The scans could not reliably distinguish atypical Parkinson disorders from IPD (62). Multiple other studies support the utility of TCU in distinguishing IPD from other disorders, including essential tremor (63,64). A three-year follow-up study reported that an enlarged echogenic area in the SN increased the risk of developing IPD by twentyfold (65). Other studies have purported to show a relationship between echogenicity and severity of neuroleptic-induced parkinsonism (66), which would imply that TCU cannot distinguish NIP from IPD, as both are associated with hyperechogenicity. In addition, about 10% of healthy controls also have large echogenic SNs, confounding specificity of the abnormality.

High magnetic field MRI (7 Tesla) may also hold promise in distinguishing IPD from NIP (67).

# Other medications causing parkinsonism

Parkinsonism is a common effect of medications used to deplete catecholamines, including reserpine, metyrosine (approved for use in pheochromocytoma), and tetrabenazine. Unlike neuroleptics, these drugs do not block the dopamine receptor but rather either interfere with synthesis (metyrosine) or vesicular packaging (reserpine and tetrabenazine). Their benefit on hyperkinetic movements, primarily chorea, are based on their ability to produce parkinsonism. Nondopaminergic drugs may cause parkinsonism but, with the exception of valproic acid and lithium, only extremely rarely. Numerous single case reports attest to very isolated occurrences with commonly used drugs that have not been associated with the syndrome, such as opiates (68) and pregabalin (69). Perhaps most important to mention are antidepressants, particularly the SSRIs which have been associated with parkinsonism in clinical trials (70–72), but several reports attest to their safety (72,73).

# References

1. Marsden CD, Mindham RHS, Mackay AVP. Extrapyramidal movement disorders produced by antipsychotic drugs. In: Bradley PB, Hirsch SR, eds. *The Psychopharmacology and Treatment of Schizophrenia*. Oxford: Oxford University Press, 1986:340–402.

2. Easterford K, Clough P, Kellett M, et al. Reversible parkinsonism with normal beta CIT in patients exposed to sodium valproate. *Neurol* 2004;**62:1435–7.**

3. Lang AE. Lithium and parkinsonism. *Ann Neurol* 1984;**15:214.**

4. Stephen PJ, Wilson J. Drug-induced parkinsonism in the elderly. *Lancet* 1984;**2:1082–3.**

5. Friedman JH. Parkinson's disease psychosis: Update. *Behav Neurol* 2013;**27:469–77.**

6. Meltzer HY, Massey BW. The role of serotonin receptors in the action of atypical antipsycotic drugs. *Curr Opin Pharmacol* 2011;**11:59–67.**

7. Kapur S, Seeman P. Antipsychotic agents differ in how fast they come off the dopamine D2 receptors. Implication for atypical antipsychotic action. *J Psychiatry Neurosci* 2000;**25:161–6.**

8. Donlon PT, Stenson RL. Neuroleptic-induced extrapyramidal symptoms. *Dis Nerv System* 1976; **7: 629–35.**

9. Gerlach J, Rasmussen T, Hansen L, Kristjansen P. Antiparkinson agents and long-term neuroleptic treatment. *Acta Psychi Neurol* 1977;**55:251–60.**

10. Klawans HL, Bergen D, Bruyn GW. Prolonged drug-induced parkinsonism. *Confinia Neurologica* 1973;**35:368–77.**

11. Negrotti A, Calzetti S. A Long-term follow-up study of cinnarizine- and flunarizine-induced parkinsonism. *Mov Disord* 1997;**12:107–10.**

12. Hardie RJ, Lees AJ. Neuroleptic-induced Parkinson's syndrome: clinical features and results of treatment with levodopa. *J Neurol Neurosurg Psychiatry* 1988;**51:850–4.**

13. Caroff SN, Hurford I, Lybrand J, Campbell EC. Movement disorders induced by antipsychotic drugs: implications of the CATIE Schizophrenia Trial. *Psychiatry for the Neurologist* 2011;**29:127–148**.

14. Halliday J, Farrington S, MacDonald S, et al. Nithsdale Schizophrenia Surveys 23: movement disorders. 20-year review. *B J Psychiatry* 2002;**181;5:422–7**.

15. Peluso MJ, Lewis SW, Barnes TRE, Jonas PB. Extrapyramidal motor side effects of first and second generation antipsychotic drugs. *Br J Psychiatry* 2012;**200:387–92**.

16. Haddad MP, Das A, Keyhanis S, Chaudhry IB. Antipsychotic drugs and extrapyramidal side effect in first episode psychosis: a systematic review. *J Psychopharmacology* 2012;**26(5Suppl):15–26**.

17. Rosebush PI, Mazurek MF. Neurologic side effects in neuroleptic naïve patients treated with haloperidol or risperidone. *Neurol* 1999;**52:782–5**.

18. Ayd FJ. A Survey of drug-induced extrapyramidal reactions. *JAMA* 1961;**175:102–8**.

19. Tinazzi M, Morgante F, Matinella A, et al. Imaging of the dopamine transporter predicts pattern of disease progression and response to levodopa in patients with schizophrenia and parkinsonism: A 2-year follow-up multicenter study. *Schizophr Res* 2014;**152:233–349**.

20. The National institute of Mental Health Psychopharmacology Service Center Collaborative Study Group. Phenothiazine treatment in acute schizophrenia. Effectiveness. *Arch Gen Psychiatry* 1964;**10:246–61**.

21. Hausner RS. Neuroleptic-induced parkinsonism and Parkinson's disease: differential diagnosis and treatment. *J Clin Psychiatry* 1993;**44:13–16**.

22. Sethi K, Zamrini EY. Asymmetry in clinical features of drug-induced parkinsonism. *J Neuropsych* 1990;**2:54–6**.

23. Hughes AJ, Daniel SE, Kilford L, Lees AJ. Accuracy of clinical diagnosis of idiopathic Parkinson's disease: A clinico-pathological study of 100 cases. *J Neurol Neurosurg Psychiatry* 1992;**55:181–4**.

24. Simpson GM, Angus JW. A rating scale for extrapyramidal side effects. *Acta Psychiatrica Scand Suppl* 1970;**212:11–19**.

25. Lou JS, Kearns G, Benice T, et al. Levodopa improves physical fatigue in Parkinson's disease: a double blind, placebo controlled crossover study. *Mov Disord* 2003;**18:1108–14**.

26. Gershanik O. Drug-Induced Parkinsonism in the aged. Recognition and prevention. *Drugs and Aging* 1994;**5:127–32**.

27. McCreadie RG, Robertson LF, Wiles DH. The Nithsdale schizophrenia surveys IX: akathisia, parkinsonism, tardive dyskinesia and plasma neuroleptic levels. *B J Psychi* 1992;**160:793–9**.

28. Van Harten PN, Matroos GE, Hoek HW, et al. The prevalence of tardive dystonia, tardive dyskinesia, parkinsonism and akathisia. The Curacao extrapyramidal syndromes study I. *Schiz Res* 1996;**19:195–203**.

29. Modestin J, Stephan PL, Erni T, et al. Prevalence of extrapyramidal syndromes in psychiatric inpatients and relation of clozapine treatment to tardive dyskinesia. *Schiz Res* 2000;**42:223–30**.

30. Muscettola G, Barbato G, Pampallona S, et al. Extrapyramidal syndromes in neuroleptic-treated patients: Prevalence, risk factors, and association with tardive dyskinesia. *J Clin Psychopharmacol* 1999;**19:203–8**.

31. Hill AL, Sun B, McDonnel DP. Incidences of extrapyramidal symptoms in patients with schizophrenia after treatment with long-acting injection (depot) or oral formulations of olanzapine. *Clin Schizophrenia and Related Psychoses*. 2014;**7:216–22**.

32. Seijo-Martinez M, Castro Del Rio M, Rodriguez Alvarez J, et al. Prevalence of parkinsonism and Parkinson's disease in the Arosa Island (Spain): a community-based door-to-door survey. *J Neurol Sci* 2011;**304:49–54**.

33. Kasten M, Bruggemann M, Konig IR, et al. Risk for antipsychotic extrapyramidal symptoms: influence of family history and genetic susceptibility. *Psychoparmalogy (Berl)* 2011;**214:729–36**.

34. Freyhan FA. Therapeutic implications of differential effects of new phenothiazine compounds. *Am J Psychiatry* 1959;**115:577–85**.

35. Medina C, Kramer MD, Kurland AA. Biperiden in the treatment of phenothiazine-induced extra-pyramidal reactions. *JAMA* 1962;**182:1127–8**.

36. Azima H, Ogle W, Effects of largactil in mental syndromes. *Can Med Assoc J*. 1954;**71:116–21**.

37. Marsden CD, Jenner P. The pathophysiology of extrapyramidal side effects of neuroleptic drugs. *Psychol Med* 1980;**10:55–72**.

38. Kennedy PF, Hershon HI. McGuire RJ. Extrapyramidal disorders after prolonged phenothiazine therapy. *Br J Psychiatry* 1971;**118:509–18**.

39. Fernandez HH, Krupp B, Friedman JH. The course of tardive dyskinesia and parkinsonism in psychiatric inpatients: a 14-year follow-up. *Neurology* 2001;**56:805–7**.

40. Tenback DE, van Harten PN. Epidemiology and risk factors for (tardive) dyskinesia. *Int Rev Neurobiol* 2011;**98:211–30**.

41. Foubert-Samier A, Helmer C, et al. Past exposure to neuroleptic drugs and risk of Parkinson's disease in an elderly cohort. *Neurol* 2012;**79:1615–21**.

42. Mindham RHS. Assessment of drug-induced extra-pyramidal reactions and of drugs given for their control. *Br J Clin Pharmac* 1976; Suppl, 395–400.

43. Magnus RV. A comparison of biperiden hydrochloride and benzhexol in the treatment of drug-induced parkinsonism. *J Int Med Res* 1980;**8:343–6**.

44. Silver H, Geraisy N, Schwartz M. No differenece in the effect of biperiden and amantadine on parkinsonism and tardive dyskinesia type involuntary movements. A double blind crossover, placebo controlled study in medicated chronic schizophrenic patients. *J Clin Psychiatry* 1995;**56:167–70**.

45. Zemishlany Z, Aizenberg D, Weiner D, Weizman A. Thrihexiphenidyl abuse in schizophrenic patients. *Int Clin Psychopharmacol* 1996;**11:199–202**.

46. Greenblatt DJ, Dimascio A, Harmatz JS, et al. Pharmacokinetics and clinical effects of amantadine in drug-induced extrapyramidal symptoms. *J Clin Pharmacol* 1977;**17:704–8**.

47. McGeer PL, Boulding JE, Gibson WC, Foulkes RG. Drug-induced extrapyramidal reactions: treatment with diphenhydramine hydrochloride and dihydroxyphenlalanine. *JAMA* 1961;**177:666–70**.

48. Fleming P, Makar H, Hunter KR. Levodopa in drug-induced extrapyramidal disorders. *Lancet* 1970; **ii:11286**.

49. Kimura N, Tsukue I. L-dopa therapy in drug-induced parkinsonism evaluated by the method of measuring the facial expression. *Hiroshima J Med Sci* 1971;**20:55–63**.

50. Friedman JH. Managing Parkinson's disease in patients with schizophrenic disorders. *Park Related Disord* 2011;**17:198–200**.

51. Sadananda SK, Holla B, Viswanath B, et al. Effectiveness of electroconvulsive therapy for drug-induced parkinsonism in the elderly. *J ECT* 2013;**29:e6–7**.

52. Friedman JH, Koller WC, Lannon MD, et al. Benztropine versus clozapine for the treatment of tremor in Parkinson's disease. *Neurol* 1997;**48:1077–81**.

53. Friedman JH, Lannon MC. Clozapine responsive tremor in Parkinson's disease. *Mov Disord* 1990;**5:225–9**.

54. Pringsheim T, Doja A, Belanger S, et al. Treatment recommendations for extrapyramidal side effects associated with second generation antipsychotics in children and adolescents. *Paed Child Health* 2011;**16:590–8**.

55. Friedman JH, Fernandez HH, Trieschmann MM. Parkinsonism in a nursing home: underrecognition. *J Ger Psychiatry Neurol* 2004;**17:39–41**.

56. Friedman JH, Skeete R, Fernandez HH. Unrecognized parkinsonism in acute care medical patients receiving neurological consultations. *J Geront A Biol Sci Med Sci* 2003;**58:94–5**.

57. Pitcairn TK, Clemie S, Gray JM, Pentland B. Non-verbal cues in the self-presentation of Parkinson patients. *Br J Clin Psychiatry* 1990;**29(Pt2):177–84**.

58. Tickle-Degnan L, Lyons KD. Practitioners' impressions of patients with Parkinson's disease: the social ecology of the expressive mask. *Soc Sci* 2004;**58:603–14**.

59. Tickle-Degnan L, Zebrowitz LA, Ha HI. Culture, gender and health care stigma: Practitioners' response to facial masking experienced by people with Parkinson's disease. *Soc Sci Med* 2011;**73:95–102**.

60. Hermanns M. The invisible and visible stigmatization of Parkinson's disease. *J Am Assoc Nurse Pract* 2013;**25:563–6**.

61. Olivares Romero J, Arjona Padilla A. Diagnostic accuracy of 123 FD-CIT SPECT in diagnosing drug-induced parkinsonism: a prospective study. *Neurologia* 2013;**28:276–82**.

62. Vlaar AM, Bouwmans A, Mess WH, et al. Transcranial duplex in the differential diagnosis of parkinsonian syndromes: a systematic review. *J Neurol* 2009;**256:530–8**.

63. Luo WF, Zhang YC, Sheng YJ, et al. Transcranial sonography on Parkinson's disease and essential tremor in a Chinese population. *Neurol Sci* 2012;**33:1005–9**.

64. Chitsa ZA, Mehrbad N, Saadatnia M, et al. Transcranial sonography on Parkinson's disease and essential tremor. *J Res Med Sci* 2013;**18(Suppl1):S28–31**.

65. Berg D, Behnke S, Seppi K, et al. Enlarged hyperechogenic substantia nigra as a risk marker for Parkinson disease. *Mov Disord* 2013;**28:216–9**.

66. Berg D, Jabs B, Merschdorf U, et al. Echogenicity of sutbstantia determined by transcranial ultrasound correlates with severity of Parkinson symptoms induced by neuroleptic. *Biol Psychiatry* 2001;**50:463–7**.

67. Kwon DH, Kim JM, Oh SH, et al. Seven Tesla magnetic resonance images of the sunstantia nigra in Parkinson's disease. *Ann Neurol* 2012;**71:267–77**.

68. Iselin-Chaves IA, Grotzsch H, Besson M, et al. Naloxone responsive acute dystonia and parkinsonism following general anesthesia. *Anaesthesia* 2009;**64:1359–62**.

69. Perez-Lloret S, Amaya M, Merello M. Pregabalin-induced parkinsonism: a case report. *Clin Neuropharmacol* 2009;**32:353–4**.

70. Miletic V, Relja M. Citalopram-induced Parkinson syndrome: case report. *Clin Neuropharmacol* 2011;**34:92–3**.

71. Draper B, Berman K. Tolerability of selective serotonin reuptake inhibitors: issues relevant to the elderly. *Drugs Aging* 2008;**25:501–19**.

72. Caley C, Friedman JH. Does fluoxetine exacerbate Parkinson's disease? *J Clin Psychiatry* 1992;**53:278–82**.

73. Pae CU. Use of antidepressants for depression in patients with Parkinson's disease. *Exp Opin Pharmacother* 2013;**14:255–7**.

# Tardive syndromes

## Clinical manifestations, pathophysiology, and epidemiology

Daniel Tarsy and Raminder Parihar

## Introduction

The tardive syndromes are a group of involuntary movement disorders which appear in delayed fashion and very often persist following prolonged exposure to dopamine receptor blocking agents (DRBA) such as the antipsychotic drugs (APDs), also known as neuroleptics, certain antiemetics such as metoclopramide and prochlorperazine, the antidepressant amoxapine, and certain calcium channel blockers not available in the United States such as cinnarizine and flunarizine. Tardive dyskinesia (TD) is the best known of the tardive syndromes and is characterized by hyperkinetic involuntary movements of the tongue, jaw, face, trunk, and extremities in the form of chorea, dystonia, athetosis, akathisia, stereotypies, and very rarely tremor. The term *tardive* was originally introduced to differentiate TD from *acute* dyskinesia (acute dystonic reactions), akathisia, and parkinsonism which were the first drug-induced extrapyramidal disorders (EPS) reported soon after the introduction of APDs in the 1950s and which were known to appear very shortly after initial exposure to an APD. TD was identified somewhat later and was initially believed to be a permanent condition. However, it was later recognized that it is often reversible and in fact occurs in several different temporal patterns including transient TD, withdrawal or withdrawal emergent TD, and persistent TD.

In this chapter, we will provide an overview of the clinical manifestations, pathophysiology, and epidemiology of TD [1–3]. Although TD will be the main focus of this review, we will also discuss other late appearing hyperkinetic as well as hypokinetic movement disorders sometimes referred to as "tardive

syndromes" such as tardive dystonia, tardive akathisia, tardive stereotypy, tardive myoclonus, tardive tic disorders, and tardive parkinsonism [4–6].

## Clinical manifestations of the tardive syndromes

TD may manifest as one or more relatively stereotyped hyperkinetic movements localized to one body region or as a complex combination of more widely distributed movements. The spectrum of movements which have been described in TD include chorea, athetosis, akathisia, stereotypy, tics, myoclonus, and rarely tremor. Collectively these hyperkinetic movements are typically referred to as "dyskinesias". "Classical TD" refers to involuntary repetitive stereotypic movements of the perioral region, such as protruding and twisting movements of the tongue; pouting, puckering, or smacking movements of the lips; retraction of the corners of the mouth; bulging of the cheeks; chewing movements; and blepharospasm [5, 6]. TD may also include stereotypic twisting, tapping, and posturing movements of the fingers and toes. Repetitive and stereotyped dyskinesias of the perioral region and limbs have been referred to by some authors as tardive stereotypy rather than TD [5, 7] although these findings overlap considerably with classic manifestations of TD and, in addition, may also lead to confusion with stereotypies sometimes associated with chronic psychosis and autism [7, 8]. Perioral movements are more prevalent in older individuals with TD while extremity and truncal involvement is often more severe in younger individuals in whom dystonic postures and even ballistic movements may also occur.

*Medication-Induced Movement Disorders*, ed. Joseph H. Friedman. Published by Cambridge University Press.
© Cambridge University Press 2015.

# Clinical subtypes and other tardive syndromes

Clinical subtypes may be based on the temporal pattern of TD including transient TD, withdrawal or withdrawal emergent TD, and persistent TD and will be discussed later in the discussion of the clinical course of TD. Several TD clinical variants or subtypes also exist based on the type of involuntary movements which predominate in these conditions. Tardive dystonia refers to TD in which more sustained dystonic manifestations such as cervical retrocollis, opisthotonus, shoulder dystonia, hyperextension of the arms or legs, blepharospasm, dystonic facial expressions, or jaw dystonia predominate. Dystonia of the trunk may include retrocollis, torticollis, axial dystonia, rocking and swaying movements of the body, and rotatory or thrusting movements of the hips. Tardive dystonia may occur at any age but is more frequent in patients under age 40 and appears to have a lower spontaneous remission rate than TD [9–11].

Tardive akathisia which means inability to sit presents as a feeling of late appearing inner restlessness which may involve the entire body or may be limited to the lower extremities [12]. Although tardive akathisia has the appearance of being uncomfortable, unlike acute akathisia it often lacks the strong subjective feeling of internal discomfort which is typical of acute akathisia. Some typical manifestations of more severe akathisia are repetitive marching movements of the legs while standing in place or repeated tapping of the feet while seated.

Other TD subtypes are much less common and include tardive tics, tardive myoclonus, tardive tremor, and tardive oral pain syndromes. However, these are often difficult to distinguish from other manifestations of classical TD or even from behavioral effects of the individual's psychosis. Tardive myoclonus presents as prominent postural myoclonic jerks of the upper extremities. Tardive tremor presents as a mixture of postural, kinetic, and rest tremor which is typically large in amplitude and low in frequency [13, 14]. Tardive pain syndromes are uncommon but may manifest as chronic pain or other unpleasant sensations in either the oral or genital regions which usually accompany the motor features of TD [4]. Many of these subtypes do not usually occur in isolation but usually coexist with the other more common manifestations of TD. This indicates that TD encompasses a mixture of motor manifestations without necessarily delineating an entirely specific or characteristic movement disorder [15].

Respiratory dyskinesia usually occurs in individuals also suffering from other dyskinetic features of TD. This often manifests as pharyngeal dyskinesia which causes dysphagia, and laryngeal dyskinesia sometimes associated with grunting noises, gasps, and interrupted speech. Typically, patients will complain of dyspnea and voice disturbance but may be unaware of its other visible and audible manifestations. Tachypnea, which often accompanies the subjective dyspnea, presents as an irregular respiratory rhythm and amplitude, to which are contributed spontaneous and uncoordinated movements of the mouth, buccal muscles, and palate moving spontaneously in an uncoordinated manner [16].

The late appearance of "tardive parkinsonism" is usually due to an increase in APD dose or a switch to a more potent DRBA but in some cases its "tardy" appearance is unexplained. In most cases, tardive parkinsonism improves and disappears after DRBAs have been discontinued, indicating that an individual has experienced temporary DIP rather than persistent or permanent parkinsonism as a complication of long-term DRBA exposure. By contrast, if DIP persists long after DRBAs have been discontinued, in most cases this is because clinical features of unsuspected, preexisting, subclinical PD have been precipitated and aggravated by exposure to DRBAs. This scenario has long been suspected, particularly since the incidence of both DIP and PD increase with age together with evidence that underlying preclinical PD is a risk factor for DIP [17–19]. More recently this has been more firmly established by the use of (123) Ioflupane DaTSCAN-SPECT brain imaging of striatal dopamine uptake [20]. Using this brain imaging technique, patients with parkinsonism on chronic APD treatment showing evidence for presynaptic dopamine terminal degeneration are presumed to have underlying PD, the symptoms of which have been aggravated by dopamine receptor blockade. By contrast, patients with normal DaTSCAN imaging are presumed to have DIP without underlying PD, which can be expected to disappear once APDs are discontinued [20]. What remains unproven is whether there are also patients proven by DaTSCAN to have no evidence of underlying PD who have permanent parkinsonism long after APDs are discontinued, which is due to long-term effects of exposure to APDs [5]. Since patients with DIP with normal DaTSCAN imaging may require as much as 6–9 months and possibly even longer after APDs are discontinued for parkinsonism to clear, caution should be exercised before concluding that DRBAs can cause permanent parkinsonism [21].

## Clinical course of TD

TD may appear as early as 1–6 months following initial exposure to DRBAs although, in the early literature, due to lack of awareness of the disorder, TD very often did not come to attention until after two or more years of treatment. Onset is usually insidious and occurs while the patient is being actively treated with a DRBA. However, TD very commonly first appears after a reduction in dose, following discontinuation of a DRBA or, as in the case of APDs, after switching to a less potent APD for psychiatric reasons or because of other adverse effects. When TD appears under these circumstances it is referred to as a "withdrawal dyskinesia" which usually makes its appearance within several weeks after stopping a DRBA [22]. TD is much less common in children where it has been called "withdrawal emergent symptoms" because they have been said to appear for the first time when APDs are discontinued [23]. This "unmasking" of TD is due to the hypokinetic parkinsonian effects of APDs which often suppress the hyperkinetic clinical manifestations of TD and thereby delay its recognition and diagnosis.

Cognitively intact and psychiatrically stable patients are usually aware of and disturbed by even mild manifestations of TD, while failure to complain of symptoms of TD more commonly occurs in chronically institutionalized or psychotic patients. In fact, however, severe orofacial dyskinesia or dystonia is often highly disfiguring and may interfere with speech, eating, swallowing, or breathing, while truncal dystonia can be extremely distressing and disabling by interfering with gait and mobility.

Remission rates in individuals with TD vary depending on a number of factors. By its definition, withdrawal dyskinesia disappears within several weeks of discontinuation of DRBAs but should be considered a precursor of more persistent forms of TD which are likely to recur if DRBAs are later resumed. In early studies, when there was much less awareness of TD, reported remission rates of TD were only 5%–40%. However, when TD is identified earlier, as in younger and less severely psychotic outpatient populations, a remission rate of 50%–90% has been observed, which usually occurs within several months but sometimes requires as long as 1–3 years after APD withdrawal [2]. In one long-term follow-up study concerning tardive dystonia, the remission rate was only 14% over a follow-up period of 8.5 years [11]. When TD persists after drug discontinuation it is referred to as persistent or permanent TD. The prognosis of TD in patients in whom continued treatment with APDs remains necessary for psychiatric indications is unknown but, in the vast majority of cases, TD either remains unchanged, is suppressed by the hypokinetic effects of APDs, or may even fluctuate in severity over time depending to some extent on changes in mood, psychosis, or variations in drugs or drug dosages [24, 25].

## Differential diagnosis of TD

It is important to identify TD as early as possible since the potential for remission appears to be related to duration of symptoms before the DRBA is discontinued. The diagnosis of TD is based on the presence of dyskinetic or dystonic involuntary movements, a history of at least three months of APD treatment, the exclusion of other causes of abnormal dyskinesias, and the persistence of abnormal movements for at least 3 months after discontinuation of DRBAs. Tongue movements are insidious in onset and at first may be limited to subtle back and forth or lateral movements of the tongue. In other patients, tic-like facial movements or increased blink frequency may be initial manifestations of TD. Although the diagnosis is usually straightforward, it is important to consider other important causes of involuntary movements in a patient being treated for a psychiatric disorder such as Wilson's disease or Huntington's disease.

Akathisia occurs both early and late in treatment with APDs and may continue to persist after cessation of APD exposure. When akathisia occurs late in treatment it is referred to as tardive akathisia and is usually associated with dyskinesias elsewhere in the body and is a coexisting manifestation of TD. Acute dyskinesias or acute dystonic reactions typically only occur immediately after introduction of APD, but may resemble TD and can sometimes occur later in treatment following switching to a more potent APD or recurrently during treatment with long-acting injectable fluphenazine esters. Acute dyskinesias may also occur after treatment with certain antidepressants but do not represent TD and, with the exception of amoxapine, which has dopamine receptor blocking properties, these remit following discontinuation of the antidepressant [26].

Tardive dystonia involving axial or cervical muscles in a relatively young individual is differentiated from primary torsion dystonia by the absence of exposure to DRBAs and a slowly progressive course. Cervical dystonia characterized by severe retrocollis is particularly common in tardive dystonia. Huntington's disease is clinically readily identified by a positive family history, a significant gait abnormality, and dementia. Tourette syndrome is easily identified by a history of fluctuating motor and vocal tics since early childhood. Other less common diagnostic possibilities include facial grimacing and choreoathetosis associated with chronic liver disease; chorea or dystonia due to antiphospholipid antibody syndrome; chorea due to hyperthyroidism or hypoparathyroidism; rheumatic or lupus chorea; acute drug-induced dyskinesias due to levodopa, amphetamines, anticholinergic drugs, antidepressants, certain calcium channel blockers, and anticonvulsants; and structural disorders of the basal ganglia.

## Spontaneous dyskinesias which resemble TD

TD must be distinguished from stereotyped movements and psychotic mannerisms which may be associated with chronic schizophrenia, as well as the spontaneous orofacial dyskinesias which often occur in elderly, edentulous, and sometimes demented individuals [8, 27]. The mean prevalence of dyskinesia among APD-treated patients has been estimated at 20% compared with a mean prevalence of 5% in untreated patients, indicating a significant background level of various spontaneous dyskinesias that must be differentiated from TD [27]. Stereotyped and manneristic movements which are observed in schizophrenia are usually less rhythmic, may appear semipurposeful, are more stereotyped and complex, and are not usually choreoathetotic or dystonic [8, 27]. Meige syndrome is an idiopathic cranial dystonia with onset in middle age which is manifested by blepharospasm and oromandibular dystonia. Meige syndrome, blepharospasm, and oromandibular dystonia are all spontaneous movement disorders which are indistinguishable in appearance from classical orofacial forms of TD so that differentiation from TD therefore depends on a thorough drug history.

## Pathophysiology of TD

The prolonged and often permanent course of TD suggests that structural alterations in the brain must be responsible for the disorder. However, standard pathological studies in laboratory animals and humans have failed to demonstrate consistent findings following chronic exposure to APDs [28]. TD is believed to result from chronic blockade of D2 dopamine receptors by DRBAs. While older first-generation APDs bind tightly to D2 receptors and remain attached for a few days, "atypical" second-generation APDs possess a lower degree of D2 receptor antagonism with rapid dissociation from the D2 receptor [29], thus possibly explaining their somewhat lower risk of TD which will be discussed later in the section on epidemiology of TD.

One theory used to explain TD pathogenesis postulates that, as demonstrated in laboratory animals, chronic exposure to DRBAs leads to upregulation of D2 receptors due to postsynaptic dopamine receptor supersensitivity [30, 31]. Although there is also evidence for upregulation of striatal dopamine receptors in humans following chronic exposure to DRBAs, this finding has not been correlated with the clinical presence of TD in these individuals [32]. Also, dopamine supersensitivity following prolonged dopamine receptor blockade in animal models is a universal and rapidly appearing pharmacologic phenomenon which lasts for only several weeks, raising some doubt about its relevance to persistent TD in humans.

Another hypothesis suggests that an imbalance between D-1 and D-2 receptor–mediated effects in basal ganglia may be responsible for TD [33]. According to this theory, classical or first-generation APDs preferentially block D-2 receptors thereby inhibiting the indirect striatopallidal outflow pathway. This results in unbalanced excessive activity of D-1 mediated striatopallidal output which causes altered firing patterns in the medial globus pallidus which in turn leads to hyperkinetic movement disorders [33]. According to this model, the ability of clozapine, a second-generation neuroleptic, to produce relatively less D-2 and relatively more D-1 blockade may account for the fact that it very uniquely does not produce TD [33].

Changes in other neuronal systems in the basal ganglia may also play a role in causing TD. In Huntington's disease, which TD closely resembles, a loss of medium spiny striatal interneurons results in choreiform dyskinesia. These striatal interneurons utilize GABA, acetylcholine, or peptides as their neurotransmitter. From this has emerged the GABA hypothesis of TD. Chronic treatment of monkeys with APDs over a period of several years produced persistent dyskinesia and reduced GABA and glutamic acid decarboxylase levels in several regions of the basal ganglia [34]. It has been proposed that excitotoxicity may account for selective destruction of a localized population of basal ganglia neurons. According to this hypothesis, chronic blockade of D-2 receptors may lead to increased glutamate release within the striatum, thereby causing excitotoxic destruction of striatopallidal GABA and peptide-containing neurons [35]. There are two potential mechanisms by which this might occur. Firstly, interference with the inhibitory action of dopamine on corticostriatal terminal D-2 receptors could cause excessive release of glutamate in the striatum leading to excitotoxic degeneration of striatopallidal GABA and peptide neurons. Secondly, blockade of nigrostriatal dopamine activity could, as in Parkinson's disease, lead to increased firing of glutamate-mediated subthalamic neurons causing excitotoxic degeneration of globus pallidus neurons.

Two other theories of TD pathogenesis have proposed the possible roles of oxidative stress and synaptic plasticity in the brain. Regarding the possible role of oxidative stress, chronic blockade of dopamine receptors leads to increased neuronal dopamine turnover, thereby generating free radicals and hydrogen peroxide [36]. This may result in neuronal damage and degeneration of multiple neurotransmitter systems. According to this hypothesis, irreversible structural changes due to neuronal loss and gliosis would occur, therefore supporting a possible "neurodegenerative" hypothesis of TD.

Regarding the possible role of synaptic plasticity, chronic blockade of D2 receptors may lead to hypersensitization of D2 receptors at both a cortical and basal ganglia level. Such hypersensitization may cause secondary effects on the synaptic plasticity of glutamatergic synapses on striatal interneurons, leading to abnormal striatopallidal output. This might be accompanied by maladaptive plasticity at the cortical level. According to this theory, the combination of maladaptive cortical synaptic plasticity and abnormal striatopallidal output produces abnormal movements [37].

# Epidemiology of tardive dyskinesia due to antipsychotic drugs

## Prevalence of TD

Prevalence estimates of TD have significant limitations when used to establish the risks of certain conditions among patient populations with different treatment exposures. APDs cause TD but can also mask its clinical manifestations by hypokinetic effects of their dopamine receptor blocking properties thereby reducing case ascertainment. In addition, the severity of TD often fluctuates with behavioral and emotional arousal so that in milder forms it may be less apparent. Differences in population age, gender, treatment duration, and type and dose of APDs also add to the complexity of determining the prevalence of TD in a particular population at a particular time.

When first described in the 1960s, the frequency of TD was widely regarded to be low due to failure of chronic psychotic patients to complain of dyskinesia, the limited familiarity of psychiatric clinicians with movement disorders in general, and the reluctance of some psychiatric clinicians to accept the possibility of a persistent disorder caused by APDs [1, 38, 39]. By the late 1970s, with greater awareness and increased vigilance, it became apparent that the prevalence of TD was substantial. Published prevalence figures varied widely between 5% and 45% among samples of hospitalized psychiatric patients and 30% among psychiatric outpatients [1, 2, 39]. Variable definitions of what was considered TD, varying ascertainment methods, patient age, and other risk factors among patient samples explain the wide variations in reported prevalence at that time. In addition, spontaneous dyskinesias independent of treatment with APDs may have inflated estimates of prevalence. Kane and colleagues analyzed 56 studies involving nearly 35,000 APD-treated patients and estimated the overall prevalence of TD to be 20%. In 19 studies involving 11,000 untreated patients not exposed to neuroleptic drugs, the prevalence of spontaneous dyskinesia was approximately 5%, suggesting a best-estimate, corrected rate for neuroleptic-associated TD of about 15% [27].

## Incidence of TD

The incidence of new cases of TD appearing in a population during a specified period of exposure is a better measure of risk than cross-sectional estimates of prevalence at a particular point in time. However, incidence data are more difficult to acquire since they require repeated prospective observations over time. In order to study prospective incidence as well as identify risk factors, Kane and colleagues at the Hillside Hospital in New York enrolled 908 consecutive patients aged 19–40 years who were admitted to a single psychiatric service and monitored them for up to 20 years for the presence of dyskinesia [40]. All patients had been treated with conventional and predominantly "high-potency" standard APDs such as haloperidol or fluphenazine. Of 908 enrolled patients, 5.6% met diagnostic criteria for TD at initial evaluation or entered with a prior diagnosis of probable TD. Cumulative new incidence of TD was 5% after one year, 27% after 5 years, 43% after 10 years, and 52% after 15 years of APD exposure [40; Kane et al. personal communication]. The cumulative incidence of persistent TD lasting for at least three months was 3% after one year, 20% after 5 years, and 34% after 10 years [40]. These rates indicate an annual new incidence of TD of about 5% per year, with about 3% for cases persisting for at least 3 months.

Similar results were obtained in other prospective studies done at Yale in patients with chronic schizophrenia [41, 42]. However, the time of antecedent exposure to APDs in these patients was much longer, with a mean of 8 years. The incidence of TD persisting for at least six months yielded a cumulative five-year total of 25%, remarkably similar to the incidence of persistent TD described above in the Hillside study.

## Incidence of TD in the elderly

In a prospective study, a population of patients never previously treated with APDs and older than 55 years, of whom 63% had dementia, had a cumulative incidence of 23% over 2.2 years. TD persisted for at least six months in 67% of these cases [43]. Another prospective study carried out for a longer period of time in older patients with a mean age of 65 years, found a cumulative TD incidence of 26.1% at one year and 59.8% after three years, or approximately 20% per year during continuous exposure to various older neuroleptics [44]. Thus, even with shorter exposure times, old age increased the risk of incidence for TD more than for younger patients.

## Risk factors for TD

Most identified risk factors for TD have been based on associations discovered in prevalence rather than

prospective incidence studies [2, 45]. Advanced age has clearly emerged as the most robust risk factor for TD [46] with the exception of the tardive dystonia subtype which occurs more often in younger individuals [9–11]. In the original Hillside study, the prospective incidence of new cases of TD in patients above age 50 was 3–5 times greater than in younger patients and the prevalence of TD in patients exposed to APDs was 5–6 times greater than among younger patients [40]. Moreover, rates of spontaneous remission decrease with increasing age [46]. Other factors such as brain injury, dementia, major affective disorder, diabetes, longer duration of APD exposure, and use of anticholinergic drugs have all been tentatively associated with greater risk for TD. Importantly, in several prospective studies previous acute EPS have been associated with a higher risk for TD [40, 47].

In some studies, female sex, being African-American, and a history of electroconvulsive treatment were also identified as risk factors for TD. Notwithstanding these possible but less well established risk factors, since TD is clearly not a universal complication of treatment with APDs it is likely that yet to be identified genetic predispositions may account for its appearance in some but not all patients with similar exposures to DRBAs. Several possible genetic candidates for TD susceptibility have been implicated but have not yet been established [48]. APD exposure by dose has long been suspected to be a risk factor for TD but this has been difficult to establish. Dosing was found to be an important risk factor in elderly patients in one prospective study [43] but other studies have reported little difference in TD prevalence or incidence between moderate and high doses of APD [39, 49].

## Epidemiology of TD in the era of modern antipsychotic drugs

With the availability of a new generation of second-generation or so-called "atypical" APDs with a presumed, but unproven, lower risk for causing acute EPS, it was hoped and even expected that TD might also prove to become a declining clinical problem. Modern second-generation APDs approved for use in the United States include aripiprazole, clozapine, olanzapine, quetiapine, risperidone, and ziprasidone. Based on their ability to produce less motor-inhibitory effects in laboratory animals as well as early and relatively short-term human clinical trials, these drugs were believed to have lower risks for causing acute EPS such as acute dystonic reactions, acute akathisia, and parkinsonism than conventional APDs. Pharmacologically, these agents are characterized by limited antagonistic actions at dopamine $D_2$-type receptors due to their relatively low affinity with and rapid dissociation from these receptors [29]. However, it currently appears that based on both prospective and retrospective studies which compare first- and second-generation APDs, with the exception of clozapine and quetiapine, the differences between these classes of medications with regard to either acute EPS or TD appears to be considerably less than was originally thought to be the case [50]. In this regard, clozapine and quetiapine are special cases, since there have been very few documented cases of TD following their chronic use, most of which have been unconvincing. Examination of many of the case reports claiming that TD has complicated the use of these two drugs indicates either that patients experienced acute rather than tardive dyskinesia without documentation that they persisted after discontinuing treatment, or that the affected patients had experienced previous exposure to other more potent first- or second-generation APDs.

## Current prevalence and incidence of TD

Several studies published between 1996 and 2002, during the time when second-generation APDs became widely available, found TD prevalence rates of 16% to 43%, suggesting that the current risk for TD may be similar to that reported earlier in association with the use of older APDs [51–54]. However, most such studies, because of the era in which they were carried out, did not separate patients exclusively treated with second-generation APDs from those also exposed to first-generation APDs either previously or concurrently. By contrast, in a later review of several prospective studies of second-generation APDs carried out through mid-2003 the annual incidence of TD associated with second-generation APDs averaged 2.1% overall, with 0.8% in adults younger than 50 years vs. 5.3% among patients over age 50 [55]. Among patients under age 50, the risk of new-onset TD was 6.8 times greater in association with haloperidol than with modern agents. Comparison of risks associated with individual second-generation APDs was difficult due to methodological differences among studies. Nevertheless, the incidence of TD varied

remarkably little among different second-generation agents, except for a greater risk with risperidone when used in relatively high doses. These findings were interpreted to indicate that in adult patients of any age treated with modern APDs the observed incidence of TD was about one-fifth the risk associated with first-generation APDs [55]. However, these findings may have been skewed by the fact that three high-dose haloperidol studies were included among the first-generation APD studies. This impression is also limited by the very few direct head-to-head comparisons of modern and older APDs. A later systematic review by the same group which evaluated several newer cross-sectional studies published between 2004 and 2007 found that the prevalence of TD was still lower among adults taking second-generation drugs than those taking first-generation APDs, but that the difference between the two groups was less than that found in the earlier study [56].

Regarding the current incidence of TD with second-generation APDs, there have been at least 19 published case reports of TD among patients never previously exposed to traditional neuroleptics and treated exclusively with modern APDs including risperidone, olanzapine, ziprasidone, and aripiprazole [2, 45, 50]. Risperidone was the APD implicated in the vast majority of these cases. This is not surprising since risperidone is no longer considered a truly atypical APD given its high affinity for D2 dopamine receptors and demonstrated potency for causing acute EPS when given in doses higher than 6mg/day [50]; but it was also the most popular and first to go generic. There have been an even larger number of published case reports of patients who had prior exposure to first-generation APDs, who developed TD for the first time only during later treatment with second-generation APDs. Despite the obvious limitations of these case report data, these reports suggest that most modern APDs other than clozapine and quetiapine carry a significant risk for causing TD and that risperidone may have a greater risk of causing TD than other modern APDs [2, 45, 50].

## Is risk of TD declining?

As reviewed above, recent estimates of TD incidence among patients treated with second-generation APDs have appeared to suggest a decline in risk compared to the prior era of traditional first-generation APDs. However, most of these recent findings have been based primarily on short-term industry sponsored studies not specifically designed to address the prospective risk of TD. Very few were blinded, randomized, or head-to-head studies designed to compare new to older APDs; most involved APD exposures of less than a year; and few included sufficiently specific neurological assessments to identify TD. In addition, the few studies that included randomization of control patients to a standard comparator used haloperidol, a first-generation high-potency APD with high risk for TD, in relatively large doses of above 12mg/day [57]. These conditions may not be representative of other less potent older agents administered in more moderate doses [50].

Another important issue is that, as already stated, prospective studies of modern APDs have included very few patients not previously exposed to older APDs, which may have contributed to their risk of developing TD on modern APDs. Moreover, for uncertain reasons the use of some second-generation APDs including clozapine, olanzapine, and risperidone has been associated with a reduction in the clinical manifestations of TD, possibly leading to a misleadingly low incidence of TD [58, 59].

In summary, the current available evidence indicates that the risk for developing TD is probably lower with most modern APDs than with older high-potency APDs, but not necessarily when compared to studies in which low potency APDs have been used in moderate doses [50]. The CATIE trial was an important independent prospective trial of patients without TD at baseline which compared the extrapyramidal effects of second-generation APDs with modest doses of perphenazine, a medium potency first-generation APD [60]. Quite remarkably, this study found no significant differences between patients treated with perphenazine compared with any of the second-generation APDs for incidence of either TD or acute EPS including parkinsonism, dystonia, or akathisia. It appears that further studies of patients never previously treated with any first-generation APDs and exposed exclusively to second-generation APDs other than risperidone will be necessary in order to establish any claims for a significant decline in the incidence of TD in association with use of second-generation drugs.

## Prevention of tardive dyskinesia

Prevention of TD rests on reducing exposure to APDs, clinical vigilance for early detection of TD,

and management of potentially reversible cases. The use of APDs for longer than three months requires careful evaluation of indications for their continued use and risks of more prolonged treatment and should be limited to situations where there is no alternative effective psychiatric therapy. Two American Psychiatric Association Task Forces on TD have published specific indications for short- and long-term APD treatment [39, 61]. Long-term use of APDs for treatment of depression, bipolar disease, neurosis, anxiety, personality disorder, and chronic pain states should be discouraged. Even in schizophrenia or related chronic psychosis, efforts should be made to maintain patients on the lowest effective APD dose while reexamining the need for continued treatment at least every six months. After remission of a first acute psychotic episode, the APD dose should be decreased and probably even carefully tapered and discontinued after treatment for 6–12 months to see if continued treatment is necessary. Any plan to continue treatment beyond six months requires careful discussion with the patient and family regarding the indication for prolonged treatment with APDs and the risks of TD. Particular care is indicated for patients above age 50 since they are well established to have a higher risk for developing TD. In appropriate cases, clozapine and quetiapine should be considered for some patients as alternatives to other second-generation APDs since, as discussed earlier in this chapter, there is little or no convincing evidence that either of these have caused persistent TD when they have been the only APD to which a patient has ever been exposed.

Since acute DIP and akathisia reflect the extent of D-2 receptor blockade, these early adverse effects, which appear to increase the risk of later appearance of TD [40, 47], should be avoided by dose reduction or by use of a less potent agent. It is prudent to use the smallest APD dose needed for effective treatment, especially since DIP may mask the signs of dyskinesia. As reviewed above, there is surprisingly little convincing evidence that second-generation APDs produce a much lower incidence of acute EPS when compared to clinically equivalent doses of first-generation drugs, and the same appears to be true for their risk of producing TD [60].

Except for prevention or treatment of acute dystonic reactions, the use of prophylactic anticholinergic drugs should be discouraged since they do not prevent TD and may actually exaggerate its manifestations once they do occur. Importantly, early APD withdrawal once TD is recognized appears to result in improved prognosis for recovery. Therefore, patients on APDs should be carefully monitored for signs of TD at regular intervals using a standard dyskinesia rating scale such as the Abnormal Involuntary Movement Scale (AIMS), which is especially useful to heighten awareness of the milder and more localized manifestations of TD. Whenever safe and feasible from a psychiatric viewpoint, APD should be tapered and discontinued as soon as the diagnosis of TD is made.

## Metoclopramide

Metoclopramide is a benzamide derivative with dopamine receptor blocking properties used for treatment of gastroparesis, gastric reflux, and chemotherapy-induced nausea and vomiting. Identical to the APDs, metoclopramide causes both acute and late appearing extrapyramidal side effects. Metoclopramide is currently a significant cause of TD, which is clinically indistinguishable from TD due to APDs [62–64]. In 2009 the FDA issued a black box warning concerning TD risk. However, no prospective data are available concerning this risk. Because there is no reliable information concerning the number of individuals taking metoclopramide on a chronic basis, the percent prevalence of metoclopramide-induced TD is not precisely known but has been estimated at 1%–15% [64]. In recent years, one large movement disorders referral center has reported that metoclopramide has replaced haloperidol in their clinic as the medication currently most commonly associated with TD [63].

Metoclopramide is a DRBA used chronically as an antiemetic and prokinetic agent for the treatment of gastroparesis, gastric reflux disorders, and more intermittently for chemotherapy-induced nausea and vomiting. Since the withdrawal of cisapride from the US market in 2000 because of serious adverse cardiac effects, metoclopramide has become the only FDA-approved drug for the treatment of gastroparesis. However, it is FDA approved only for short-term treatment of less than 12 weeks. If it appears to be clinically indicated for more than 12 weeks and, as in the case for persistent gastroparesis, no effective substitute is available, then patients should be treated with the lowest effective dose and carefully educated regarding its risk for causing TD. The risk-benefit ratio of using metoclopramide in elderly patients, women, individuals taking APDs, and individuals with preexisting movement disorders must be carefully considered. Patients taking metoclopramide chronically should be carefully examined for early signs of TD on a regular basis, and discontinuing of its use should periodically be considered if clinically feasible. In the case of gastric reflux, for which metoclopramide is often used chronically, alternative treatment with proton pump inhibitors, 5-HT3 inhibitors such as ondansetron, NK1 receptor antagonists, and, where available, domperidone should be considered instead.

## Conclusions

Given the risks involved, it is clear that DRBAs should be used very selectively and with great attention to minimize the risk of causing TD, a permanent and disfiguring neurological disorder. Unfortunately, in psychiatric practice, the widespread use of second-generation APDs and the perception that they may be safer, at least from the viewpoint of acute extrapyramidal reactions, has resulted in their more widespread use, much of which has been for expanding off-label indications, for some of which there is insufficient research support [50]. In medical and gastroenterologic practice there has been an unfortunate lack of awareness of the risk for TD with long-term use of metoclopramide. Although it appears that the incidence of TD appears to be somewhat lower than it was in the era of the first-generation APDs, the risk reduction is surprisingly modest and less than has generally been assumed. Moreover, the risk of TD may in fact not be substantially lower than with some of the older relatively lower potency APDs such as perphenazine, thioridazine, and molindone, especially when they have been used in moderate doses [50].

## References

1. Tarsy D. History and definition of tardive dyskinesia. *Clin Neuropharmacol* 1983; **6**: 91–99.

2. Tarsy D. Tardive dyskinesia. In: Hurtig HI, Dashe JF, eds. *UpToDate*. Wolters Kluwer 2014.

3. Tarsy D, Baldessarini RJ. Tardive dyskinesia. *Ann Rev Med* 1984; **35**:605–623.

4. Jankovic J. Tardive syndromes and other drug-induced movement disorders. *Clin Neuropharmacol* 1995; **18**: 197–214.

5. Waln O, Jankovic J. An update on tardive dyskinesia: From phenomenology to treatment. *Tremor Other*

*Hyperkinet Mov* 2013; http://tremorjournal.org/article/view/161.

6.  Bhidayasiri R, Boonyawairoj S. Spectrum of tardive syndromes: Clinical recognition and management. *Postgrad Med J* 2011;**87**:132–141.

7.  Stacy M, Cardoso F, Jankovic J. Tardive stereotypy and other movement disorders in tardive dyskinesia. *Neurology* 1993;**43**:937–941.

8.  Marsden CD, Tarsy D, Baldessarini RJ. Spontaneous and drug-induced movement disorders in psychotic patients. In: *Psychiatric Aspects of Neurologic Disease.* Benson DF, Blumer D (Eds) Grune and Stratton, New York, 1975. p. 219–265.

9.  Tarsy D, Granacher R, Bralower M. Tardive dyskinesia in young adults. *Am J Psychiatry* 1977;**134**:1032–1034.

10. Burke RE, Fahn S, Jankovic J et al. Tardive dystonia: Late-onset and persistent dystonia caused by antipsychotic drugs. *Neurology* 1982; **32**: 1335–1346.

11. Kiriakakis V, Bhatia KP, Quinn NP, et al. The natural history of tardive dystonia. *Brain* 1998;**121**:2053–2066.

12. Tarsy D. Akathisia. In: Joseph AB, Young RR, eds. *Movement Disorders in Neurology and Neuropsychiatry*, Joseph AB, Young RR (Eds) Blackwell, Boston 1999; 75–83.

13. Stacy M, Jankovic J. Tardive tremor. *Mov Disord* 1992;**7**:53–57.

14. Tarsy D, Indorf G. Tardive tremor due to metoclopramide. *Mov Disord* 2002;**17**:620–621.

15. Tarsy D. Baldessarini RJ. The tardive dyskinesia syndrome. In: *Clinical Neuropharmacology*, Klawans HL (Ed) Raven Press, New York, 1976. p. 29–61.

16. Rich MW, Radwany, SM. Respiratory dyskinesia. *An under-recognized phenomenon. Chest* 1994; **105**: 1826–1832.

17. Playford ED, Britton TC, Thompson PD, et al. Exacerbation of postural tremor with emergence of parkinsonism after treatment with neuroleptic drugs. *J Neurol Neurosurg Psychiatry* 1995;**58**:487–489.

18. Goetz CG. Drug-induced parkinsonism and idiopathic Parkinson's disease. *Arch Neurol* 1983;**40**:325–326.

19. Chabolla DR, Maraganore DM, Ahlskog JE. Drug-induced parkinsonism as a risk factor for Parkinson's disease: A historical cohort study in Olmsted County, Minnesota. *Mayo Clin Proc* 1998;**73**:724–727.

20. Lorberboym M, Treves TA, Melamed E, et al. [123]-FP/CIT SPECT imaging for distinguishing drug-induced parkinsonism from Parkinson's disease. *Mov Disord* 2006;**21**:510–514.

21. Lim TT, Ahmed A, Itin I, et al. Is 6 months of neuroleptic withdrawal sufficient to distinguish drug-induced parkinsonism from Parkinson's disease? *Intern J Neuroscience* 2013;**123**(3):170–4.

22. Gardos G, Cole JO, Tarsy D. Withdrawal syndromes associated with antipsychotic drugs. *Am J Psychiatry* 1978;**135**:1321–1324.

23. Polizos P, Engelhardt DM, Hoffman SP, et al. Neurological consequences of psychotropic drug withdrawal in schizophrenic children. *J Autism Child Schizo* 1973;**3**:247–253.

24. Gardos G, Casey DE, Cole JO, et al. Ten-year outcome of tardive dyskinesia. *Am J Psychiatry* 1994; **151**: 836–841.

25. Fernandez HH, Krupp B, Friedman JJ. The course of tardive dyskinesia and parkinsonism in psychiatric patients: 14-year follow-up. *Neurology* 2001;**56**:805–807.

26. Yassa R, Camille Y, Belzile L. Tardive dyskinesia in the course of antidepressant therapy: A prevalence study and review of the literature. *J Clin Psychopharm* 1987;**7**:243–246.

27. Kane JM, Smith JM. Tardive dyskinesia. Prevalence and risk factors, 1959–1979. *Arch Gen Psychiatry* 1982; **39**: 473–481.

28. Harrison PJ. The neuropathological effects of antipsychotic drugs. *Schizophrenia Res* 1999; **40**:87–99.

29. Kapur S, Seeman P. Does fast dissociation from the dopamine d(2) receptor explain the action of atypical antipsychotics: A new hypothesis. *Am J Psychiatry* 2001;**158**:360–369.

30. Tarsy D, Baldessarini RJ. Pharmacologically induced behavioral sensitivity to apomorphine. *Nature (New Biol)* 1973;**245**:262–263.

31. Tarsy D, Baldessarini RJ. Behavioral supersensitivity to apomorphine following chronic treatment with drugs which interfere with the synaptic function of catecholamines. *Neuropharmacology* 1974; **13**: 927–940.

32. Lee T, Seeman P, Tourtelotte WW, et al. Binding of $^3$H-neuroleptic and $^3$H-apomorphine in schizophrenic brains. *Nature* 1980; **274**: 897–900.

33. Gerlach J, Hansen L. Clozapine and D-1/D-2 antagonism in extrapyramidal functions. *Br J of Psychiatry* 1992; **160** (Suppl 17) 34–37.

34. Gunne LM, Haggstrom JE, Sjoquist B. Association with persistent neuroleptic-induced dyskinesia of regional changes in brain GABA synthesis. *Nature* 1984; **309**: 347–349.

35. De Keyser J. Excitotoxic mechanisms may be involved in the pathophysiology of tardive dyskinesia. *Clin Neuropharmacol* 1991;**14**:562–565.

36. Lohr JB, Kuczenski R, Niculescu AB. Oxidative mechanisms and tardive dyskinesia. *CNS Drugs* 2003;**17**:47–62.

37. Teo JT, Edwards MJ, Bhatia K. Tardive dyskinesia caused by maladaptive synaptic plasticity: a hypothesis. *Mov Disord* 2012;**27**:1205–15.

38. Weiden PJ, Mann J, Hass G, et al. Clinical nonrecognition of neuroleptic-induced movement disorders: a cautionary study. *Am J Psychiatry* 1987; **144**:1148–1153.

39. Baldessarini RJ, Cole JO, Davis JM, Gardos G, Preskorn HS, Simpson GM, Tarsy D. *Tardive dyskinesia. American Psychiatric Association Task Force on Late Effects of Antipsychotic Drugs.* American Psychiatric Association, Washington, 1980. *Am J Psychiatry* 1980; 137:1163–1172.

40. Kane JM, Woerner M, Weinhold P, Wegner J, Kinon D. A prospective study of tardive dyskinesia development: Preliminary results. *J Clin Psychopharmacol* 1982; **2**:345–349.

41. Morgenstern H, Glazer WM. Identifying risk factors for tardive dyskinesia among long-term outpatients maintained with neuroleptic medications. Results of the Yale tardive dyskinesia study. *Arch Gen Psychiatry* 1993; **50**:723–733.

42. Glazer WM, Morgenstern H, Doucette JT. Predicting the long-term risk of tardive dyskinesia in outpatients maintained on neuroleptic medications. *J Clin Psychiatry* 1993;54:133–139.

43. Woerner MG, Alvir JMJ, Saltz BL, Lieberman JA, Kane JM. Prospective study of tardive dyskinesia in the elderly: rates and risk factors. *Am J Psychiatry* 1998; **155**:1521–1528.

44. Jeste DV, Carigiuri NP, Paulsen JS, Heaton RK, Lacro JP, Harris MJ, Bailey A, Fell RL, McAdams LA. Risk of tardive dyskinesia in older patients. A prospective longitudinal study of 266 outpatients. *Arch Gen Psychiatry* 1995; **52**:756–765.

45. Tarsy D, Baldessarini RJ. Epidemiology of tardive dyskinesia: Is risk declining with modern antipsychotics? *Mov Dis* 2006;2:589–598.

46. Smith JM, Baldessarini RJ. Changes in prevalence, severity, and recovery in tardive dyskinesia with age. *Arch Gen Psychiatry* 1980; 37:1368–1373.

47. Tenback DE, van Harten PN, Sloof CJ, et al. Evidence that early extrapyramidal symptoms predict later tardive dyskinesia: a prospective analysis of 10,000 patients in the European Schizophrenia Outpatient Health Outcomes (SOHO) study. *Am J Psychiatry* 2006;**163**:1438–1440.

48. Muller DJ, Shinkai T, De Luca V, et al. Clinical implications of pharmacogenetics for tardive dyskinesia. *The Pharmacogenomic Journal* 2004; **4**:77–87.

49. Oosthuizen PP, Emsley R, Stephanus Maritz J, Turner JA, Keyter N. Incidence of tardive dyskinesia in first-episode psychosis patients treated with low-dose haloperidol. *J Clin Psychiatry* 2003; **64**:1075–1080.

50. Tarsy D, Lungo C, Baldessarini RJ. In: Weiner WJ, Tolosa E, eds. *Epidemiology of tardive dyskinesia.*

51. Van Os J, Fahy T, Jones P, Harvey I, Toone B, Murray R. Tardive dyskinesia: who is at risk? *Acta Psychiatr Scand* 1997; **96**:206–216.

52. Van Harten PN, Hoek HW, Matroos GE, Koeter M, Kahn RS. Intermittent neuroleptic treatment and risk for tardive dyskinesia: Curacao extrapyramidal syndromes study III. *Am J Psychiatry* 1998; **155**:565–567.

53. Muscettola G, Barbato G, Pampallona S, Casiello M, Bollini P. Extrapyramidal syndromes in neuroleptic-treated patients: prevalence, risk factors, and association with tardive dyskinesia. *J Clin Psychopharmacol* 1999; **19**:203–208.

54. Halliday J, Farrington S, MacDonald S, MacEwan, Sharkey V, McCreadie R. Nithsdale schizophrenia surveys 23: Movement disorders. *Br J Psych* 2002;**181**:422–427.

55. Correll CU, Leucht S, Kane JM. Reduced risk for tardive dyskinesia associated with second generation antipsychotics: Systematic review of one-year studies. *Am J Psychiatry* 2004; **161**:414–425.

56. Correll CU, Schenk EM. Tardive dyskinesia and new antipsychotics. *Curr Opin Psychiatry* 2008;**21**:151–156.

57. Baldessarini RJ, Tarazi FI. Drugs and the treatment of psychiatric disorders: antipsychotic and antimanic agents. In: Hardman JG, Limbird LE, Gilman AG, eds. *Goodman and Gilman's The Pharmacologic Basis of Therapeutics,* 11th ed. New York, McGraw-Hill Press, 2005;461–500.

58. Tarsy D, Baldessarini RJ, Tarazi FI. Effects of newer antipsychotics on extrapyramidal function. *CNS Drugs* 2002; **16**:23–45.

59. Caroff SN, Mann SC, Campbell EC, et al. Movement disorders associated with atypical antipsychotic drugs. *J Clin Psychiatry* 2002;**63** (Suppl 4):12–19.

60. Miller del D, Eudicone JM, Pikalov A, et al. Comparative assessment of the incidence and severity of tardive dyskinesia in patients receiving ariprazole or haloperidol for the treatment of schizophrenia: post hoc analysis. *J Clin Psychiatry* 2007;**68**:1901–1906.

61. *Tardive dyskinesia: a Task Force Report of the American Psychiatric Association.* Washington, DC: American Psychiatric Association Press. 1992.

62. Miller LG, Jankovic J. Metoclopramide-induced movement disorders. Clinical findings with a review of the literature. *Arch Int Med* 1989;**149**:2486–2492.

63. Kenney C, Hunter C, Davidson A, et al. Metoclopramide, an increasingly recognized cause of tardive dyskinesia. *J Clin Pharmacol* 2008;**48**:379–384.

64. Rao AS, Camilleri M. Review article: metoclopramide and tardive dyskinesia. *Aliment Pharmacol Ther* 2010;**31**:11–19.

*Handbook of Clinical Neurology*, 32d edition. Amsterdam, Elsevier, 2011; 601–616.

# Tardive dyskinesia treatment

Tracy M. Jones, Israt Jahan, and Theresa A. Zesiewicz

## Introduction

Tardive syndromes (TS) are characterized by abnormal, involuntary movements, and are typically caused by exposure to dopamine receptor blocking agents (DRBAs). The original description of TS was that of Schonecker in 1957, following the introduction of neuroleptics to treat psychiatric conditions (1). The term "tardive" was first used by Faurbye et al. in 1964, and refers to the delayed onset of the movements in relation to the DRBA exposure (2,3). TS consist of several subgroups, including tardive dyskinesia, dystonia, akathisia, myoclonus, stereotypy, tremor, and tourettism (4,5).

One form of TS, tardive dyskinesia (TD), is characterized by repetitive, stereotypic, involuntary, choreiform movements of the face, tongue, and jaw (oro-buccal-lingual dyskinesia), torso, and extremities. Symptoms of TD may include lip smacking, tongue twisting and thrusting, lip pursing, cheek puffing, grimacing, chewing, pelvic thrusting, piano-playing movements of the hands, foot tapping, and bridling (retraction of corners of the mouth) (6,7). TD may severely impact quality of life, leading to speaking and chewing difficulty, and may cause embarrassment (8). It is estimated to affect approximately 20% to 50% of patients who have been exposed to DRBAs, with a yearly incidence ranging from 5% in younger patients to 12% in older patients (9). Risk factors are thought to include older age, female gender, drug or alcohol addiction, preexisting brain damage, diabetes mellitus, and negative schizophrenic symptoms (5,10). The exact etiology of TD is unknown, but hypotheses include dopaminergic receptor hypersensitivity, upregulation of dopamine (D) 2 receptors, overactivity of striatal dopamine transmission, cerebral imbalance of dopaminergic and cholinergic activity, gamma-aminobutyric acid depletion, and oxidative stress (11–14).

The following criteria are necessary to meet the diagnosis of TS: 3 months total cumulative neuroleptic exposure during which it can be continuous or discontinuous, the presence of at least moderate abnormal involuntary movements in one or more body area or at least mild movements in 2 or more body areas, and the absence of other conditions that might produce abnormal involuntary movements (15). Criteria of TD diagnosis according to the American Psychiatric Association includes at least 3 months of DRBA exposure, or 1 month exposure in persons over age 60 years (4), dyskinesia that occurs during exposure to a DRBA or within 6 months of discontinuation of the DRBA, and movements that must persist for at least one month following DRBA withdrawal (16).

Treatment of TD may be challenging. It may be prevented by avoiding DRBAs, but these medications are often necessary to manage psychiatric conditions. Second-generation antipsychotics have generally replaced the use of first-generation antipsychotics for treatment of psychosis, due to their more favorable side effect profile for extrapyramidal symptoms compared to first-generation antipsychotics. However, second-generation agents may also cause TD, in rates similar to those of first-generation agents (17–19). Little evidence exists that discontinuation of neuroleptics actually results in resolution of TD (20). Although the most common cause of TD is exposure to neuroleptics, an initial reduction in neuroleptic dose often worsens TD symptoms (21) by "unmasking" the underlying disorder.

The risk of TD versus the benefit of using neuroleptics must be considered individually. Before

*Medication-Induced Movement Disorders*, ed. Joseph H. Friedman. Published by Cambridge University Press.
© Cambridge University Press 2015.

prescribing DRBAs, patients should be advised of the possible risk of TD, and the American Psychiatric Association recommends evaluation for the presence of TD at least every 3 to 6 months using the Abnormal Involuntary Movement Scale (AIMS) (16), which is mandated by some states' laws. Health care providers may consider a slow reduction or discontinuation of DRBAs if TD occurs, but frequent mental health monitoring must occur. In cases of gastrointestinal dysfunction, ondansetron (Zofran) may be used rather than conventional DRBA antinausea agents, including metoclopramide, prochlorperazine, and promethazine (22).

# Treatment with pharmaceutical agents

## Anticholinergics

Anticholinergic medications have been considered as treatment of TD based on the hypothesis that DRBA exposure contributes to a reduction in the number of acetylcholine-containing cells in the striatal and accumbal subregions (23). However, there are currently no convincing controlled trials that suggest that anticholinergic medications effectively treat TD. One systematic review of anticholinergic treatment of TD concluded that, "no confident statement can be made about the effectiveness of anticholinergics to treat people with neuroleptic-induced tardive dyskinesia" (24). Pretreatment with anticholinergic agents prior to use of DRBAs is not recommended, as these medications may actually worsen cognition, particularly in the elderly (21). Trihexyphenidyl and ethopropazine have shown some efficacy in the treatment of tardive dystonia (4). We think that anticholinergics are contraindicated in dyskinetic forms of TD, especially the most common, oral-buccal-lingual.

## Antiepileptics

Several antiepileptics have been evaluated as possible treatments for TD, including levetiracetam, piracetam, and zonisamide. *Levetiracetam* (LEV) is a stereoisomer of piracetam, and is approved by the United States Food and Drug Administration (FDA) to treat partial and generalized seizures in adults and absence seizures in children (25). LEV has shown promise in ameliorating symptoms of TD, although research is limited (26,27). One double blind, placebo controlled trial randomized 50 TD patients to receive LEV 500–3000mg/day or placebo for 12 weeks, followed by an additional 12-week open-label extension phase, using the AIMS as the primary endpoint (28). Patients receiving LEV experienced a mean 43.5% improvement in total AIMS scores compared to 18.3% improvement in the placebo arm (p = 0.022).

*Piracetam* is an antiepileptic medication chemically related to LEV that has been used to treat myoclonus and other movement disorders (27). Libov et al. performed a 9-week double blind, placebo controlled, crossover study in 40 TD patients with schizophrenia or schizoaffective disorder (29). Patients were randomized to receive either piracetam (4800 mg/day) or placebo for two 4-week periods, separated by a 1-week washout phase. A mean reduction of three points was reported in the Extrapyramidal Symptom Rating Scale (ESRS) in patients treated with piracetam. The ESRS includes all the extrapyramidal syndromes so an improvement by three points is not clinically interpretable.

*Zonisamide* is an antiepileptic drug that was tested in a four-week, open-label study using the AIMS as a primary endpoint (30). The study reported a significant decrease in the AIMS score from 24.1 to 19.5 in 11 patients treated with zonisamide. Approximately 36% of study participants experienced a decrease of 20% or more in the AIMS scale, with a mean dose of zonisamide of 81.2 mg/day +/− 25.2 mg/day.

## Antihypertensives

There are suggestions that *propranolol*, a beta blocker, may improve oral-buccal dyskinesia and respiratory dyskinesia in low doses (31–33). Propranolol was first proposed as a possible treatment for TD in the 1980s (32), and was recently revisited by Factor in the presentation of two cases (34). The first patient was a 67-year-old female with metoclopramide-induced TD who was treated with 20mg propranolol three times a day. The patient experienced a reduction in orofacial dyskinesia and complete remission of respiratory dyskinesia after 8 months of therapy. The second patient was a 77-year-old male with neuroleptic-induced TD who showed improvement of buccal and respiratory dyskinesia with propranolol 80mg/day. As with any antihypertensive agent, caution is recommended with use in depressed patients, and blood pressure should be monitored periodically.

Additional antihypertensive agents have also been identified as potential treatments of TD. *Acetazolamide* is a carbonic anhydrase inhibitor that was evaluated in a controlled trial in 8 elderly and 25 younger patients (35). Patients older than 73 years received acetazolamide 1.5 g/day in 3 divided doses, while younger patients received 2 g/day along with thiamine administration for 3 weeks. Thiamine was added to the treatment to decrease the risk of kidney stones that may occur with acetazolamide use. AIMS scores decreased at endpoint relative to baseline by 46% in the elderly patients and 41% in younger patients. *Diltiazem,* a calcium channel blocker, failed to show significant improvement in TD in a controlled trial, and received a Level B recommendation from the AAN guideline ("probably does not treat") (36). In another trial, *nifedipine* was reported to have improved TD symptoms in doses up to 90 mg/day (37). Double blind, randomized, placebo controlled trials should be undertaken to further evaluate the efficacy of propranolol in the treatment of TD.

# Antioxidants

Antioxidants have been considered as possible treatments for TD, including ginkgo biloba, vitamin E, vitamin B6, melatonin, branched chain amino acids, resveratrol, essential fatty acids, omega 3, and eicosapentaenoic acid (11,23,38).

*EGb-761,* an extract from Ginkgo biloba, was evaluated in a double blind, placebo controlled clinical trial in 157 TD patients with schizophrenia (39). Patients were randomized to 240 mg/day of Egb-761 or placebo for 12 weeks. The primary outcome measures were the AIMS score, and the proportion of patients who experienced greater than 30% improvement in TD symptoms. There were significant improvements in the AIMS score in patients taking Egb-761 compared to placebo, and 51% of patients treated with Egb-761 showed improvement of 30% or more in the AIMS score. Egb-761 received a Level B recommendation ("probably improves TD") according to the AAN guideline, but it should be noted that the data on Egb-761 exists for schizophrenic patients only (36).

*Vitamin E* is a potent antioxidant that has been evaluated as treatment for TD in several studies. One metaanalysis of 221 patients found significant improvements in the AIMS scores in patients treated with vitamin E 400–1600IU compared to those who received placebo (28.4% in patients treated with vitamin E versus 4.6% in those given placebo, p = 0.004) (38). Other clinical trials have failed to replicate these findings (40–43). A double blind, placebo controlled trial randomized 158 patients to receive either vitamin E 1,600 IU/day or placebo for at least one year and up to two years, but there were no significant effects of vitamin E on AIMS scores or additional outcome measures (40). Due to the variability in study outcomes, vitamin E received a Level U recommendation from the AAN guideline (Data insufficient to support or refute benefit) (36).

*Melatonin,* a naturally occurring antioxidant, is a neurohormone secreted by the pineal gland and is six- to tenfold more potent than vitamin E (44). Melatonin in doses of 2 mg/day was evaluated in a short duration study, but no differences were noted in outcome measures with its use (45). Another study that utilized higher doses of melatonin (10 mg/day) for a longer duration of 16 weeks found >30% of improvement in TD symptoms (46). Seventy-seven percent of patients (n = 17) reported higher AIMS score reductions that those taking placebo.

*Branch Chain Amino Acids* (BCAAs, leucine, isoleucine, valine) have also been studied as possible treatments for TD. In one study, 6 children with TD who had been previously or currently taking neuroleptics, were treated with 222 mg/kg BCAA in 148 ml water three times/day for two weeks (47). The clinical diagnosis of TD was made through the use of the Simpson Abbreviated Dyskinesia Scale (SADS). TD symptoms reportedly improved about 50%–60% in five out of six children, although one child showed increased symptoms. In another study, 36 male patients with TD were randomized to receive BCAAs in a dose of 222 mg/kg (high; N = 18), 167mg/kg (medium), or 56mg/kg (low) three times daily or placebo (N = 18) for 3 weeks (48). A 36.5% (p = 0.0009) mean improvement was noted in patients treated with BCAAs compared to 3.4% mean improvement in the placebo group.

*Vitamin B6.* In one double blind, placebo controlled, crossover clinical trial, 15 TD patients with schizophrenia or schizoaffective disorder were randomized to receive vitamin B6 or placebo for 4 weeks with crossover phase following a 1 week washout period (49). Patients treated with 400 mg daily experienced greater improvements in the TD subscale of the Extrapyramidal Symptom Rating Scale than those patients who received placebo (68.6% versus 32.8%, respectively). Another double blind, placebo controlled trial randomized 50 patients to receive vitamin B6 1200 mg/day or placebo for a 12-week crossover study (50). There was a significant reduction in the ESRS clinical global impression scores of 2.4 units in patients treated with vitamin B6 compared to 0.2 units in the placebo group (p < 0.001).

*Essential fatty acids (EFAs, omega-3):* A double blind, placebo controlled trial compared EPA 2g/day and placebo in TD patients, but failed to find any significant improvements in outcome measures (23).

## First generation antipsychotics

First-generation antipsychotics (FGAs) may improve TD symptoms for short periods, but they are not recommended to treat TD, as they may mask symptoms while worsening the underlying condition. Side effects of FGAs may include parkinsonism and rigidity (51–54).

## Second-generation antipsychotics

*Risperidone:* Several controlled trials have studied the effect of risperidone on TD. In one study, 135 schizophrenic patients were randomized to receive risperidone (6–16 mg/day) or placebo for 8 weeks (55). Patients treated with risperidone had lower Extrapyramidal Symptom Rating Scale (ESRS) scores (p < 0.05) than those receiving placebo. A randomized, double blind, placebo controlled trial in 49 TD patients with schizophrenia assigned patients to receive risperidone 6mg/day or placebo for 12 weeks (56). There was a mean AIMS reduction of 5.5+/−3.8 in the risperidone group versus a score of 1.1+/−4.8 in the placebo group (p < 0.05). More significant improvements in lingual-facial-buccal movements were observed in the risperidone group starting in the 8th week of the study. Another controlled trial compared the effects of risperidone and olanzapine in patients with schizophrenia with TD (57). AIMS scores decreased significantly in both groups (risperidone: −7.4+/−6.9, P < 0.0001; olanzapine: −6.2+/−8.0, P = 0.0002), but more so in patients taking risperidone (P = 0.0001). Risperidone is probably effective in reducing TD short term, but is also a cause for TD, and is not generally recommended as treatment, particularly long term.

Clozapine is a weak blocker of D2 receptors, and its administration carries a lower risk of TD than other FGAs (4,58). There have been reports that clozapine may even improve TD symptoms. In one study, 12 TD patients who were treated with clozapine (dose range of 20–900mg) for 18 weeks experienced

improvement in the mean Tardive Dyskinesia Rating Scale (TDRS) score (decrease from 26 to 12)(59). Five patients dropped out of the study—two due to non–study-associated issues and three due to clozapine side effects (new onset grand mal seizures [1 patient] and leukopenia [2 patients]). In another 6-month study, patients with severe TD were treated with clozapine for at least 6 months and also had marked improvement in symptoms (60). Bassitt et al. conducted a 6-month, open-label study evaluating the effects of clozapine in 7 patients with schizophrenia and severe TD. There was a 52% improvement in Extrapyramidal Symptom Rating Scale (ESRS) and a 41% mean improvement in the AIMS score was noted with mean clozapine dose of 393 mg/day (61). Alternatively, Gerlach et al. compared clozapine and haloperidol in a single-blind, crossover trial of eight schizophrenic patients, and found no effect (62).

Clozapine may be an attractive option for patients with psychiatric illness, as it offers antipsychotic benefit with limited risk of extrapyramidal symptoms. However, a potentially serious side effect of clozapine is agranulocytosis, and patients who take Clozaril must undergo periodic blood count monitoring (76).

Olanzapine: One controlled trial compared the effects of risperidone and olanzapine in patients with schizophrenia and TD, and found that AIMS scores improved significantly in both groups (risperidone: −7.4+/−6.9, P < 0.0001; olanzapine: −6.2+/−8.0, P = 0.0002). Patients taking olanzapine showed approximately 30% improvement in the AIMS score relative to baseline scores (57). In another 8-month open-label study of 95 patients with schizophrenia, olanzapine significantly reduced the mean AIMS score from baseline of 11.8 to 7.3 (p < 0.001) at a mean dose of 12mg/day (63). Olanzapine received a Level U rating by the AAN (possibly effective in reducing TD) (36).

The pharmacology of *quetiapine* is similar to clozapine without the risk of agranulocytosis, and its associated risk of TD is lower than that of FGAs (4). Further research is warranted regarding its effect on TD.

*Aripiprazole* is an atypical antipsychotic that acts as a partial $D_2$ receptor agonist, $5-HT_{2A}$ receptor antagonist, and $5-HT_{1A}$ receptor partial agonist. Multiple case reports have demonstrated a modest reduction to full remission of TD with the institution of aripiprazole in doses ranging from 5–30mg per day (64). However, at present, no randomized, double blind, placebo controlled trials testing the efficacy of aripiprazole have been completed.

## Cholinergics

According to the cholinergic deficiency theory, TD may be associated with an imbalance between cerebral acetylcholine and dopamine (23). A systematic review including studies that investigated the anticholinergics such as lecithin containing phosphatide choline, cetanol, and meclofenoxate concluded that the use of cholinergics in the treatment of TD was unclear since sample sizes were small (5–20) (65).

One open-label, pilot study of donepezil in the treatment of tardive dyskinesia was conducted on ten patients with schizophrenia or schizoaffective disorder. The patients were administered donepezil, 5–10mg/day for six weeks after a two-week baseline. The AIMS scale was conducted at two-week intervals. The study reported statistically significant improvement (p = 0.0009) in overall AIM scores, with the most substantial reductions in orofacial movement and upper arm movement (66).

## Dopamine-depleting agents

Dopamine-depleting agents are used in the treatment of TD in response partially to the proposed hypothesis of dopamine receptor hypersensitivity, and partially to the observation that drugs that cause parkinsonism reduce choreic movements. Hyperactive dopamine receptors produce the movement of tardive dyskinesia, and the continued blockade of these receptors may be useful to treat TD.

Tetrabenazine (TBZ) is a dopamine-depleting agent that inhibits vesicular monoamine transporter 2 (VMAT2). It is approved by the FDA as an orphan drug for the treatment of chorea in Huntington's disease. Open-label and controlled trials indicate that TBZ has efficacy in treating TD. One double blind, placebo controlled trial evaluated the effect of TBZ in 24 hospitalized patients by testing the frequency of movements in a 3-minute time period (67). Antipsychotics were withdrawn in a run-in phase, and TBZ (up to 150 mg/day) was administered for 14 weeks, followed by a placebo period for 2 weeks. Patients treated with TBZ experienced a 60% reduction in TD. Ondo et al. performed a 20-week open-label study of TBZ in TD patients using blinded video for AIMS rating (68). There was a 54% decrease in AIMS scores from 17.9 to 8.2 (p < 0.001) in patients treated with TBZ at a mean dose of 58 mg/day. Guay et al. retrospectively reviewed ten trials that cumulatively enrolled a total of 1,142 patients who received TBZ for TD, and found that approximately 70% of patients showed marked, excellent, or complete improvement in TD symptoms (69). Side effects of TBZ include parkinsonism, depression, akathisia, nausea, vomiting, nervousness, anxiety, insomnia, and rarely, hyperthermia and neuroleptic malignant syndrome (11,69,70).

*Reserpine* is an irreversible, dopamine-depleting agent that inhibits vesicular monoamine transporter (VMAT1) (5). Due to untoward side effects such as depression and hypotension, its use as treatment for TD has been limited (4,70). In a double blind, controlled study of reserpine, 30 patients received reserpine 0.75–1.5mg daily, alpha-methyldopa 750–1,500mg daily, or placebo for two weeks. Reserpine improved TD about 50%, on a scale that rated TD from 0 (absent) to 3(severe) (71).

# Dopamine agonists

Dopamine agonists are used in the treatment of TD due to the theory of dopamine system supersensitivity, which suggests that dopamine antagonists produce hypersensitivity of dopamine receptors (23). One dopamine agonist, bromocriptine, has not been found to be effective in treating TD, and there is little data (72,73).

# GABA agonists

*Baclofen* is a GABA$_B$ agonist and its efficacy has been analyzed in several RCTs. One double blind trial randomized 33 TD patients to receive baclofen in doses up to 90mg/day or placebo (74). Sixty-seven percent of patients treated with baclofen had a 25% or greater reduction in the AIMS score compared to 47% of patients on placebo. Another double blind, crossover trial (3 weeks in each period) evaluated baclofen in 20 patients with TD, using increasing doses over 2 weeks up to 120 mg/day (mean dose 75mg/day).There was a significant reduction in the hyperkinesia score (P < 0.05) with complete remission of movement in three patients (75). Another controlled trial was conducted on 31 psychiatric outpatients using 30–90mg per day of baclofen or placebo for 6 weeks (76). The results showed no statistical difference between the AIMS score in the treatment group versus the placebo group, leading the authors to conclude no treatment effect.

*Benzodiazepines* are indirect GABA agonists. A 12-week double blind placebo controlled, randomized, crossover trial to evaluate the effect of clonazepam on

TD was conducted on 19 TD patients who were concurrently being treated with neuroleptics, using a maximum clonazepam dose of 4.5mg/day (mean dose 3.9mg/day) (77). Results indicated a 37.1% improvement in dyskinesia ratings in patients treated with clonazepam. The effect of clonazepam was greater in patients with dystonic features (41.5% improvement, p < 0.001) versus choreoathetoid features (26.5% improvement, p < 0.001). Clonazepam received a Level B status by the AAN (probably effective in reducing TD symptoms short term) (36).

## Glutamateric medications

Amantadine has shown some promise in the reduction of TD possibly due to its ability to block N-methyl-D-aspartate) NMDA receptors (78). One double blind, placebo controlled trial randomized 16 TD patients to receive amantadine up to 300mg/day or placebo, and found an overall significant improvement in AIMS scores with amantadine use (p = 0.05) (79). Another double blind study randomized 22 patients with schizophrenia to receive amantadine (400 mg/day) or placebo for 5 weeks (80). Significant improvements (P = 0.000) in the mean AIMS score (decrease from baseline of 13.5 to 10.5) and a 21.3% reduction in AIMS severity were reported in patients treated with amantadine, while patients treated with placebo showed no improvement or reduction in mean AIMS score. Amantadine received a Level C recommendation from the AAN guideline ("possibly effective")(36).

## Botulinum toxin

Botulinum toxin is an established therapy for both blepharospasm and cervical dystonia. The use of botulinum toxin as a therapy for TD with dystonic features has shown some promise. A case report of an 81-year-old female with tongue protrusion, pain, and pruritus had a greater than ten-year history of orofacial dyskinesia. Twenty-five units of Botox were administered in each side of the tongue in the genioglossus muscle. The results were an absence of orolingual movements as well as a reduction in the pruritus and pain in the tongue. The maximum benefit lasted approximately two months (81). A single blind study was used to test botulinum toxin A in 12 patients with orofacial dyskinesia for 33 weeks and showed a significant decrease (p = 0.035) in AIMS scores when antipsychotic dose was kept constant, but not when

the dose was allowed to fluctuate due to changing symptoms (82).

## Conclusion

TD is often challenging to control. This review indicates that clonazepam, TBZ, ginkgo biloba, and amantadine have some efficacy in improving TD. SGAs, such as risperidone, may improve TD, but are generally not recommended, as they may mask TD symptoms. Current research is hampered by nonuniformity in trials, including variability in patient selection, concomitant use of neuroleptics, severity of TD, and heterogeneity of psychiatric illness. Further well-controlled trials are needed to determine therapy for TD.

## References

1. Schonecker M. Paroxysmal dyskinesia as the effect of megaphen. *Nervenarzt.* 1957;**28**:550–553.

2. Goldberg RJ. Tardive dyskinesia in elderly patients: an update. *J Am Med Dir Assoc.* 2002;3(3):152–161.

3. Faurbye A, Rash PJ, Petersen PB, et al. Neurological symptoms in pharmacotherapy of psychoses. *Acta Psychiatr Scan.* 1964;**40**:10–27.

4. Fernandez HH, Friedman JH. Classification and treatment of tardive syndromes. *Neurologist.* 2003;9:16–27.

5. Waln O, Jankovic J. An update on tardive dyskinesia: from phenomenology to treatment. *Tremor Other Hyperkinet Mov.* 2013;3:1–10.

6. Bhidayasiri R, Boonyawairoj S. Spectrum of tardive syndromes: clinical recognition and management. *Postgrad Med J.* 2011;87:132–141.

7. Orti-Pareja M, Jimenez-Jimenez FJ, Vasquez A, et al. Drug-induced tardive syndromes. *Parkinsonism Relat Disord.* 1999;5:59–65.

8. Mehanna R, Jankovic J. Respiratory disorders associated with dystonia. *Mov Disord.* 2012;27:1816–1819.

9. Kane JM, Smith JM. Tardive dyskinesia: Prevalence and risk factors 1959–1979. *Arch Gen Psychiatry.* 1982;**39**:473–481.

10. Tarsy D, Baldessarini RJ. Epidemiology of tardive dyskinesia: is risk declining with modern antipsychotics? *Mov Disord.* 2006;**21**:589–598.

11. Ragheb MM, Goldberg RJ. Tardive Dyskinesia in geriatric patients. *Aging Health.* 2006;2(5):833–849.

12. Dilsaver SC, Greden JF. Possible cholinergic mechanism in reserpine and tardive dyskinesia. *Am J Psychiatry.* 1984 Jan;**141**(1):151–2.

13. Tamminga CA, Thaker GK, Nguyen JA. GABAmimetic treatments for tardive dyskinesia:

efficacy and mechanism. *Psychopharmacol Bull.* 1989;**25**(1):43–6 (Review).

14. Lister J, Nobrega JN, Fletcher PJ, Remington G. Oxidative stress and the antipsychotic-induced vacuous chewing movement model of tardive dyskinesia: evidence for antioxidant-based prevention strategies. *Psychopharmacology (Berl).* 2014 Jun;**231**(11):2237–49.

15. Schooler NR, Kane JM. Research diagnoses for tardive dyskinesia. *Arch Gen Psychiatry.* 1982 Apr;**39**(4):486–7.

16. American Psychiatric Association. Differential diagnosis of tardive dyskinesia. In: *Tardive Dyskinesia: A Task Force Report of the American Psychiatric Association.* Washington DC: The Association; 1980:21–22.

17. Correll CU, Schenk EM. Tardive dyskinesia and new antipsychotics. *Curr Opin Psychiatry* 2008;**21**:151–156.

18. Bakker PR, de Groot IW, van Os J, et al. Long-stay psychiatry patients: a prospective study revealing persistent antipsychotic-induced movement disorder. *PLoS One* 2011;**6**:e25588.

19. Miller DD, Caroff SN, Davis SM, et al. Extrapyramidal side-effects of antipsychotics in a randomized trial. *Br J. Psychiarty* 2008;**193**:279–288.

20. Glazer WM, Morgenstern H, Schooler N, et al. Predictors of improvement in tardive dyskinesia following discontinuation of neuroleptic medication. *Br J. Psychiatry* 1990;**157**:585–592.

21. Egan MF, Apud J, Wyatt RJ. Treatment of tardive dyskinesia. *Schizophrenia Bulletin.* 1997;**23**(4):583–609.

22. Pantanwala AE, Amini R, Hays DP, et al. Antiemetic therapy for nausea and vomiting in the emergency department. *J Emerg Med* 2010;**39**(3):330–336.

23. Rana AQ, Chaudry ZM, Blanchet PJ. New and emerging treatments for symptomatic tardive dyskinesia. *Drug, Design, Development and Therapy.* 2013;**7**:1329–1340.

24. Soares-Weiser K, Mobsy C, Holliday E. Anticholinergic medication for neuroleptic-induced tardive dyskinesia (Review). *The Cochrane Library.* 1997:**2**. Retrieved from www.thecochrane library.com.

25. DeSmedt T, Raedt R, Vonck K, Boon P. Levetiracetam: Part II, the clinical profile of a novel anticonvulsant drug. *CNS Drug Reviews.* 2007;**13**(1):57–78.

26. Jankelowitz SK. Treatment of neurolept-induced tardive dyskinesia. *Neuropsychiatr Dis Treat.* 2013;**9**:1371–1380.

27. Cloud LJ, Zutshi D, Factor S. Tardive dyskinesia: Therapeutic options for an increasingly common disorder. *Neurotherapeutics.* 2014;**11**:166–176.

28. Woods SW, Saksa JR, Baker CB, Chen SJ, Tek C. Effects of levetiracetam on tardive dyskinesia: a randomized, double-blind, placebo controlled study. *J Clin Psychiatry.* 2008: **69**(4):546–554.

29. Libov I, Miodownik C, Bersudsky Y, Dwolatzky T, Lerner V. Efficacy of piracetam in the treatment of tardive dyskinesia in schizophrenic patients: A randomized, double-blind, placebo-controlled crossover study. *J Clin Psychiatry.* 2007;**68**(7):1031–1037.

30. Iwata, Y, Irie, S, Ulchida, H, Suzuki T, Watanabe K, Iwashita S, Mimura M. Effects of zonisamide on tardive dyskinesia: A preliminary open-label trial. *J Neurol Sci.* 2012;**315**:137–140.

31. Schrodt GR, Wright JH, Simpson R, Moore DP, Chase S. Treatment of tardive dyskinesia with propranolol. *J Clin Psychiatry.* 1982;**43**(8):328–331.

32. Wilbur R, Kulik F. Propranolol (inderal) for tardive dyskinesia and extrapyramidal side effects from neuroleptics: Possible involvement of beat – adrenergic mechanisms. *Prog Neuropsychopharmacol.* 1981;**4**(6):627–632.

33. Perenyi A, Farkas A. Propranolol in the treatment of tardive dyskinesia. *Biol Psychiatry.* 1983;**18**:391–394.

34. Factor SA. Propranolol therapy for tardive dyskinesia revisited. *Mov Dis.* 2012;**27**(13):1703.

35. Cowen MA, Green M, Bertollo DN, Abbott K. A treatment for tardive dyskinesia and some other extrapyramidal symptoms. *J Clin Psychopharmacol.* 1997;**17**(3):190–193.

36. Bhidayasiri R, Fahn S, Weiner WJ, Gronseth GS, Sullivan K, Zesiewicz T. Evidence-based guideline: Treatment of tardive syndromes. Report of the guideline development subcommittee of the American Academy of Neurology. *Neurology.* 2013;**81**:463–469.

37. Suddath RL, Straw GM, Freed WJ, Bigelow LLB, Kirch D, Wyatt RJ. A clinical trial of nifedipine in schizophrenia and tardive dyskinesia. *Pharmacol Biochem Behav.* 1991;**39**:743–745.

38. Pham DQ, Plakogiannis R. Vitamin E supplementation in Alzheimer's disease, Parkinson's disease, tardive dyskinesia, and cataract: Part 2. *Ann Pharmacother* 2005;**39**:2066–2068.

39. Zhang WF,Tan YL, Zhang XY, Chan RC, Wu HR, Zhou DF. Extract of ginkgo biloba treatment for tardive dyskinesia in schizophrenia a randomized, double blind, placebo-controlled trial. *J Clin Psychiatry.* 2011;**72**(5):615–621.

40. Adler LA, Rotrosen J, Edson R, et al. Vitamin E treatment for tardive dyskinesia. Veterans Affairs Cooperative Study #394 Study Group. *Arch Gen Psychiatry.* 1999;**56**:836–841.

41. Lam LC, Chiu HF, Hung SF. Vitamin E in the treatment of tardive dyskinesia: a replication study. *J Nerv Ment Dis.* 1994;**182**:113–114.

42. Shriqui CL, Bradwejn J, Annable L, Jones BD. Vitamin E in the treatment of tardive dyskinesia: A double-blind placebo-controlled study. *Am J Psychiatry*. 1992;**149**:391–393.

43. Schmidt M, Meister P, Baumann P. Treatment of tardive dyskinesia with vitamin E. *Eur Psychiatry*. 1991;**6**:201–207.

44. Nelson LA, McGuire JM, Hausafus SN. Melatonin for the treatment of tardive dyskinesia. *Ann Pharmacother* 2003;**37**:1128–1131.

45. Shamir E, Barak Y, Plopsky I, Zisapel N, Elizur A, Weizman A. Is melatonin effective for tardive dyskinesia? *J Clin Psychiatry*. 2000;**61**:556–558.

46. Shamir E, Barak Y, Shalman I, et al. Melatonin treatment for tardive dyskinesia: A double-blind, placebo-controlled, crossover study. *Arch Gen Psychiatry*. 2001;**58**:1049–1052.

47. Richardson MA, Small AM, Read LL, Chao HM, Clelland JD. Branched chain amino acid treatment of tardive dyskinesia in children and adolescents. *J Clin Psychiatry* 2004;**65**(1):92–96.

48. Richardson MA, Bevans ML, Read LL, et al. Efficacy of the branch chain amino acids in the treatment of tardive dyskinesia in men. *Am J Psychiatry*. 2003;**160**(6):1117–1124.

49. Lerner V, Miodownik C, Kaptsan A, Cohen H, Matar M, Lowenthal U, Kolter M. Vitamin B6 in the treatment of tardive dyskinesia: A double blind placebo-controlled crossover study. *Am J Psychiatry* 2001;**158**:1511–1514.

50. Lerner V, Miodownik C, Kaptsan A, et al. Vitamin B6 treatment for tardive dyskinesia: a randomized, double-blind, placebo-controlled, crossover study. *J Clin Psychiatry*. 2007;**68**(11):1648–1654.

51. Grohmann R, Koch R, Schmidtd LG. Extrapyramidal symptoms in neuroleptic recipients. *Agents Actions Suppl.* 1990;**29**:71–82.

52. Ross RT. Drug-induced parkinsonism and other movement disorders. *Can J Neurol Sci.* 1990 May;**17**(2):155–162.

53. Cookson JC. Side effects during long-term treatment with depot anti-psychotics *Clin Neuropharm.* 1991;**14**(S2):S24-S30.

54. Lauterbach EC. Haloperidol-induced dystonia and parkinsonism in discontinuing metoclopramide: implications for differential thalamocortical activity. *J Clin Psychopharmacol.* 1992;**12**(6):442–443.

55. Chouinard G. Effects of risperidone in tardive dyskinesia: An analysis of the Canadian multicenter risperidone study. *J Clin Psychopharmacol.* 1995;**15**: (Suppl 1):36S-44S.

56. Bai YM, Yu SC, Lin CC. Risperidone for severe tardive dyskinesia: A 12-week randomized, double-blind, placebo-controlled study. *J Clin Psychiatry.* 2003;**64**:1342–1348.

57. Chan HY, Chiang SC, Chang CJ, et al. A randomized controlled trial of risperidone and olanzapine for schizophrenic patients with neuroleptic-induced tardive dyskinesia. *J Clin Psychiatry.* 2010;**71**:1226–1233.

58. Dalack GW, Becks L, Meador-Woodruff JH. Tardive dyskinesia, clozapine and treatment response. *Prog Neuropsychopharmacol Biol Psychiatry.* 1998;**22**(4):567–573.

59. Simpson GM, Lee JH, Shrivastava RK. Clozapine in tardive dyskinesia. *Psychopharmacology.* 1978;**56**:75–80.

60. Littrel K, Magill AM. The effect of clozapine on preexisting tardive dyskinesia. *J Psychosoc Nurs Ment Health Serv.* 1993;**31**(9):14–18.

61. Bassitt DP, Louza Neto MR. Clozapine efficacy in tardive dyskinesia in schizophrenic patients. *Eur Arch Psychiatry Clin Neurosci* 1998;**248**:209–211.

62. Gerlach J, Koppelhus P, Helweg E, Monrad A. Clozapine and haloperidol in a single-blind cross-over trial: Therapeutic and biochemical aspects in the treatment of schizophrenia. *Acta Psychiatr Scand.* 1974;**50**:410–424.

63. Kinon BJ, Jeste DV, Kollack-Walker S, Stauffer V, Liu-Seifert H. Olanzapine treatment for tardive dyskinesia in schizophrenia patients: a prospective clinical trial with patients randomized to blinded dose reduction periods. *Prog Neuropsychopharmacol Biol Psychiatry* 2004;**28**:985–996.

64. Na-Ri K, Moon-Doo K. Tardive dyskinesia: Treatment with aripiprazole. *Clin Psychopharmacol Neurosci.* 2011;**9**(1):1–8.

65. Tammenmaa IA, Sailas E, McGrath JJ, Soares-Weiser K, Wahlbeck K. Systematic review of cholinergic drugs for neuroleptic-induced tardive dyskinesia: a meta-analysis of randomized controlled trials. *Prog Neuropsychopharmacol Biol Psychiatry.* 2004;**28**:1099–1107.

66. Caroff SN, Campbell EC, Havey JC, SullivanKA, Katz IR, Mann SC. Treatment of tardive dyskinesia with donepezil. *J Clin Psychiatry.* 2001;**62**(2):128–129.

67. Kazamatsuri H, Chien CP, Cole JO. Treatment of tardive dyskinesia: clinical efficacy of a dopamine-depleting agent, tetrabanzine. *Arch Gen Psychiatry.* 1972;**27**:95–99.

68. Ondo WG, Hanna PA, Jankovic J. Tetrabenzine treatment for tardive dyskinesia: Assessment by randomized videotape protocol. *Am J Psychiatry.* 1999;**156**(8):1279–1281.

69. Guay DR. Tetrabenzaine, a monoamine-depleting drug used in the treatment of hyperkinetic movement disorders. *Am J Geriatr Pharmacother.* 2010;**8**(4):331–373.

70. Chen JJ, Ondo WG, Dashtipour K, Swope, DM. Tetrabenazine for the treatment of hyperkinetic movement disorders: a review of the literature. *Clin Ther.* 2012;**34**(7):1487–1504.

71. Huang CC, Wang RIH, Hasegawa A, et al. Reserpine and alpha-methyldopa in the treatment of tardive dyskinesia. *Psychopharmacology.* 1981;**73**:359–362.

72. Goff DC, Renshaw PF, Sarid-Segal O, Dreyfuss DA, Amico ET, Ciraulo DA. A placebo-controlled trial of selegiline (L-deprenyl) in the treatment of tardive dyskinesia. *Biol Psychiatry.* 1993;**33**(10):700–706.

73. Lieberman JA, Alvir J, Mukherjee S, Kane JM. Treatment of tardive dyskinesia with bromocriptine. A test of the receptor modification strategy. *Arch Gen Psychiatry.* 1989;**46**(10):908–913.

74. Stewart RM, Rollins J, Beckham B, Roffman M. Baclofen in tardive dyskinesia patients maintained on neuroleptics. *Clin Neuropharmacol* 1982;**5**:365–373.

75. Gerlach J, Rye T, Kristjansen P. Effect of baclofen on tardive dyskinesia. *Psychopharmacology (Berl).* 1978;**56**:145–151.

76. Glazer WM, Moore DC, Bowers MB, Bunney BS, Roffman M. The treatment of tardive dyskinesia with baclofen. *Psychopharmacology (Berl).* 1985;**87**:480–483.

77. Thaker GK, Nguyen JA, Strauss ME, Jacobson R, Kaup BA, Tamminga CA. Clonazepam treatment of tardive dyskinesia: A practical GABA mimetic strategy. *Am J Psychiatry.* 1990;**147**(7):445–451.

78. Yung C. Case vignettes of movement disorders. *Brain Res Bull.* 1983;**11**:191–194.

79. Angus S, Sugars J, Boltezar R, Koskewich S, Schneider N. A Controlled trial of amantadine hydrochloride and neuroleptics in the treatment of tardive dyskinesia. *J Clin Psychopharmacol.* 1997;**17**(2):88–91.

80. Pappa S, Tsouli S, Apostolou G, et al. Effects of amantadine on tardive dyskinesia: a randomized, double-blind, placebo-controlled study. *Clin Neuropharmacol.* 2010;**33**(6):271–275.

81. Tschopp L, Salazar Z, Micheli F. Botulinum toxin in painful tardive dyskinesia. *Clin Neuropharmacol.* 2009;**32**(3):165–166.

82. Slotema CW, van Harten PN, Bruggeman R, et al. Botulinum toxin in the treatment of orofacial tardive dyskinesia: a single blind study. *Prog Neuropsychopharmacol Biol Psychiatry.* 2008;**32**(2):507–509.

# Atypical antipsychotics and movement disorders

Rob M.A. de Bie

## Introduction

The term atypical antipsychotics alludes to the existence of a class of drugs which are supposed to be at least as effective as the old, typical antipsychotics for antipsychotic effect but are less likely to cause severe side effects, especially fewer extrapyramidal symptoms (EPS), including tardive dyskinesia.(1–3) Atypical antipsychotics are also referred to as second-generation antipsychotics.

The term atypical antipsychotic met widespread acceptance in the 1990s when clozapine was reintroduced in Europe and North America for the treatment of "treatment-resistant schizophrenia," that is, schizophrenia not responding to typical, first-generation antipsychotics.(4,5) Two decades earlier, clozapine had already been used as a first-line treatment for schizophrenia, but in 1975, it was withdrawn due to the occurrence of agranulocytosis. Clozapine's mode of action is different from other antipsychotics in that its clinical potency does not correlate with its ability to block dopamine D2 receptors.(4,6) Also, the lower rate of EPS matched the idea of a different mode of action.

Subsequently, the "new" and "atypical" mode of action of clozapine was attributed to several new drugs.(1,2) At the moment, the following drugs are considered "atypical" antipsychotic agents: clozapine (marketed as Clozaril), quetiapine (Seroquel), risperidone (Risperdal), olanzapine (Zyprexa), ziprasidone (Geodon), aripiprazole (Abilify), melperone (Buronil), asenapine (Saphris), blonanserin (Lonasen), iloperidone (Fanapt), lurasidone (Latuda), and sertindole (Serdolect). However, there is no universally accepted definition of "atypical" and some of these drugs are clinically indistinguishable in their movement side effects from first-generation antipsychotics.

Meltzer, Matsubara, and Lee hypothesized that the favorable clinical characteristic of clozapine, that is, the low risk for EPS, is due to the relatively stronger 5-$HT_{2A}$-receptor affinity compared with that for the dopamine D2 receptor.(7) This concept largely contributed to the development of the leading atypical antipsychotics such as risperidone, olanzapine, quetiapine, and ziprasidone.(6) Aripiprazole is different in this respect because it is a partial dopamine D2 receptor agonist (and thus a weak D2 receptor agonist) and also a 5-$HT_{2A}$-antagonist.(8) Kapur and Remington challenged this hypothesis and suggested that the factor responsible for atypical antipsychotics being atypical is "fast dissociation" from the D2 receptor, leading to transient or easily displaceable occupancy.(9) Westerink proposed moderate dopamine D2 receptor occupancy as another key feature.(10) This might be the case for clozapine and quetiapine, which have low affinities for the D2 receptor.(6,11)

When analyzing or comparing studies of movement disorders associated with atypical antipsychotics, it is important to consider several methodological issues that potentially limit conclusions. For example, the incidence and severity of movement disorders can be affected by the following: drug dose, concomitant administration of antiparkinsonian drugs, the duration of treatment and observation, the extent of prestudy washout periods and carryover effects of prior drug treatment, and the susceptibility of the patient sample (e.g., the elderly, drug-naïve or treatment refractory patient).(12) Another important factor to consider is the number of dropouts, which, in general, is large in these kinds of studies.(13)

When assessing the effect of atypical antipsychotics in comparison with typical agents, it is important to consider studies using low- as well as high-potency drugs as comparators, because side effects of first-generation antipsychotics typically vary with the potency of the agent. Whether a drug is classified as high or low-potency is determined by its relative antipsychotic effectiveness compared to "chlorpromazine."(14,15) Examples of high-potency drugs are fluphenazine and haloperidol. High-potency antipsychotics are associated with more frequent EPS and less histaminic effects (e.g., sedation), alpha-adrenergic effects (e.g., orthostatic hypotension), and anticholinergic effects.(16) In contrast, low-potency agents have fewer EPS, a high risk of sedation, a high risk of orthostatic hypotension and tachycardia, and a high risk of anticholinergic and antiadrenergic effects.(16)

Early randomized trials suggested that atypical antipsychotics are superior to first-generation antipsychotics in the treatment of schizophrenia.(17–20) More recent studies, however, largely conducted by independent investigators, have found less substantial differences in EPS between these two classes of drugs.(21,22) The differences between the earlier studies and more recent studies may be related to the earlier studies commonly utilizing the high-potency haloperidol, often at higher doses, as the comparator.(22,23) For example, in clinical trials risperidone resulted in a significantly lower incidence of acute EPS, greater reductions in EPS rating scores, fewer dropouts, and less frequent use of anticholinergic drugs compared with haloperidol.(24–27) In a small study of first-episode schizophrenics, risperidone-treated patients experienced one-fourth the incidence of parkinsonism and concurrent anticholinergic use compared with patients receiving typical antipsychotics.(28) However, postmarketing studies and closer inspection of trial data show that the occurrence of EPS is dose dependent. Advantages of risperidone disappear if doses above 6 mg per day are used or if lower doses of haloperidol or less potent drugs are used in comparison.(22,29) The CATIE trial found no differences in EPS between typical and atypical antipsychotics.(21)

Over time, it has become clear that the atypical antipsychotics are not a homogeneous class and differ in many properties. With the exception of clozapine, olanzapine, and risperidone, atypical antipsychotics are not better than low-potency first-generation antipsychotic drugs.(30) Nevertheless, the distinguishing features that are attributed to clozapine seem to withstand the current debate about whether atypical antipsychotic drugs are better than first-generation antipsychotics.

# Atypical antipsychotics and tardive syndromes

In concordance with the above, the risk for late or tardive dyskinesias appears to be lower with atypical antipsychotics than with the older antipsychotics. However, risks of tardive syndromes with atypical antipsychotics have been reduced much less than expected.(31) In a review of 12 trials involving 28,051 patients (followed for 463,925 person-years) the annualized tardive dyskinesia incidence was 3.9% for atypical antipsychotics and 5.5% for typical antipsychotics.(32) Stratified by age, annual tardive dyskinesia incidence rates were 3.0% with atypical antipsychotics versus 7.7% with typical antipsychotics in adults, and 5.2% for both atypical and typical antipsychotics in the elderly (based almost exclusively on one retrospective cohort study). A cautious interpretation of these results is warranted because the review was based on a mix of controlled and uncontrolled studies and blinded and open-label studies, as well as historical and limited direct comparisons with typical antipsychotics (the latter unfortunately exclusively with medium to high doses of haloperidol).(32,33)

Optimistic expectations for the efficacy and neurological safety of atypical antipsychotics have encouraged their wide use in many conditions, sometimes off-label or in combinations, increasing the chance of a higher prevalence of tardive syndromes, especially in older ages.(31) The risk for tardive syndromes is low with clozapine.(34) Data are insufficient to support or refute use of atypical antipsychotics to improve tardive syndromes.(35)

# Atypical antipsychotics and neuroleptic malignant syndrome

Although neuroleptic malignant syndrome (NMS) is historically associated with the typical antipsychotic drugs, it is also a potential adverse effect of atypical antipsychotics. Troller et al. reviewed published cases of NMS with the following atypical antipsychotics: clozapine, quetiapine, risperidone, olanzapine, ziprasidone, and aripiprazole.(36) The majority of cases of NMS induced by atypical antipsychotics present with the typical NMS features. There appears to be one major exception, clozapine-induced NMS is significantly less likely than NMS induced by risperidone, olanzapine, and typical antipsychotics to manifest with rigidity.(36) Incidence estimates for NMS vary widely, and it remains uncertain whether atypical drugs are less likely to cause NMS than the typical antipsychotics. Caroff and Mann have estimated the incidence of NMS with typical antipsychotics to be approximately 0.2%.(37) This low incidence makes it unlikely that comparative studies will be adequately powered to detect real differences in the incidence of NMS induced by atypical versus typical antipsychotics.

## Clozapine

Clozapine is a dibenzodiazepine derivate that was developed in the 1950s. Its clinical use had been delayed because of an associated risk of agranulocytosis.(12) Following the publication by Kane et al. in 1988 of a multicenter clinical trial that assessed clozapine's efficacy compared to chlorpromazine in the treatment of patients who were refractory to typical neuroleptics, clozapine received renewed attention.(38) In this study, 30% of the clozapine-treated patients were categorized as responders compared with 4% of chlorpromazine-treated patients. The authors also found a reduction of EPS, which was significantly greater in the clozapine group compared to the patients receiving chlorpromazine combined with benztropine mesylate.(38) Although not a study of new onset or actual incidence of EPS, this report supported a more favorable reduction in the prevalence of preexisting EPS with clozapine.(12)

## Extrapyramidal symptoms

In a Cochrane review of randomized controlled trials (RCT) comparing clozapine with typical antipsychotics for schizophrenia, the risk ratio for the development of motor adverse effects with clozapine was 0.57 (95%CI 0.50 to 0.65) when compared to typical antipsychotics.(39) For children and adolescents this ratio was 0.77 (95%CI 0.67 to 0.90) and for the elderly 0.75 (95%CI 0.22 to 2.60). The study included 52 trials (4,746 participants). Forty-four of the included studies were less than 13 weeks in duration, and, overall, trials were at a significant risk of bias.(39) In a Cochrane review of clozapine versus the other atypical antipsychotics, clozapine tended to cause less EPS than the other atypical antipsychotics, but this was only significant compared to risperidone for parkinsonism with a risk ratio of 0.39 (95%CI 0.22 to 0.68) and to zotepine with a risk ratio of 0.05 (95%CI 0.00 to 0.86).(40)

## Parkinson's disease

A very common nonmotor symptom of Parkinson's disease is visual hallucinations, with prevalence rates ranging from 22%–38% and a lifetime prevalence of up to 70%.(41) Less common, but more troubling, are delusions, which are usually paranoid in nature, and affect about 5% of drug-treated PD patients. Unfortunately, all of the drugs available for treating motor symptoms in Parkinson's disease worsen the psychotic symptoms. Levodopa, which is the most potent and least expensive antiparkinson drug, is least likely to contribute to the hallucinations.(41)

When visual hallucinations become troublesome—due to loss of insight—antipsychotic drugs are prescribed. In spite of the established effectiveness of clozapine, proven by two multicenter, double blind, placebo controlled studies for the treatment of Parkinson's disease psychosis, several drawbacks limit the earlier use when hallucinations are still minor.

In the 4-week double blind RCT, conducted by the Parkinson Study Group, 60 patients with Parkinson's disease and psychosis were randomized to low doses of clozapine or placebo.(42) The patients in the clozapine group had significantly more improvement than those in the placebo group on all three of the measures used to determine the severity of psychosis. Clozapine treatment had no deleterious effect on the severity of parkinsonism and even improved tremor. In a subsequent 12-week, open-label extension of the study there was an unexpectedly high death rate.(43) The authors state that the death of six patients was a result of the nature of the advanced disease and not of clozapine. In 2004, Pollak et al. conducted a 4-week, double blind RCT of clozapine and placebo, followed by a 12-week clozapine open phase.(44) This was then followed by a 1-month washout period. At the end of the 12-week open period, 25 of the initial 55 patients had completely recovered from delusions and hallucinations and of these, 19 experienced a relapse within 1 month of the clozapine washout period.

Cumbersome monitoring, consisting of frequent white blood cell counts, is required when using clozapine because of the 1%–5% incidence of agranulocytosis in the elderly.(40,45–47) This hematological problem is not dose related and therefore frequent monitoring needs to be done, even with doses as low as 6.25 mg per day (N.B.—usually clozapine doses in schizophrenia are 300–900 mg per day). Weight gain and the metabolic syndrome are not a problem in Parkinson's disease patients, probably because of the low doses.(40,44) Other side effects such as sedation and orthostatic hypotension are frequently observed and may be a dose-limiting factor. The sedating effect of clozapine may be used in an advantageous way because many psychotic patients with Parkinson's disease are awake at night when their symptoms worsen. As a result, clozapine is typically administered at bedtime. This is sometimes supplemented with a lower dose in the morning. A normal starting dose is 6.25 mg at bedtime, which then may be increased every one to two weeks with 6.25 mg or 12.5 mg per day. On average, doses are between 12.5 mg and 50 mg per day.

## Quetiapine

Quetiapine, a dibenzothiazepine compound, was developed specifically to have a profile similar to clozapine with respect to EPS, but without the risk of hematological problems. Like clozapine, it has a greater affinity for $5\text{-HT}_{2A}$ than dopamine D2 receptors.(6,12)

## Extrapyramidal symptoms

In patients with schizophrenia, quetiapine causes fewer EPS compared with typical antipsychotics (risk ratio 0.17; 95%CI 0.09 to 0.32), including less akathisia, parkinsonism, dystonia, and tremor.(48) When compared to clozapine, there is no difference regarding the frequency of akathisia, rigidity, tremor, or use of antiparkinson medication.(49) In comparison to olanzapine, fewer patients on quetiapine need to take antiparkinson medication at least once (risk ratio 0.51, 95%CI 0.32 to 0.81), but apart from this, there are no significant differences in EPS. Quetiapine produces fewer EPS than risperidone when assessed with the Simpson-Angus Scale. There are no significant differences regarding dyskinesia and akathisia. When compared to ziprasidone, significantly fewer people in the quetiapine group use antiparkinson medication at least once. The frequency of akathisia or "any EPS" are the same. Studies comparing quetiapine with aripiprazole do not show a difference regarding frequency of EPS, but there are only a few studies, and those comprise small sample sizes.(49)

## Parkinson's disease

The first successful report on quetiapine use in parkinsonian patients was published in 1996.(50) More open studies of patients with Parkinson's disease

followed and these suggested an advantage of quetiapine in this population; that is, improvement in psychosis was seen in more than 80% of patients, and motor worsening in only 13%.(51,52) Consistently reported side effects of quetiapine include sedation and hypotension.(53)

In 2005, Ondo et al. published the results of a double blind RCT of quetiapine for hallucinations in Parkinson's disease.(54) Follow-up was 12 weeks. Among the 31 patients originally included in the trial, there were six dropouts. Compared to placebo, none of the hallucinations, psychosis, or motor impairment assessments changed significantly on quetiapine. Rabey et al. conducted a double blind 12-week RCT investigating a total of 58 Parkinson's disease patients of whom 29 were demented.(55) The study was characterized by a high dropout rate of 45% (n = 26) primarily due to lack of efficacy. Compared to placebo no outcome variable changed significantly with quetiapine. This was also true when considering only the demented or the nondemented patients. Shotbolt et al. published the results of their RCT of quetiapine in 24 subjects in 2009.(56) Thirteen patients completed 6 weeks of the study and eight completed the 12-week double blind phase. There was no significant difference in time-to-dropout between patients receiving quetiapine or placebo. No significant changes were found for any of the endpoints in either group. Fernandez et al. (2009) conducted a 1-month double blind RCT of quetiapine for the treatment of visual hallucinations, using changes in REM sleep architecture (assessed with polysomnography) as the primary endpoint.(57) Eleven of the 16 patients randomized completed the study. There was no statistically significant difference in change of REM sleep duration in either arm.

Two studies compared quetiapine with clozapine for the treatment of psychosis in patients with Parkinson's disease. Morgante et al. (2004) conducted a 12-week rater-blinded RCT to compare quetiapine and clozapine in 20 patients.(58) No significant differences were found in the psychosis and motor scores between the two groups. In 2006, Merims et al. published the results of a 22-week RCT.(59) Only seven of the 14 patients randomized to receive clozapine and nine of the 13 randomized to quetiapine completed the study. Compared to baseline, clozapine, but not quetiapine, significantly improved the frequency scores of the categories "hallucinations" and "delusions" of the neuropsychiatric inventory (NPI). The severity scores of hallucinations and delusions in either group did not change significantly. There was no worsening in parkinsonian symptoms.

For some time, quetiapine had been the treatment of first choice for Parkinson's disease psychosis because of ease of use, lack of compulsory blood monitoring, and consistently encouraging results in open-label studies.(51) But because of the not so positive efficacy data in recent RCTs and several methodological concerns of these studies (e.g., small sample size, low quality rating), there is insufficient evidence to strongly support the use of quetiapine for the treatment of psychosis in Parkinson's disease. Importantly, there are no new safety concerns identified in the new studies.(53)

For psychosis in Parkinson's disease, quetiapine can be started at, for example, 12.5 mg per day (bedtime) and then increased with, for example, 25 mg per day each week until it causes either symptomatic effects or adverse effects. In general, dosages range from 25 to 200 mg per day.

## Risperidone

Risperidone, a benzisoxazole, was introduced in 1994. As with the other "atypicals" it was initially hoped that risperidone would have the same favorable EPS profile as clozapine. And although risperidone is an effective and widely used antipsychotic agent, it has not lived up to the expectation that it would provide an alternative to clozapine.

## Extrapyramidal symptoms

Initial studies with risperidone for schizophrenia were quite promising, with lower rates of EPS, decreased dropout rates, and a reduction in the concomitant use of anticholinergics compared with haloperidol treatment.(26,27,60–64) These benefits were soon found to be highly dose dependent; that is, the advantages of risperidone were greatly diminished at doses greater than 6 mg per day.(26,27,60–64) This dose dependency was also seen in drug-naïve patients, and not only with respect to the occurrence of EPS, but also regarding the use of anticholinergic medications. When lower doses of haloperidol or low-potency typical antipsychotics were compared to risperidone, the EPS liability of risperidone was similar.(26,27,60–65)

There are not enough data available to allow for a reliable comparison of risperidone and clozapine regarding EPS.(66) When risperidone is compared to olanzapine, those taking olanzapine have slightly fewer EPS in the medium term (risk ratio 1.67, 95%CI 1.14 to 2.46), have fewer new episodes of parkinsonism (risk ratio 1.73, 95%CI 1.07 to 2.81), and need less antiparkinsonian medication (risk ratio 1.67, 95%CI 1.15 to 2.41).(66) In comparison to amisulpride, there are no significant differences with risperidone in terms of either the number of patients who reported EPS or received antiparkinsonian medication.(66)

## Parkinson's disease

Risperidone reduces hallucinations and psychosis in Parkinson's disease. However, several open-label series have demonstrated consistently that the drug worsens motor features of Parkinson's disease.(67,68) One double blind RCT compared clozapine and risperidone in 10 patients with Parkinson's disease.(69) The study demonstrated similar efficacy in both treatment groups for psychiatric symptoms, but there was nonsignificant worsening of motor symptoms in the risperidone treatment group compared to improvement of motor symptoms in the clozapine group. In conclusion, risperidone is not useful for the treatment of psychosis in Parkinson's disease.

## Olanzapine

Olanzapine, a thienobenzodiazepine derivative, is the next atypical antipsychotic agent introduced after risperidone. Patients with schizophrenia taking olanzapine experience fewer EPS than those given typical antipsychotics.[70] Olanzapine may be associated with slightly more extrapyramidal side effects than quetiapine, but less than risperidone and ziprasidone.(71)

## Parkinson's disease

In 2002, Breier et al. reported two double blind, placebo controlled RCTs that examined the efficacy of low-dose olanzapine for psychosis in patients with Parkinson's disease.(72) Both studies, one in the United States (n = 83) and the other in Europe (n = 77), were reported in one publication. Although no significant treatment group differences regarding psychosis were observed, motor function worsened significantly in patients on olanzapine compared to placebo in both trials. In the U.S. study, patients in the olanzapine group showed significantly higher rates of EPS (olanzapine, 24.4%; placebo, 2.4%; P = .003), hallucinations (olanzapine,

24.4%; placebo, 4.8%; P = .013), and increased salivation (olanzapine, 22.0%; placebo, 4.8%; P = .026).(72)

In the same year, Ondo et al. published a smaller double blind, placebo controlled RCT.(73) Thirty patients with Parkinson's disease and hallucinations underwent nine weeks of treatment with olanzapine or placebo (2:1 ratio). This study also failed to detect significant differences between olanzapine and placebo in any of the psychosis measures. Again, there was significant worsening of motor symptoms in the olanzapine group, mainly through the worsening of gait and bradykinesia.

In conclusion, olanzapine is not useful for the treatment of psychosis in Parkinson's disease.

## Ziprasidone

Ziprasidone, a benzothiazolylpiperazine derivative, was introduced in the United States in 2001. In schizophrenia, the antipsychotic effect of ziprasidone is equal to that of haloperidol, but with less EPS.(74) It also, however, causes more nausea and vomiting than the typical drugs, and, at present, there is no data suggesting that it is very different from other atypical compounds.(74) Ziprasidone produces slightly more EPS than olanzapine, but less EPS than risperidone.(75)

## Parkinson's disease

Schindehütte and Trenkwalder report on four patients with Parkinson's disease and psychosis who received treatment with ziprasidone after clozapine and quetiapine had failed.(76) Three patients showed a significant improvement of psychosis, without deterioration of motor function. In one case, ziprasidone considerably increased decline in off-periods. Two patients developed pathological laughing as a possible side effect of ziprasidone.(76) Pinter et al. compared ziprasidone with clozapine in a 4-week, single blind, open-label, RCT.(77) Fourteen of the 16 recruited patients completed the study, eight patients on clozapine and six patients on ziprasidone. Throughout the study, there were no statistical differences between both groups regarding motor symptoms. Psychotic symptoms were reduced in both groups but with more intensity in the ziprasidone group than in the clozapine group.(77) All in all, because data are limited, reliable advice regarding the usefulness of ziprasidone for the treatment of psychosis in Parkinson's disease cannot be given.

## Aripiprazole

Aripiprazole is a relatively new antipsychotic drug. In schizophrenia, aripiprazole differs little from typical antipsychotic drugs with respect to the antipsychotic effects, but it is associated with fewer EPS, particularly akathisia.(78) When compared with clozapine and with quetiapine, the occurrence of EPS is not different. Risperidone is more likely to give EPS than aripiprazole.(79)

## Parkinson's disease

Friedman et al. conducted an open-label flexible-dose pilot study to evaluate the safety and tolerability of aripiprazole in patients with Parkinson's disease and psychosis.(80) Although some patients had a favorable response, aripiprazole was associated with an exacerbation of motor symptoms. The authors concluded that aripiprazole did not appear promising for psychosis in Parkinson's disease.(80)

## Melperone

The results of an open-label study suggested that melperone could be very helpful for Parkinson's disease psychosis without having a deleterious effect on motor function.(81) One double blind RCT assessed the efficacy of melperone for the treatment of psychosis in Parkinson's disease.(82) There were four arms in the study: placebo, 20 mg, 40 mg, and 60 mg, given daily. Ninety subjects were randomized (30 placebo and 20 in each active arm). Seventy-five subjects completed the 8-week study. The main outcome variable for psychosis showed no significant benefit at any dose. The main safety outcome variable was the UPDRS motor score, which showed no differences in outcome. In conclusion, melperone is not effective for the treatment of Parkinson's disease psychosis, but joins clozapine and quetiapine as the only antipsychotics that do not worsen motor function in people with Parkinson's disease.(82)

## Asenapine, blonanserin, iloperidone, lurasidone, and sertindole

Recently, the US Food and Drug Administration approved iloperidone (2009), asenapine (2009), and lurasidone (2010). Sertindole and blonanserin are approved and used outside the United States for treatment of schizophrenia. Sertindole, after being voluntarily suspended by the manufacturer in 1998 because of the potential risk of cardiovascular-related death, was relaunched in Europe in 2005. Due to the recent introduction of these compounds, limited evidence comparing these antipsychotics exists, and all the pivotal RCTs were sponsored by the industry. Thus, further well-controlled, adequately powered, head-to-head clinical trials are required in the nearest future.(83)

## Conclusions

Currently, the concept of atypical antipsychotics as a class of drugs which are equally effective when compared to the typical antipsychotics, considering the antipsychotic effect, but are less likely to cause EPS has led to debate about its validity. Over time, it has become clear that the atypical antipsychotics are not a homogeneous class and differ in many properties. Nevertheless, based on the studies reviewed above, the risk of EPS is best represented as risperidone>ziprasidone>olanzapine>quetiapine>clozapine. There are not enough data available to reliably determine the order of the other atypical antipsychotics in this list.

The risks of tardive syndromes with the atypical antipsychotics have been reduced, but much less than expected (annualized tardive dyskinesia incidence of 3.9% for atypical antipsychotics and 5.5% for typical antipsychotics).

For patients with Parkinson's disease and when visual hallucinations become troublesome—due to loss of insight—antipsychotic drugs are prescribed. The preferred antipsychotic is clozapine in a low dose. The use of clozapine for the treatment of Parkinson's disease psychosis is supported by the results of two multicenter, double blind, placebo controlled studies. There is insufficient evidence to strongly support the use of quetiapine for the treatment of psychosis in Parkinson's disease, because of the not so positive efficacy data in recent RCTs and several methodological concerns of these studies. The other atypical antipsychotics are not useful for the treatment of psychosis in Parkinson's disease because the antipsychotic effect is not clear (i.e., olanzapine, melperone), motor features worsen (i.e., risperidone, olanzapine, aripiprazole), or data are limited (e.g., ziprasidone).

## References

1. Leucht S, Pitschel-Walz G, Abraham D, Kissling W. Efficacy and extrapyramidal side-effects of the new antipsychotics olanzapine, quetiapine, risperidone, and sertindole compared to conventional antipsychotics and placebo. A meta-analysis of randomized controlled trials. *Schizophr Res.* 1999; **35**: 51–68.

2. Geddes J, Freemantle N, Harrison P, Bebbington P. Atypical antipsychotics in the treatment of schizophrenia: systematic overview and meta-regression analysis. *BMJ.* 2000; **321**: 1371–6.

3. Glazer WM. Extrapyramidal side effects, tardive dyskinesia, and the concept of atypicality. *J Clin Psychiatry.* 2000; **61** (Suppl 3): 16–21.

4. Hippius H. The history of clozapine. *Psychopharmacology.* 1989; **99**: S3-S5.

5. Meltzer H. Introduction. *Psychopharmacology.* 1989; **99**: S1-S2.

6. Meltzer HY. What's atypical about atypical antipsychotic drugs? *Curr Opin Pharmacol.* 2004; **4**: 53–7.

7. Meltzer HY, Matsubara S, Lee J-C. Classification of typical and atypical antipsychotic drugs on the basis of dopamine D-1, D-2 and serotonin2 pKi values. *J Pharmacol Exp Ther.* 1989; **251**: 238–46.

8. Burris KD, Molski TF, Xu C, Ryan E, Tottori K, Kikuchi T, Yocca FD, Molinoff PB. Aripiprazole, a novel antipsychotic, is a high affinity partial agonist at human dopamine D2 receptors. *J Pharmacol Exp Ther.* 2002; **302**: 381–9.

9. Kapur S, Remington G. Dopamine D(2) receptors and their role in atypical antipsychotic action: still necessary and may even be sufficient. *Biol Psychiatry.* 2001; **50**: 873–83.

10. Westerink BHC. Can antipsychotic drugs be classified by their effects on a particular group of dopamine neurons in the brain? *Eur J Pharmacol.* 2002; **455**: 1–18.

11. Kapur S, Zipursky RB, Remington G. Clinical and theoretical implications of 5-HT2 and D2 receptor occupancy of clozapine, risperidone, and olanzapine in schizophrenia. *Am J Psychiatry.* 1999; **156**: 286–93.

12. Caroff SN, Mann SC, Campbell EC, Sullivan KA. Movement disorders associated with atypical antipsychotic drugs. *J Clin Psychiatry.* 2002; **63** (Suppl 4): 12–9.

13. Hutton P, Morrison AP, Yung AR, Taylor PJ, French P, Dunn G. Effects of drop-out on efficacy estimates in five Cochrane reviews of popular antipsychotics for schizophrenia. *Acta Psychiatr Scand.* 2012; **126**: 1–11.

14. Woods SW. Chlorpromazine equivalent doses for the newer atypical antipsychotics. *J Clin Psychiatry.* 2003; **64**: 663–7.

15. Rijcken CA, Monster TB, Brouwers JR, de Jong-van den Berg LT. Chlorpromazine equivalents versus defined daily doses: how to compare antipsychotic drug doses? *J Clin Psychopharmacol.* 2003; **23**: 657–9.

16. Lehman AF, Lieberman JA, Dixon LB, et al. American Psychiatric Association; Steering Committee on

Practice Guidelines. Practice guideline for the treatment of patients with schizophrenia, second edition. *Am J Psychiatry.* 2004; **161** (2 Suppl): 1–56.

17. Jeste DV, Okamoto A, Napolitano J, Kane JM, Martinez RA. Low incidence of persistent tardive dyskinesia in elderly patients with dementia treated with risperidone. *Am J Psychiatry.* 2000; **157**: 1150–5.

18. Dolder CR, Jeste DV. Incidence of tardive dyskinesia with typical versus atypical antipsychotics in very high risk patients. *Biol Psychiatry.* 2003; **53**: 1142–5.

19. Grant MJ, Baldessarini RJ. Possible improvement of neuroleptic-associated tardive dyskinesia during treatment with aripiprazole. *Ann Pharmacother.* 2005; **39**: 1953.

20. Kinon BJ, Jeste DV, Kollack-Walker S, Stauffer V, Liu-Seifert H. Olanzapine treatment for tardive dyskinesia in schizophrenia patients: a prospective clinical trial with patients randomized to blinded dose reduction periods. *Prog Neuropsychopharmacol Biol Psychiatry.* 2004; **28**: 985–96.

21. Miller DD, Caroff SN, Davis SM, et al. Extrapyramidal side-effects of antipsychotics in a randomised trial. *Brit J Psychiat.* 2008; **193**: 279–88.

22. Kane JM, McGlashan TH. Treatment of schizophrenia. *Lancet.* 1995; **346**: 820–5.

23. Hugenholtz GW, Heerdink ER, Stolker JJ, Meijer WE, Egberts AC, Nolen WA. Haloperidol dose when used as active comparator in randomized controlled trials with atypical antipsychotics in schizophrenia: comparison with officially recommended doses. *J Clin Psychiatry.* 2006; **67**: 897–903.

24. Simpson GM, Lindenmayer JP. Extrapyramidal symptoms in patients treated with risperidone. *J Clin Psychopharmacol.* 1997; **17**: 194–201.

25. Castelao JF, Ferreira L, Gelders YG, et al. The efficacy of the D2 and 5-HT2 antagonist risperidone (R64,766) in the treatment of chronic psychosis. An open dose-finding study. *Schizophr Res.* 1989; **2**: 411–5.

26. Peuskens J. Risperidone in the treatment of patients with chronic schizophrenia: a multinational, multi-centre, double-blind, parallel group study versus haloperidol. Risperidone Study Group. *Br J Psychiatry.* 1995; **166**:712–33.

27. Lemmens P, Brecher M, Van Baelen B. A combined analysis of double-blind studies with risperidone vs. placebo and other antipsychotic agents: factors associated with extra pyramidal symptoms. *Acta Psychiatr Scand.* 1999; **99**: 160–70.

28. Kopala LC, Good KP, Honer WG. Extrapyramidal signs and clinical symptoms in first-episode schizophrenia: response to low-dose risperidone. *J Psychopharmacol.* 1997; **17**: 308–13.

29. Rosebush PI, Mazurek MF. Neurologic side effects in neuroleptic-naive patients treated with haloperidol or risperidone. *Neurology.* 1999; **52**: 782–5.

30. Leucht S, Corves C, Arbter D, Engel RR, Li C, Davis JM. Second-generation versus first-generation antipsychotic drugs for schizophrenia: a meta-analysis. *Lancet.* 2009; **373**: 31–41.

31. Tarsy D, Lungu C, Baldessarini RJ. Epidemiology of tardive dyskinesia before and during the era of modern antipsychotic drugs. *Handb Clin Neurol.* 2011; **100**: 601–16.

32. Correll CU, Schenk EM. Tardive dyskinesia and new antipsychotics. *Curr Opin Psychiatry.* 2008; **21**: 151–6.

33. Correll CU, Leucht S, Kane JM, Lower risk for tardive dyskinesia associated with second-generation antipsychotics: a systematic review of 1-year studies. *Am J Psychiatry.* 2004; **161**: 414–25.

34. Ye M, Tang W, Liu L, et al. Prevalence of tardive dyskinesia in chronic male inpatients with schizophrenia on long-term clozapine versus typical antipsychotics. *Int Clin Psychopharmacol.* 2014 May 16 [Epub ahead of print].

35. Bhidayasiri R, Fahn S, Weiner WJ, et al. Evidence-based guideline: treatment of tardive syndromes: report of the Guideline Development Subcommittee of the American Academy of Neurology. *Neurology.* 2013; **81**: 463–9.

36. Trollor JN, Chen X, Sachdev PS. Neuroleptic malignant syndrome associated with atypical antipsychotic drugs. *CNS Drugs.* 2009; **23**: 477–92.

37. Caroff SN, Mann SC. Neuroleptic malignant syndrome. *Med Clin North Am.* 1993; **77**: 185–202.

38. Kane J, Honigfeld G, Singer J, Meltzer H. Clozapine for the treatment-resistant schizophrenic. A double-blind comparison with chlorpromazine. *Arch Gen Psychiatry.* 1988; **45**: 789–96.

39. Essali A, Al-Haj Haasan N, Li C, Rathbone J. Clozapine versus typical neuroleptic medication for schizophrenia (Review). *Cochrane Database Syst Rev.* 2009; **1**: CD000059.

40. Asenjo Lobos C, Komossa K, Rummel-Kluge C, Hunger H, Schmid F, Schwarz S, Leucht S. Clozapine versus other atypical antipsychotics for schizophrenia. *Cochrane Database Syst Rev.* 2010; **11**: CD006633.

41. Diederich NJ, Fénelon G, Stebbins G, Goetz CG. Hallucinations in Parkinson disease. *Nat Rev Neurol.* 2009; **5**: 331–42.

42. The Parkinson Study Group. Low-dose clozapine for the treatment of drug-induced psychosis in Parkinson's disease. *N Eng J Med.* 1999; **340**: 757–63.

43. Factor SA, Friedman JH, Lannon MC, Oakes D, Bourgeois K, and The Parkinson Study Group. Clozapine for the treatment of drug-induced psychosis

in Parkinson's disease: Results of the 12 week open label extension in the PSYCLOPS trial. *Mov Disord.* 2001; **16**: 135–9.

44. Pollak P, Tison F, Rascol O, et al. Clozapine in drug induced psychosis in Parkinson's disease: a randomised, placebo controlled study with open follow up. *J Neurol Neurosurg Psychiatry.* 2004; **75**: 689–95.

45. Alvir JMJ, Lieberman JA, Safferman AZ, Schwimmer JL, Schaaf JA. Clozapine-induced agranulocytosis: incidence and risk factors in the United States. *N Engl J Med.* 1993; **329**: 162–7.

46. Barak Y, Wittenberg N, Naor S, Kutzuk D, Weizman A. Clozapine in elderly psychiatric patients: tolerability, safety, end efficacy. *Compr Psychiatry.* 1999; **40**: 320–5.

47. Snowdon J, Halliday G. A study of the use of clozapine in old age psychiatry. *Int Clin Psychopharmacol.* 2011; **26**: 232–5.

48. Suttajit S, Srisurapanont M, Xia J, Suttajit S, Maneeton B, Maneeton N. Quetiapine versus typical antipsychotic medications for schizophrenia. *Cochrane Database Syst Rev.* 2013; **5**: CD007815.

49. Asmal L, Flegar SJ, Wang J, Rummel-Kluge C, Komossa K, Leucht S. Quetiapine versus other atypical antipsychotics for schizophrenia. *Cochrane Database Syst Rev.* 2013; **11**: CD006625.

50. Evatt ML, Jewart D, Juncos JL. 'Seroquel' treatment of psychosis in parkinsonism. *Mov Disord.* 1996; **11**: 595.

51. Friedman JH, Factor SA. Atypical antipsychotics in the treatment of drug-induced psychosis in Parkinson's disease. *Mov Disord.* 2000; **15**: 201–11.

52. Henderson MJ, Mellers JDC. Psychosis in Parkinson's disease: `between a rock and a hard place'. *Int Rev Psychiatry.* 2000; **12**: 319–34.

53. Seppi K, Weintraub D, Coelho M, et al. The Movement Disorder Society Evidence-Based Medicine Review Update: Treatments for the non-motor symptoms of Parkinson's disease. *Mov Disord.* 2011; **26** (Suppl 3): S42–80.

54. Ondo WG, Tintner R, Voung KD, Lai D, Ringholz G. Double-blind, placebo-controlled, unforced titration parallel trial of quetiapine for dopaminergic-induced hallucinations in Parkinson's disease. *Mov Disord.* 2005; **20**: 958–63.

55. Rabey JM, Prokhorov T, Miniovitz A, Dobronevsky E, Klein C. Effect of quetiapine in psychotic Parkinson's disease patients: a double-blind labeled study of 3 months' duration. *Mov Disord.* 2007; **22**: 313–8.

56. Shotbolt P, Samuel M, David A. Quetiapine in the treatment of psychosis in Parkinson's disease. *Ther Adv Neurol Disord.* 2010; **3**: 339–50.

57. Fernandez HH, Friedman JH, Jacques C, Rosenfeld M. Quetiapine for the treatment of drug-induced psychosis in Parkinson's disease. *Mov Disord.* 1999; **14**: 484–7.

58. Morgante L, Epifanio A, Spina E, et al. Quetiapine and clozapine in parkinsonian patients with dopaminergic psychosis. *Clin Neuropharmacol.* 2004; **27**: 153–6.

59. Merims D, Balas M, Peretz C, Shabtai H, Giladi N. Rater-blinded, prospective comparison: quetiapine versus clozapine for Parkinson's disease psychosis. *Clin Neuropharmacol.* 2006; **29**: 331–7.

60. Simpson GM, Lindenmayer JP. Extrapyramidal symptoms in patients treated with risperidone. *J Clin Psychopharmacol.* 1997; **17**: 194–201.

61. Castelão JF, Ferreira L, Gelders YG, Heylen SL. The efficacy of the D2 and 5-HT2 antagonist risperidone (R 64,766) in the treatment of chronic psychosis. An open dose-finding study. *Schizophr Res.* 1989; **2**: 411–5.

62. Marder SR, Meibach RC. Risperidone in the treatment of schizophrenia. *Am J Psychiatry.* 1994; **151**: 825–35.

63. Claus A, Bollen J, De Cuyper H, et al. Risperidone versus haloperidol in the treatment of chronic schizophrenic inpatients: a multicentre double-blind comparative study. *Acta Psychiatr Scand.* 1992; **85**: 295–305.

64. Min SK, Rhee CS, Kim CE, Kang DY. Risperidone versus haloperidol in the treatment of chronic schizophrenic patients: a parallel group double-blind comparative trial. *Yonsei Med J.* 1993; **34**: 179–90.

65. Hunter RH, Joy CB, Kennedy E, Gilbody SM, Song F. Risperidone versus typical antipsychotic medication for schizophrenia. *Cochrane Database Syst Rev.* 2003; **2**: CD000440.

66. Gilbody SM, Bagnall AM, Duggan L, Tuunainen A. Risperidone versus other atypical antipsychotic medication for schizophrenia. *Cochrane Database Syst Rev.* 2000; **3**: CD002306.

67. Ford B, Lynch T, Greene P. Risperidone in Parkinson's disease. *Lancet.* 1994; **344**: 681.

68. Rich SS, Friedman JH, Ott BR. Risperidone versus clozapine in the treatment of psychosis in six patients with Parkinson's disease and other akinetic-rigid syndromes. *J Clin Psychiatry.* 1995; **56**: 556–9.

69. Goetz CG, Blasucci LM, Leurgans S, Pappert EJ. Olanzapine and clozapine. Comparative effects on motor function in hallucinating PD patients. *Neurology.* 2000; **55**: 789–94.

70. Duggan L, Fenton M, Rathbone J, Dardennes R, El-Dosoky A, Indran S. Olanzapine for schizophrenia. *Cochrane Database Syst Rev.* 2005; **2**: CD001359.

71. Komossa K, Rummel-Kluge C, Hunger H, et al. Olanzapine versus other atypical antipsychotics for schizophrenia. *Cochrane Database Syst Rev.* 2010; **3**: CD006654.

72. Breier A, Sutton VK, Feldman PD, et al. Olanzapine in the treatment of dopamimetic-induced psychosis in

patients with Parkinson's disease. *Biol Psychiatry.* 2002; **52**: 438–45.

73. Ondo WG, Levy JK, Vuong KD, Hunter C, Jankovic J. Olanzapine treatment for dopaminergic induced hallucinations. *Mov. Disord.* 2002; **17**: 1031–5.

74. Bagnall A, Lewis RA, Leitner ML, Kleijnen J. Ziprasidone for schizophrenia and severe mental illness. *Cochrane Database Syst Rev.* 2000; **2**: CD001945.

75. Komossa K, Rummel-Kluge C, Hunger H, et al. Ziprasidone versus other atypical antipsychotics for schizophrenia. *Cochrane Database Syst Rev.* 2009; **4**: CD006627.

76. Schindehütte J, Trenkwalder C. Treatment of drug-induced psychosis in Parkinson's disease with ziprasidone can induce severe dose-dependent off-periods and pathological laughing. *Clin Neurol Neurosurg.* 2007; **109**: 188–91.

77. Pintor L, Valldeoriola F, Baillés E, Martí MJ, Muñiz A, Tolosa E. Ziprasidone versus clozapine in the treatment of psychotic symptoms in Parkinson disease: a randomized open clinical trial. *Clin Neuropharmacol.* 2012; **35**: 61–66.

78. Bhattacharjee J, El-Sayeh HG. Aripiprazole versus typical antipsychotic drugs for schizophrenia. *Cochrane Database Syst Rev.* 2008; **3**: CD006617.

79. Khanna P, Suo T, Komossa K, et al. Aripiprazole versus other atypical antipsychotics for schizophrenia. *Cochrane Database Syst Rev.* 2014; **1**: CD006569.

80. Friedman JH, Berman RM, Goetz CG, et al. Open-label flexible-dose pilot study to evaluate the safety and tolerability of aripiprazole in patients with psychosis associated with Parkinson's disease. *Mov Disord.* 2006; **21**: 2078–81.

81. Barbato L, Monge A, Stocchi F, Nordera G. Melperone in the treatment of iatrogenic psychosis in Parkinson's disease. *Funct Neurol.* 1996; **11**: 201–7.

82. Friedman JH. Melperone is ineffective in treating Parkinson's disease psychosis. *Mov Disord.* 2012; **27**: 803–4.

83. Wang SM, Han C, Lee SJ, Patkar AA, Masand PS, Pae CU. Asenapine, blonanserin, iloperidone, lurasidone, and sertindole: distinctive clinical characteristics of 5 novel atypical antipsychotics. *Clin Neuropharmacol.* 2013; **36**: 223–38.

# Restless legs syndrome

Roongroj Bhidayasiri and Pattamon Panyakaew

Restless legs syndrome (RLS), recently renamed Willis-Ekbom disease (WED), is a sensorimotor disorder with a primary sensory symptom of a strong, often irresistible urge to move the legs. The operational diagnostic criteria for RLS of the International RLS Study Group (IRLSSG) rely on the presence of four essential clinical features, including 1) an urge to move the legs caused by uncomfortable and unpleasant sensations; 2) the symptoms begin or worsen during rest or inactivity; 3) the symptoms are partially or totally relieved by movements; and 4) the symptoms only occur or are worse in the evening or night than during the day.(1) The symptoms are not solely accounted for as being primary to another condition, such as leg cramps or positional discomfort.(2) In addition to the essential criteria, three supportive factors have been identified: 1) a positive family history of RLS; 2) a positive response to dopaminergic drugs; and 3) periodic limb movements during wakefulness and sleep.(1) Recent epidemiologic surveys of RLS in the general population reported a prevalence of 7.2% for any form of RLS (primary or secondary) and 2.4% for primary RLS, making it the most common movement disorder and among the most common of the sleep disorders.(3, 4)

A large number of disorders have been suggested to be associated with RLS. The evidence for some is stronger than for others, which poses the important question of whether these disorders are comorbid, coincidental, or secondary causes of RLS. Indeed, many of these conditions share an association with depleted iron stores (iron deficiency and anemia), renal failure, pregnancy, rheumatoid arthritis, peripheral neuropathies, Parkinson's disease, and liver disease, while others cannot yet be explained on the basis of a single pathophysiological mechanism.(5) In

addition to the above causes, there are many reports in the literature asserting pharmacologically induced RLS. One of the earliest reports of medication-induced RLS was one of Ekbom's original descriptions of a survey of his 175 personal cases that RLS can be caused by the intake of certain drugs including promethazine and prochlorperazine.(6) Early studies also suggested that RLS can be induced by certain substances and medications, such as caffeine and beta-blockers.(7, 8) Caffeine was claimed as a cause of RLS due to its propensity to increase nervous system arousal and the direct peripheral contractile effect on the striated muscle.(8) However, it is difficult to determine the true causation of those medications in the early reports since the information on the diagnosis of RLS and the temporal associations were often incomplete.(9, 10) Following the early descriptions, there has continued to be a flow of publications that have identified a variety of medications that can induce or aggravate RLS. Some drugs used to treat RLS, especially dopaminergic medications, can also aggravate the symptoms in the form of what we now know as augmentation. However, the vast majority of the literature on medication-induced RLS are case reports and the quality of available evidence varies. In order to establish true causation for medication-induced RLS, there should be no history of RLS prior to drug initiation, secondary causes should be excluded, dosage timing close to bedtime to explain nocturnal symptoms, endorsement of all four 2003 National Institute of Health (NIH) criteria for definitive diagnosis of RLS, and a polysomnogram (PSG) should be administered to rule out sleep-disordered breathing as a cause of nocturnal disturbance that may be associated with RLS.(11) The most important evidence for etiologic determination comes from

*Medication-Induced Movement Disorders*, ed. Joseph H. Friedman. Published by Cambridge University Press.
© Cambridge University Press 2015.

trials on and off the offending medication with clinical reassessments for changes in RLS. Despite the large number of studies, very few articles applied the above criteria to determine the true causation of RLS.

Awareness of the medications that can potentially lead to RLS is crucial because it changes treatment strategies. Instead of starting another medication such as a dopamine agonist to treat iatrogenic RLS, it may be more prudent to withdraw the potentially offending medication as the first line intervention. In general, medication-induced RLS should resolve when the dosage is reduced or the drug is withdrawn. A new dose increase, or rechallenge with the same drug should be followed by symptom recurrence.

## Which medications can cause RLS? Pharmacological perspectives

A basic understanding of the possible mechanisms involved in RLS will help us understand why certain classes of medications are more likely to induce or precipitate RLS than others. Although the exact mechanism of RLS is still unknown, several lines of evidence from neuroimaging, neuropathology, CSF, and genetic linkage studies favor altered brain iron-dopamine mechanisms. This association is supported by human studies of striatal $D_2$ receptors and iron reduction, increased nigral tyrosine hydroxylase, reduced CSF ferritin, and human genome-wide association studies implicating linkages to several susceptible loci. Abnormal iron stores have been correlated with altered central neurotransmitter systems, as dopamine production requires ferritin as a cofactor for tyrosine hydroxylase, the rate-limiting enzyme in dopamine production.(12) Furthermore, recent evidence also suggests that there is a probable association of peripheral tissue hypoxia and dopaminergic neurons outside of the blood-brain barrier and RLS.(13, 14) The above evidence supports the understanding that RLS is a network disorder that involves many regions of the nervous system, from the periphery to the cortex, and contains structures that are involved in somatosensory perception as well as the generation of movement.(12)

Since the impressive efficacy of dopaminergic drugs for the treatment of RLS supports the dysfunction of the dopaminergic system in the pathophysiology of RLS, it is reasonable to assume that dopamine receptor blocking agents (DRBAs), which are primarily antipsychotics, can induce RLS. On the

other hand, the mechanism of antidepressant-induced RLS is more difficult to explain since most antidepressants process $\alpha_1$-adrenoreceptor blockade (mainly the tricyclic antidepressants), $\alpha_2$-adrenoreceptor blockade (mirtazapine), and very weak $D_2$-receptor antagonistic activity. Some antidepressants also exhibit histamine $H_1$, muscarinic, and $5\text{-}HT_{2A}$ receptor blockades. Therefore, none of these actions would be expected to provoke RLS through the dopaminergic system directly. Drugs that selectively inhibit serotonin transporters have been shown to downregulate dopaminergic and norepinephric neurons and this mechanism may be partly responsible for the development of extrapyramidal syndromes associated with the use of these medications.(15) Nevertheless, the exact mechanism in which each class of medications contributes to RLS is largely unknown and it is likely that more than one mechanism is involved which facilitates abnormal dopamine/serotonin interactions. In addition, individual susceptibility, as well as pharmacologic profiles of individual medications, needs to be considered as not all patients who are exposed to these medications will develop RLS. Detailed discussions are provided below on each class of drugs.

Among various medications that have been shown to cause RLS, two separate systematic reviews have identified similar groups of medications that have been frequently associated with RLS. The first study evaluated the evidence with the least amount of confounding by rating the quality of individual articles according to strict inclusion and exclusion criteria. It identified strong evidence for medication-induced RLS for the following drugs: escitalopram; fluoxetine; L-dopa/carbidopa and pergolide; L-thyroxine; mianserin; mirtazapine; olanzapine; and tramadol.(11) Another systematic review identified medications that induced RLS as an adverse reaction from the French pharmacovigilance database. The most reported drugs were antidepressants (amitriptyline, escitalopram, mianserin, mirtazapine, duloxetine), antipsychotics (thioridazine, loxapine, risperidone, and aripiprazole), and tramadol.(16) The common occurrence of these medications to induce RLS may give us some insights into the pathophysiological mechanism of RLS. For the purpose of the review in this chapter, we have categorized the medications that can cause RLS into five main groups: 1) antidepressants, 2) antipsychotics, 3) antiepileptic drugs, 4) opioids and opioid receptor agonists, and 5)

**Table 9.1** Medications that have been reported to induce/exacerbate restless legs syndrome (RLS)

**1) Antidepressants**

– Mirtazapine
– Mianserin
– Amitriptyline
– Fluoxetine
– Paroxetine
– Citalopram/escitalopram
– Duloxetine

**2)  Dopamine receptor blocking agents**

2.1) *Antipsychotics*

– Levomepromazine
– Haloperidol
– Pimozide
– Thioridazine
– Loxapine
– Risperidone
– Olanzapine
– Quetiapine
– Aripiprazole
– Clozapine

2.2) *Nonantipsychotics*

– Prochlorperazine
– Metoclopramide
– Clebopride

miscellaneous (Table 9.1). In this chapter, we also review the issue of augmentation, which is the progressive exacerbation of RLS earlier in the day after administration of dopaminergic medication in the afternoon or evening.(17)

# Antidepressants

Antidepressant medications constitute different classes of medications but the frequently used groups in clinical practice are tricyclic antidepressants (TCAs), selective serotonin reuptake inhibitors (SSRIs), serotonin-norepinephrine reuptake inhibitors (SNRIs), alpha 2 antagonists as serotonin and norepinephrine disinhibitors (SNDIs), and monoamine oxidase inhibitors (MAOIs). The principle mechanism of all effective antidepressants involves boosting the synaptic action of one or more of the monoamines, mainly dopamine, serotonin, and norepinephrine. This action is often but not exclusively conducted by acutely blocking one or more of the

presynaptic transporters of these monoamines.(18) MAOIs were the first class of antidepressants to be developed, but fell out of favor because of concerns about interactions with certain foods and numerous drug interactions. RLS has been reported as a possible side effect in a number of TCAs (amitriptyline), SSRIs (fluoxetine, paroxetine, sertraline, citalopram escitalopram), SNRIs (venlafaxine, duloxetine), and others (mianserin, mirtazapine), but the majority of evidence is in the form of case reports.(19–32) Among those reports, frequent associations were observed on mirtazapine and mianserin, which share similar 5-$HT_2$ antagonistic activity, supporting the possibility that the different effects of noradrenergic and serotonergic transmission are involved in the development of RLS.(26, 28, 30–32) One retrospective chart review indicated that the risk of developing RLS among mirtazapine users was approximately 8% and the concomitant use of medication with tramadol, fluoxetine, or dopamine receptor blocking agents (DRBAs, including domperidone which is a peripheral dopamine $D_2$ receptor antagonist) could potentially increase the risk.(26, 27, 33) To the best of our knowledge, no cases of RLS have been reported as an adverse event of reboxetine or bupropion.

Despite a number of case reports suggesting that some antidepressants may induce RLS, a few systematic studies reported contradictory results. In a retrospective study looking at the association between the clinical diagnosis of RLS and the use of antidepressants in 200 patients who presented for the evaluation of sleep initiation insomnia, while 45% of the patients met clinical diagnostic criteria for RLS and 38% were treated with antidepressants, there were no statistical associations between RLS and antidepressant use or the use of any specific class of antidepressants.(34) However, only two patients in this study were on mirtazapine. Moreover, another study found that SSRIs improved preexisting RLS in 70% of patients, in contrast with 9% of patients who were free of RLS prior to treatment but developed RLS during treatment.(35) A separate study even argued that neither antidepressants nor neuroleptics but nonopioid analgesics are associated with an increased risk of RLS, but this claim has been rebutted based on methodological limitations.(36, 37)

Data that support an association come from a large European epidemiological study involving 18,980 subjects on the study of the prevalence of RLS that reported an increased risk (OR=3.11) in patients taking SSRIs, but not for TCAs or other types of antidepressants.(38) As mentioned earlier, the French pharmacovigilance database also found RLS to be an adverse reaction to antidepressants (OR=15.9; amitriptyline, escitalopram, mianserin, mirtazapine, and duloxetine). In addition, another systematic review provided strong supporting evidence for drug-induced RLS on similar medications. (11, 16) One prospective study evaluated patients who were treated for the first time with antidepressants and sought to answer the question of whether RLS occurred or preexisting RLS worsened as a result of the medication.(39) Although the medications were limited to second-generation antidepressants (fluoxetine, paroxetine, citalopram, sertraline, escitalopram, venlafaxine, duloxetine, reboxetine, and mirtazapine), 9% of patients reported RLS as a side effect of the administration of these drugs, of which mirtazapine represented the most frequent medication causing RLS (28%). Importantly, the symptoms usually occurred during the initial days of treatment with these medications, and abated in the further course of therapy. The co-medication with benzodiazepines, neuroleptics, and TCAs did not pose additional risk of RLS and no case occurred while using reboxetine in this study.

The issue of whether antidepressants can increase the risk of developing RLS is clinically relevant since many RLS patients suffer from depression, and vice versa RLS also occurs more frequently among patients with depression and anxiety.(40, 41) Therefore, the association, if demonstrated, has important clinical implications for how physicians would consider antidepressants in the general population, among whom RLS is a very common disorder, and how they would modify their treatment recommendations in patients who already suffer from RLS and need to start on antidepressants. Even though the evidence is contradictory, the association between RLS and antidepressants is likely to be substantial with considerable differences observed between various agents. While an average risk of SSRIs and SNRIs to induce RLS is about 5%, the risk is probably highest in mirtazapine (28%) and is negligible in reboxetine and bupropion. No studies have specifically determined the risk of RLS in TCAs. Based on the above information, physicians should differentiate the risk of RLS in individual patients who are to be started on antidepressants. In those who are susceptible to RLS due to coexisting risk factors including old age, female, and the presence of chronic diseases (e.g., musculoskeletal disease, iron deficiency, heart disease, obstructive sleep apnea, peripheral neuropathies, Parkinson's disease), careful considerations should be made when starting antidepressants in these patients, particularly with mirtazapine and mianserin. Once started, physicians should specifically ask the patient for RLS symptoms at the first visit. If no symptoms have occurred by then, RLS is unlikely to appear in the further course of treatment. If the symptoms are not too pronounced, the medication can be maintained with a chance of abatement of RLS in the short term but a close follow-up is recommended. If RLS symptoms are intolerable, physicians may consider switching to another antidepressant with less of a likelihood of precipitating RLS. The most appropriate options include reboxetine and bupropion. A recent double-blinded, randomized controlled trial of 29 moderate to severe RLS patients suggested that bupropion does not exacerbate RLS symptoms and may be a reasonable choice if an antidepressant is needed in individuals with RLS.(42) If a patient who is already on antidepressants complains of RLS symptoms, physicians should determine if a causal relationship with an antidepressant is based on a close temporal association between the start of the antidepressant and the onset of symptoms.

## Antipsychotics

Since a positive therapeutic response to levodopa or a dopamine agonist is considered as a supportive clinical feature of IRLSSG, it seems logical that patients who take antipsychotics may be at risk of developing RLS. Antipsychotics are a class of drugs used to control symptoms in patients with psychotic disorders, such as schizophrenia and delusional disorders. A key pharmacological property of all antipsychotics is their ability to block dopamine-2 ($D_2$) receptors. Distinguished from typical or conventional antipsychotics, "atypical" antipsychotics may be associated at a clinical level with diminished extrapyramidal syndrome, a reduced capacity to elevate plasma prolactin, and less severe negative symptoms.(43) From a pharmacological perspective, the mechanisms of atypical antipsychotics vary depending on individual agents but generally fall into one of four categories: 1) serotonin dopamine antagonists, 2) $D_2$ antagonist with rapid dissociation, 3) $D_2$ partial agonists, and 4) serotonin partial agonists at $5HT_{1A}$ receptors. These mechanistic properties may be involved in the pathogenesis of RLS in susceptible individuals.(44)

Similar to antidepressants, the majority of the evidence of antipsychotic-induced RLS is in the form of case reports and very few have reported the association of RLS with typical antipsychotics, including levomepromazine, pimozide, haloperidol, and sulpiride.(45–47) The French pharmacovigilance database identified thioridazine and loxapine as the offending agents.(16) Among those atypical antipsychotics, risperidone, olanzapine, aripiprazole, quetiapine, and clozapine are the frequent suspects.(48–59) Olanzapine, risperidone, and aripiprazole were also identified as the frequent causes of drug-induced RLS in two systematic reviews.(11, 16) The low number of reports of RLS in patients taking typical antipsychotics may be due to several causes, such as low awareness of this association when typical antipsychotics were introduced, and does not necessarily imply that atypical antipsychotics are at greater propensity to induce RLS in comparison with typical antipsychotics. Interpretations of those case reports should be made with caution since patients were often co-medicated with other medications, particularly antidepressants and other antipsychotics, and the possibility of either medication or both as a cause of RLS should be considered. Despite some suggestions on the likelihood of various antipsychotics to induce RLS based on their pharmacological profiles, there is currently no published study that specifically evaluates or compares the propensity of different antipsychotics to induce RLS.

The prevalence of RLS in patients taking antipsychotics is expected to be higher than in the normal population. In a study involving 182 hospitalized schizophrenic patients, the prevalence of RLS was significantly higher in the schizophrenia group (21.4%) than in the control group (9.3%).(60) Moreover, the IRLS score of the patients was higher than that of the normal control subjects, indicating that the RLS symptoms were more severe in the patients' group. The number and dosages of antipsychotics, and co-medications with antidepressants and anxiolytics, were not related to the severity of RLS. A separate study, which determined the prevalence of primary RLS in 100 patients taking antipsychotics for various disorders, found no differences in the prevalence in comparison with the healthy age- and sex-matched controls and only one patient was diagnosed with RLS. The patient developed symptoms four years after taking perphenazine for depression and the association

was presumed to be coincidental.(61) The differences in the reported prevalence among these two studies may be due to different methodologies, study populations, and designs. Interestingly, the most common RLS complaints in schizophrenic patients were restlessness and fidgeting, which was different from the control group who reported paresthesia and tingling.(60) Although restlessness and fidgeting could be symptoms of akathisia, these symptoms were very mild or absent during the daytime, posing the possibility that the characters of RLS in schizophrenic patients may be different than idiopathic patients. In most reports, patients developed RLS within hours to days after starting antipsychotics or an increase in the dosage. Symptoms usually disappeared in a matter of hours to days after stopping the medications.(48–51, 53, 54)

The contribution of genetic susceptibility in antipsychotic-induced RLS has been explored in several candidate genes including G protein $\beta_3$ subunit, $D_{1-4}$ receptor, $MAO_A$, and $MAO_B$ genes.(44, 62, 63) A probable association has been established between antipsychotic-induced RLS and G protein $\beta_3$ subunit gene and the interaction between the variable number of tandem repeat polymorphisms in the promoter region of the $MAO_A$ gene and the A644 G single nucleotide polymorphism in intron 13 of the $MAO_B$ gene. This dynamic has been reported to show a significant influence on the RLS scores of patients with schizophrenia.(44)

When considering dopamine receptor blocking agents (DRBAs) as a probable cause of RLS, it is important to evaluate the possibilities of other drugs in addition to antipsychotics that also block dopamine receptors. Among those, calcium channel blockers (cinnarizine, flunarizine), metoclopramide, prochlorperazine, clebopride, domperidone, and melatonin also share at least in part a DRBA action in addition to specific pharmacologic profiles of the individual agents. Prochlorperazine was mentioned as a possible cause of RLS in the original description of Ekbom.(6) Although there was no specific case report of metoclopramide-induced RLS, metoclopramide was tested as a drug challenge in untreated RLS patients with the aim of understanding the dopaminergic mechanism in RLS. Following a 10-mg infusion of metoclopramide, both sensory and motor symptoms of RLS as monitored by suggested immobilization test (SIT) could not be provoked.(64) Both prochlorperazine and metoclopramide can commonly induce akathisia and the clinical differentiation from RLS can be difficult if the symptoms occur in the evening or at night.(65, 66) Interestingly, there was a recent case of idiopathic RLS that dramatically worsened with the addition of domperidone, which is a peripheral $D_2$ receptor antagonist.(14) This possible link was later supported by a study showing that 48% of PD patients who were taking domperidone had RLS, compared with 21% not taking domperidone ($p=0.01$).(14) As this study determined the prevalence of RLS in PD patients, a true causation between domperidone and RLS in normal populations needs to be evaluated in future studies. One case report of hemi-RLS was induced by clebopride, which is a substituted benzamide with dopamine antagonistic and prokinetic actions similar to metoclopramide.(67) Since melatonin has been shown to inhibit dopamine release in the striatum and there is a temporal relationship between the onset of melatonin secretion at night and the onset or worsening of RLS symptoms, melatonin may theoretically play a role in the genesis of RLS.(68, 69) One small study evaluated the effects of the administration of exogenous melatonin and, conversely, the suppression of endogenous melatonin secretion by bright light exposure in eight RLS patients.(70) Exogenous melatonin significantly increased RLS symptoms while bright light exposure improved leg discomfort slightly. We are not aware of any reports of cinnarizine- and flunarizine-induced RLS in the medical literature.

The above evidence suggests that the associations between RLS and these medications are limited to theoretical possibilities, supported by a few case reports or specific experimental situations. Therefore, a definite conclusion cannot be made as to whether RLS can be a consequence of the use of nonantipsychotic DRBAs.

## Antiepileptic drugs

Evidence on antiepileptic-induced RLS in the medical literature is limited to a few case reports. The first report was from two epileptic patients who developed RLS while taking methsuximide and phenytoin.(71) While the diagnosis of RLS in these two patients was based only on clinical descriptions of creeping sensations in the legs in association with insomnia, the symptoms abated once medications were discontinued. Subsequently, there were reports of RLS as a consequence of topiramate and zonisamide use and the symptoms rapidly resolved as soon as the treatments

were suspended.(72–75) The possibility that both topiramate and zonisamide may induce RLS is possibly attributable to their multiple mechanisms of action, including blockage of sodium and T-type calcium channels, inhibition of carbonic anhydrase, inhibition of glutamate release, and dopaminergic activity. Specifically, zonisamide is considered to have biphasic effects on the dopaminergic system in which therapeutic doses have been found to increase intracellular and extracellular dopamine in the rat striatum, while supratherapeutic doses reduce intracellular dopamine.(76) Topiramate has recently been shown to reduce levodopa-induced dyskinesias in MPTP-lesioned primates and modulate cortico-mesolimbic dopamine function.(77, 78) It is not known if these observations are relevant to the occurrence of RLS.

In contrast to a possibility of antiepileptic-induced RLS in very few reported patients, certain antiepileptic drugs have been shown to be efficacious in the treatment of RLS, particularly pregabalin, gabapentin, gabapentin enacarbil, oxcarbazepine, lamotrigine, and levetiracetam. Recent European guidelines on the management of RLS have recommended the use of pregabalin and gabapentin enacarbil as an effective treatment of primary RLS.(79)

## Opioids and opioid receptor agonists

While opioids and opioid receptor agonists, including tramadol, methadone, oxycodone-naloxone, and intrathecal morphine, may be considered as alternative medications in the treatment of RLS following unsuccessful treatment with dopaminergic medications, a number of recent reports have highlighted the possibility of tramadol inducing or exacerbating RLS.(11, 16, 80, 81) The French pharmacovigilance database identified three cases of RLS as being attributable to an adverse reaction to tramadol (OR=13.05).(16) Similarly, a recent systematic review with qualitative scoring and comparative analysis suggested that tramadol was among the potential agents that could induce or exacerbate RLS.(11) However, details were unavailable in these two studies as to whether the identified cases were patients with de novo RLS or with augmentation. Two separate case reports suggested the possibility that long-term use of tramadol may augment RLS symptoms.(82, 83)

The combination of dopaminergic agents and an opioid is frequently used in clinical practice, particularly in severe cases, but this approach has never been investigated with respect to efficacy or adverse events.

This seems to be a reasonable option for short-term use in severe intractable RLS patients who do not respond to dopaminergic treatment, but physicians should be aware of the possibility of at least augmentation with tramadol. Two recent guidelines have not supported the use of opioids in the treatment of RLS due to insufficient evidence.(79, 84)

## Miscellaneous

There were three case reports of lithium-induced RLS in which the possibility of co-medication with levomepromazine was not excluded in one of the two cases. (46, 85, 86) Although the mechanism of lithium-induced RLS is unclear, the possibility of lithium enhancing noradrenergic functions while reducing dopamine synthesis has been suggested.(85) RLS has been included as a potential side effect among different types of movement disorders in association with interferon-α by exerting complex interactions between dopaminergic transmission and opioid receptors.(87) Methoxy polyethylene glycol-epoetin beta (CERA), a recombinant erythropoietics-stimulating agent without reported mechanism on dopaminergic activity, was recently claimed to induce RLS in one patient with chronic renal failure.(88) However, the possibility of secondary RLS as a result of renal failure and anemia cannot be entirely excluded in this patient. RLS symptoms may also complicate thyroxine replacement in at-risk hypothyroid patients with low serum ferritin.(89) Interestingly, there has been a single case report of one patient with periodic limb movements in sleep (PLMS) with a relatively low ferritin level who developed severe diurnal RLS symptoms a few months after starting a controlled-release levodopa.(90) The symptoms subsided once levodopa was discontinued. This finding may be considered to be a form of augmented RLS symptoms, previously described in patients with PLMS.(17)

It is likely that there will be an increasing number of reports suggesting the association between RLS and various classes of medications in which some of them may share, at least in part, a dopaminergic modulation. At this point, there is insufficient evidence to determine if these medications (in the miscellaneous section) are able to solely induce RLS as an adverse reaction. More likely, the incidence occurs in patients who are posed to be at risk, i.e., those with anemia, low ferritin, or chronic renal failure. Therefore, physicians should be aware of this potential association and exercise caution

when these patients return back to them with suggestive RLS symptoms or new-onset insomnia.

## Augmentation

Augmentation is the development of progressively more severe RLS earlier in the day after the administration of dopaminergic medications in the afternoon or evening.(17) It may take the form of earlier onset of symptoms (100% of patients), and increasing severity of preexisting symptoms (96%). In addition, patients may experience a spread of symptoms to different body parts, usually the arms, and a shorter duration of the effect of the medication.(91) Moreover, patients with augmentation frequently have an increase in severity with increased doses of medication, and an improvement following a decrease in medication. This paradoxical response to treatment whereby symptoms improve following discontinuation of medication is useful for distinguishing augmentation from disease progression.(92) In the original description, 82% of RLS patients and 31% of PLMS patients developed augmentation following the treatment with levodopa/carbidopa.(17) Augmentation was severe enough to warrant a change in medication in 50% of RLS patients and 13% of PLMS patients. In a recent US community study, estimated prevalence of augmentation in all patients with RLS treated with a dopaminergic medication was 75%, with an annual rate increase of 8%.(93) Four factors were considered to increase the risk of augmentation: 1) dosage and half-life of medications, 2) duration of treatment, 3) low serum ferritin levels, and 4) positive family history of RLS.(94) Subsequent studies have reported different prevalence of augmentation ranging from 27%–82% of patients on long-term levodopa, 8%–56% for those on pramipexole, 3%–9% for those on cabergoline, 9.7% for those on rotigotine, and 4% for patients using ropinirole on a long-term basis.(92, 95–99) An overall augmentation rate of 48% was observed in a study involving 83 patients on a variety of dopamine agonists, with a mean follow-up of 39 months. (100) With levodopa, augmentation may occur within 2 to 4 months.(94) However, it is difficult to compare augmentation rates across drugs, as they have not been adequately evaluated using standardized tools. Nevertheless, it appears that augmentation is more common with levodopa and shorter-acting dopamine agonists and is progressive.(84) Therefore, long-term trials are needed to estimate its real incidence. A recent prospective study specifically designed to determine the incidence of augmentation found that it starts to emerge with a 3.5% incidence of augmentation for ropinirole.(92) With the exception of a case series on the use of tramadol, no cases of augmentation have been reported using nondopaminergic medications.(82, 83)

A consensus on the standardized operational definition of augmentation has been established. The first NIH-sponsored consensus defined the primary feature of augmentation as a drug-induced shift of symptoms to a period of time two hours earlier than was the typical time of daily onset prior to pharmacological intervention.(1) A more refined European RLS study group–sponsored consensus, the Max Planck Institute (MPI) criteria, indicated that reliable detection of augmentation can be obtained based on a four-hour time advance of symptoms, or a smaller (two to four hours) advance of symptoms expressed along with other required clinical indications, including a shorter latency of symptoms at rest, a spread of symptoms to other body parts in addition to the lower limbs, or a greater intensity of symptoms.(101) In addition, the augmentation severity rating scale was developed to measure the severity of augmentation in clinical trials.(101)

Augmentation must be differentiated from conditions that it may closely resemble, including tolerance, early morning rebound, progression of RLS, fluctuations in disease severity, and neuroleptic-induced akathisia.(91) Tolerance occurs when the effectiveness of a medication decreases over time necessitating an increase in dosage in order to maintain the initial relief of symptoms. Therefore, tolerance symptoms do not appear earlier in the day as observed in augmentation. In addition, symptoms do not become more severe than at baseline. As the name suggests, "rebound" refers to the reappearance of symptoms in the early morning, which corresponds to the time when the half-life of the medication has expired.(102) The natural progression of RLS usually takes years to develop, as opposed to augmentation, where symptoms worsen within months. In contrast to augmentation, symptoms of neuroleptic-induced akathisia lack circadian nature and patients often complain of inner restlessness rather than limb restlessness and paresthesia as observed in RLS.(103) Importantly, patients with neuroleptic-induced akathisia usually have a history of neuroleptic exposure and there is usually no family history.

Several mechanisms explaining augmentation have been proposed, including dopamine hyperstimulation,

overstimulation of $D_1$ receptors compared with $D_2$ receptors, brain iron deficiency, a genetic predisposition, and changes in neuroendocrine secretion and the chronobiotic system.(91, 94) The full discussion of these mechanisms is beyond the scope of this chapter. However, it is generally believed that small doses of levodopa over a long period of time may result in an increase in the dopamine concentrations in the CNS; and that in the absence of down-regulation, repeated doses can lead to increased dopamine concentrations over a short time frame.(104)

The risk of augmentation will be minimized by treating any possible factors that may contribute to RLS symptoms, such as low ferritin level, and by maintaining the minimal dose of the dopaminergic medications, with the maximal possible effects. The dose increases should be carefully considered, particularly if they exceed usually accepted levels. They should be limited to a breakthrough of clinically important symptoms that cannot be managed behaviorally and should be balanced against the option of adding an alternative medication.(84) When serum ferritin is < 50 μg/L, an oral iron supplement should be considered. Any drugs that potentially exacerbate RLS symptoms, including antidepressants and antipsychotics, should be avoided. Augmentation only requires treatment when it is clinically significant. In very mild cases, patients may increase their daytime activities to diminish the symptoms.(91, 94) If the patient is bothered by symptoms earlier in the daytime, one strategy is to split the medication dose into two or add an additional very small dose of a dopamine agonist.(91, 94) However, this strategy is unlikely to last that long and patients may later develop even earlier symptoms requiring earlier medications. When the symptoms become severe, the approach is to gradually reduce dopaminergic medications and at the same time, add either an $\alpha_2\delta$ anticonvulsant (e.g., gabapentin enacarbil, pregabalin, or gabapentin), or an opioid.(79) For further details on the management of augmentation, please consult the RLS treatment algorithm and the recent evidence-based guidelines on the long-term management of RLS.(84, 101)

## Conclusion

RLS is a very common disorder affecting 5% to 10% of the general population, and it causes sleep disruption, impaired quality of life, and reduced daytime productivity. Although in the majority of patients the cause is primary or familial, evaluations for secondary causes need to be performed if patients have atypical presentations or there is a temporal association with the offending illness or medications. A variety of medications are reported to exacerbate or trigger RLS symptoms. The most cited classes of drugs are antidepressants and antipsychotics. Since not all patients who are exposed to these medications develop RLS, it is likely that other factors are involved in the generation of RLS, including specific pharmacologic profiles of individual medications, genetic predisposition, co-medications, and comorbidities, such as low ferritin. It is also likely that the list of responsible medications will continue to grow. Therefore, treating physicians should be aware of the medications that can potentially lead to RLS because it can change treatment strategies. Instead of starting another medication such as a dopamine agonist to treat RLS symptoms, it may be more appropriate to consider reducing the dose or withdrawing the offending medication as the first line of intervention. Another important clinical scenario is when physicians consider adding another medication to treat a coexisting disorder in RLS patients, for example, depression or insomnia. Physicians need to exercise careful consideration with the aspects of possible RLS exacerbations and drug interactions, particularly in those who are at risk. Given the lack of evidence, it is important to evaluate and monitor each patient carefully.

For RLS patients who are already on dopaminergic therapy, the dose should be kept at the minimal effective level to avoid the possible risk of augmentation. Although the mechanism of augmentation is unclear, it appears that augmentation is more common with levodopa and shorter-acting dopamine agonists and is progressive. While the best approach is prevention, physicians should reevaluate all concomitant medications, and address any possible factors that may worsen RLS symptoms. Should augmentation require treatment, physicians have options to split the doses of dopaminergic medication, add nondopaminergic medication, or increase daytime physical activities.

## References

1. Allen RP, Picchietti D, Hening WA, Trenkwalder C, Walters AS, Montplaisi J. Restless legs syndrome: diagnostic criteria, special considerations, and epidemiology. A report from the restless legs syndrome diagnosis and epidemiology workshop at the National Institutes of Health. *Sleep Med.* 2003 Mar;4(2):101–19. PubMed PMID: 14592341.

2. American Academy of Sleep Medicine. *International classification of sleep disorders.* 2nd ed. Westchester, IL.: American Academy of Sleep Medicine; 2005.

3. Allen RP, Walters AS, Montplaisir J, Hening W, Myers A, Bell TJ, et al. Restless legs syndrome prevalence and impact: REST general population study. *Arch Intern Med.* 2005 Jun 13;**165**(11):1286–92. PubMed PMID: 15956009.

4. Allen RP, Bharmal M, Calloway M. Prevalence and disease burden of primary restless legs syndrome: results of a general population survey in the United States. *Mov Disord.* 2011 Jan;**26**(1):114–20. PubMed PMID: 21322022.

5. Chokroverty S. Introduction: Comorbid disorders and special populations. In: Hening W, Allen RP, Chokroverty S, Earley CJ, editors. *Restless legs syndrome.* Philadelphia: Saunders, Elsevier; 2009. p. 161–6.

6. Ekbom KA. Restless legs syndrome. *Neurology.* 1960 Sep;**10**:868–73. PubMed PMID: 13726241.

7. Morgan LK. Letter: Restless legs: precipitated by beta blockers, relieved by orphenadrine. *Med J Aust.* 1975 Nov 8;**2**(19):753. PubMed PMID: 1214686.

8. Lutz EG. Restless legs, anxiety and caffeinism. *J Clin Psychiatry.* 1978 Sep;**39**(9):693–8. PubMed PMID: 690085.

9. Ginsberg HN. Propranolol in the treatment of restless legs syndrome induced by imipramine withdrawal. *Am J Psychiatry.* 1986 Jul;**143**(7):938. PubMed PMID: 3717447.

10. Derom E, Elinck W, Buylaert W, van der Straeten M. Which beta-blocker for the restless leg? *Lancet.* 1984 Apr 14;**1**(8381):857. PubMed PMID: 6143173.

11. Hoque R, Chesson AL, Jr. Pharmacologically induced/exacerbated restless legs syndrome, periodic limb movements of sleep, and REM behavior disorder/REM sleep without atonia: literature review, qualitative scoring, and comparative analysis. *J Clin Sleep Med.* 2010 Feb 15;**6**(1):79–83. PubMed PMID: 20191944. Pubmed Central PMCID: 2823282.

12. Trenkwalder C, Paulus W. Restless legs syndrome: pathophysiology, clinical presentation and management. *Nat Rev Neurol.* 2010 Jun;**6**(6):337–46. PubMed PMID: 20531433.

13. Salminen AV, Rimpila V, Polo O. Peripheral hypoxia in restless legs syndrome (Willis–Ekbom disease). *Neurology.* 2014 Apr 30. PubMed PMID: 24789861.

14. Rios Romenets S, Dauvilliers Y, Cochen De Cock V, Carlander B, Bayard S, Galatas C, et al. Restless legs syndrome outside the blood–brain barrier-exacerbation by domperidone in Parkinson's disease.

*Parkinsonism Relat Disord*. 2013 Jan;**19**(1):92–4. PubMed PMID: 22922159.

15. Blier P, El Mansari M. Serotonin and beyond: therapeutics for major depression. *Philos Trans R Soc Lond B Biol Sci*. 2013;**368**(1615):20120536. PubMed PMID: 23440470. Pubmed Central PMCID: 3638389.

16. Perez–Lloret S, Rey MV, Bondon–Guitton E, Rascol O, Montastruc AJ, French Association of Regional Pharmacovigilance C. Drugs associated with restless legs syndrome: a case/noncase study in the French Pharmacovigilance Database. *J Clin Psychopharmacol*. 2012 Dec;**32**(6):824–7. PubMed PMID: 23131889.

17. Allen RP, Earley CJ. Augmentation of the restless legs syndrome with carbidopa/levodopa. *Sleep*. 1996 Apr;**19**(3):205–13. PubMed PMID: 8723377.

18. Stahl SM. *Antidepressants*. In: Stahl SM, editor. *Stahl's essential psychopharmacology: Neuroscientific basis and practical applications*. New York: Cambridge University Press; 2008. p. 511–666.

19. Sanz–Fuentenebro FJ, Huidobro A, Tejadas–Rivas A. Restless legs syndrome and paroxetine. *Acta Psychiatr Scand*. 1996 Dec;**94**(6):482–4. PubMed PMID: 9021005.

20. Page RL, 2nd, Ruscin JM, Bainbridge JL, Brieke AA. Restless legs syndrome induced by escitalopram: case report and review of the literature. *Pharmacotherapy*. 2008 Feb;**28**(2):271–80. PubMed PMID: 18225972.

21. Chou KJ, Chen PY, Huang MC. Restless legs syndrome following the combined use of quetiapine and paroxetine. *Prog Neuropsychopharmacol Biol Psychiatry*. 2010 Aug 16;**34**(6):1139–40. PubMed PMID: 20470847.

22. Buskova J, Vorlova T, Pisko J, Sonka K. Severe sleep-related movement disorder induced by sertraline. *Sleep Med*. 2012 Jun;**13**(6):769–70. PubMed PMID: 22440086.

23. Belli H, Akbudak M, Ural C. Duloxetine-related galactorrhea and restless legs syndrome: a case report. *Psychiatr Danub*. 2013 Sep;**25**(3):266–7. PubMed PMID: 24048395.

24. Perroud N, Lazignac C, Baleydier B, Cicotti A, Maris S, Damsa C. Restless legs syndrome induced by citalopram: a psychiatric emergency? *Gen Hosp Psychiatry*. 2007 Jan-Feb;**29**(1):72–4. PubMed PMID: 17189751.

25. Ozturk O, Eraslan D, Kumral E. Oxcarbazepine treatment for paroxetine-induced restless leg syndrome. *Gen Hosp Psychiatry*. 2006 May-Jun;**28**(3):264–5. PubMed PMID: 16675374.

26. Chang CC, Shiah IS, Chang HA, Mao WC. Does domperidone potentiate mirtazapine-associated restless legs syndrome? *Prog Neuropsychopharmacol Biol Psychiatry*. 2006 Mar;**30**(2):316–8. PubMed PMID: 16309808.

27. Prospero-Garcia KA, Torres-Ruiz A, Ramirez-Bermudez J, Velazquez-Moctezuma J, Arana-Lechuga Y, Teran-Perez G. Fluoxetine-mirtazapine interaction may induce restless legs syndrome: report of 3 cases from a clinical trial. *J Clin Psychiatry*. 2006 Nov;**67**(11):1820. PubMed PMID: 17196069.

28. Agargun MY, Kara H, Ozbek H, Tombul T, Ozer OA. Restless legs syndrome induced by mirtazapine. *J Clin Psychiatry*. 2002 Dec;**63**(12):1179. PubMed PMID: 12530413.

29. Hargrave R, Beckley DJ. Restless leg syndrome exacerbated by sertraline. *Psychosomatics*. 1998 Mar-Apr;**39**(2):177–8. PubMed PMID: 9584547.

30. Bahk WM, Pae CU, Chae JH, Jun TY, Kim KS. Mirtazapine may have the propensity for developing a restless legs syndrome? A case report. *Psychiatry Clin Neurosci*. 2002 Apr;**56**(2):209–10. PubMed PMID: 11952928.

31. Bonin B, Vandel P, Kantelip JP. Mirtazapine and restless leg syndrome: a case report. *Therapie*. 2000 Sep-Oct;**55**(5):655–6. PubMed PMID: 11201984.

32. Pae CU, Kim TS, Kim JJ, Chae JH, Lee CU, Lee SJ, et al. Re-administration of mirtazapine could overcome previous mirtazapine-associated restless legs syndrome? *Psychiatry Clin Neurosci*. 2004 Dec;**58**(6):669–70. PubMed PMID: 15601394.

33. Kim SW, Shin IS, Kim JM, Park KH, Youn T, Yoon JS. Factors potentiating the risk of mirtazapine-associated restless legs syndrome. *Hum Psychopharmacol*. 2008 Oct;**23**(7):615–20. PubMed PMID: 18756499.

34. Brown LK, Dedrick DL, Doggett JW, Guido PS. Antidepressant medication use and restless legs syndrome in patients presenting with insomnia. *Sleep Med*. 2005 Sep;**6**(5):443–50. PubMed PMID: 16084763.

35. Dimmitt SB, Riley GJ. Selective serotonin receptor uptake inhibitors can reduce restless legs symptoms. *Arch Intern Med*. 2000 Mar 13;**160**(5):712. PubMed PMID: 10724062.

36. Leutgeb U, Martus P. Regular intake of non-opioid analgesics is associated with an increased risk of restless legs syndrome in patients maintained on antidepressants. *Eur J Med Res*. 2002 Aug 30;**7**(8):368–78. PubMed PMID: 12204845.

37. Berger K. Non-opioid analgesics and the risk of restless leg syndrome-a spurious association? *Sleep Med*. 2003 Jul;**4**(4):351–2. PubMed PMID: 14592311.

38. Ohayon MM, Roth T. Prevalence of restless legs syndrome and periodic limb movement disorder in the general population. *J Psychosom Res*. 2002 Jul;**53**(1):547–54. PubMed PMID: 12127170.

39. Rottach KG, Schaner BM, Kirch MH, Zivotofsky AZ, Teufel LM, Gallwitz T, et al. Restless legs syndrome as side effect of second generation antidepressants.

*J Psychiatr Res.* 2008 Nov;**43**(1):70–5. PubMed PMID: 18468624.

40. Winkelmann J, Prager M, Lieb R, Pfister H, Spiegel B, Wittchen HU, et al. "Anxietas tibiarum". Depression and anxiety disorders in patients with restless legs syndrome. *J Neurol.* 2005 Jan;**252**(1):67–71. PubMed PMID: 15654556.

41. Picchietti D, Winkelman JW. Restless legs syndrome, periodic limb movements in sleep, and depression. *Sleep.* 2005 Jul;**28**(7):891–8. PubMed PMID: 16124671.

42. Bayard M, Bailey B, Acharya D, Ambreen F, Duggal S, Kaur T, et al. Bupropion and restless legs syndrome: a randomized controlled trial. *J Am Board Fam Med.* 2011 Jul-Aug;**24**(4):422–8. PubMed PMID: 21737767.

43. Goldstein JM. The new generation of antipsychotic drugs: how atypical are they? *Int J Neuropsychopharmacol.* 2000 Dec;**3**(4):339–49. PubMed PMID: 11343614.

44. Kang SG, Park YM, Choi JE, Lim SW, Lee HJ, Lee SH, et al. Association study between antipsychotic-induced restless legs syndrome and polymorphisms of monoamine oxidase genes in schizophrenia. *Hum Psychopharmacol.* 2010 Jul;**25**(5):397–403. PubMed PMID: 20589923.

45. Horiguchi J, Yamashita H, Mizuno S, Kuramoto Y, Kagaya A, Yamawaki S, et al. Nocturnal eating/drinking syndrome and neuroleptic-induced restless legs syndrome. *Int Clin Psychopharmacol.* 1999 Jan;**14**(1):33–6. PubMed PMID: 10221640. Epub 1999/04/30. eng.

46. Terao T, Yoshimura R, Terao M, Yasumatsu S, Ohmori O, Shiratsuchi T, et al. Restless legs syndrome induced by psychotropics. *Ann Clin Psychiatry.* 1992;**4**(2):127–30.

47. Akpinar S. Treatment of restless legs syndrome with levodopa plus benserazide. *Arch Neurol.* 1982 Nov;**39**(11):739. PubMed PMID: 7126008.

48. Duggal HS, Mendhekar DN. Clozapine-associated restless legs syndrome. *J Clin Psychopharmacol.* 2007 Feb;**27**(1):89–90. PubMed PMID: 17224721. Epub 2007/01/17. eng.

49. Kraus T, Schuld A, Pollmacher T. Periodic leg movements in sleep and restless legs syndrome probably caused by olanzapine. *J Clin Psychopharmacol.* 1999 Oct;**19**(5):478–9. PubMed PMID: 10505594. Epub 1999/10/03. eng.

50. Wetter TC, Brunner J, Bronisch T. Restless legs syndrome probably induced by risperidone treatment. *Pharmacopsychiatry.* 2002 May;**35**(3):109–11. PubMed PMID: 12107855. Epub 2002/07/11. eng.

51. Pinninti NR, Mago R, Townsend J, Doghramji K. Periodic restless legs syndrome associated with quetiapine use: a case report. *J Clin Psychopharmacol.* 2005 Dec;**25**(6):617–8. PubMed PMID: 16282854. Epub 2005/11/12. eng.

52. Urbano MR, Ware JC. Restless legs syndrome caused by quetiapine successfully treated with ropinirole in 2 patients with bipolar disorder. *J Clin Psychopharmacol.* 2008 Dec;**28**(6):704–5. PubMed PMID: 19011442. Epub 2008/11/18. eng.

53. Kang SG, Lee HJ, Kim L. Restless legs syndrome and periodic limb movements during sleep probably associated with olanzapine. *J Psychopharmacol.* 2009 Jul;**23**(5):597–601. PubMed PMID: 18562412. Epub 2008/06/20. eng.

54. Khalid I, Rana L, Khalid TJ, Roehrs T. Refractory restless legs syndrome likely caused by olanzapine. *J Clin Sleep Med.* 2009 Feb 15;**5**(1):68–9. PubMed PMID: 19317385. Pubmed Central PMCID: 2637170. Epub 2009/03/26. eng.

55. Rittmannsberger H, Werl R. Restless legs syndrome induced by quetiapine: report of seven cases and review of the literature. *Int J Neuropsychopharmacol.* 2013 Jul;**16**(6):1427–31. PubMed PMID: 23331473.

56. Bolanos-Vergaray J, Obaya JC, Gonzalez R, Echeverri C, Piquer P. Restless legs syndrome due to aripiprazole. *Eur J Clin Pharmacol.* 2011 May;**67**(5):539–40. PubMed PMID: 21104073.

57. Webb J. Co-occurring akathisia and restless legs syndrome likely induced by quetiapine. *J Neuropsychiatry Clin Neurosci.* 2012 Spring;**24**(2):E46–7. PubMed PMID: 22772702.

58. Raveendranathan D, Shiva L, Venkatasubramanian G, Rao MG, Varambally S, Gangadhar BN. Clozapine-induced restless legs syndrome treated with aripiprazole. *J Neuropsychiatry Clin Neurosci.* 2013 Spring;**25**(2):E62–3. PubMed PMID: 23686071.

59. Aggarwal S, Dodd S, Berk M. Restless leg syndrome associated with olanzapine: a case series. *Curr Drug Saf.* 2010 Apr;**5**(2):129–31. PubMed PMID: 20406161.

60. Kang SG, Lee HJ, Jung SW, Cho SN, Han C, Kim YK, et al. Characteristics and clinical correlates of restless legs syndrome in schizophrenia. *Prog Neuropsychopharmacol Biol Psychiatry.* 2007 Jun 30;**31**(5):1078–83. PubMed PMID: 17459547.

61. Jagota P, Asawavichienjinda T, Bhidayasiri R. Prevalence of neuroleptic-induced restless legs syndrome in patients taking neuroleptic drugs. *J Neurol Sci.* 2012 Mar 15; **314** (1–2): 158–60. PubMed PMID: 22099638.

62. Kang SG, Lee HJ, Choi JE, Park YM, Park JH, Han C, et al. Association study between antipsychotics-induced restless legs syndrome and polymorphisms of dopamine D1, D2, D3, and D4 receptor genes in schizophrenia. *Neuropsychobiology.* 2008; **57** (1–2): 49–54. PubMed PMID: 18451638.

63. Desautels A, Turecki G, Montplaisir J, Brisebois K, Sequeira A, Adam B, et al. Evidence for a genetic association between monoamine oxidase A and restless legs syndrome. *Neurology*. 2002 Jul 23;**59**(2):215–9. PubMed PMID: 12136060.

64. Winkelmann J, Schadrack J, Wetter TC, Zieglgansberger W, Trenkwalder C. Opioid and dopamine antagonist drug challenges in untreated restless legs syndrome patients. *Sleep Med*. 2001 Jan;**2**(1):57–61. PubMed PMID: 11152983.

65. Drotts DL, Vinson DR. Prochlorperazine induces akathisia in emergency patients. *Ann Emerg Med*. 1999 Oct; **34** (4 Pt 1): 469–75. PubMed PMID: 10499947.

66. Parlak I, Atilla R, Cicek M, Parlak M, Erdur B, Guryay M, et al. Rate of metoclopramide infusion affects the severity and incidence of akathisia. *Emerg Medicine J*. 2005 Sep;**22**(9):621–4. PubMed PMID: 16113179. Pubmed Central PMCID: 1726928.

67. Erro R, Amboni M, Allocca R, Santangelo G, Barone P, Vitale C. Hemi-restless legs syndrome induced by clebopride. *Eur J Neurol*. 2012 Jun;**19**(6):e59. PubMed PMID: 22577755.

68. Tosini G, Dirden JC. Dopamine inhibits melatonin release in the mammalian retina: in vitro evidence. *Neurosci Lett*. 2000 Jun 2;**286**(2):119–22. PubMed PMID: 10825651.

69. Lewy AJ, Wehr TA, Goodwin FK, Newsome DA, Markey SP. Light suppresses melatonin secretion in humans. *Science*. 1980 Dec 12;**210**(4475):1267–9. PubMed PMID: 7434030.

70. Whittom S, Dumont M, Petit D, Desautels A, Adam B, Lavigne G, et al. Effects of melatonin and bright light administration on motor and sensory symptoms of RLS. *Sleep Med*. 2010 Apr;**11**(4):351–5. PubMed PMID: 20226733.

71. Drake ME. Restless legs with antiepileptic drug therapy. *Clin Neurol Neurosurg*. 1988;**90**(2):151–4. PubMed PMID: 3145164.

72. Chen JT, Garcia PA, Alldredge BK. Zonisamide-induced restless legs syndrome. *Neurology*. 2003 Jan 14;**60**(1):147. PubMed PMID: 12525743.

73. Velasco PE, Goiburu JA, Pinel RS. Restless legs syndrome induced by zonisamide. *Mov Disord*. 2007 Jul 30;**22**(10):1517–8. PubMed PMID: 17486608.

74. Romigi A, Izzi F, Placidi F, Sperli F, Cervellino A, Marciani MG. Topiramate-induced restless legs syndrome: a report of two cases. *J Neurol*. 2007 Aug;**254**(8):1120–1. PubMed PMID: 17473947.

75. Bermejo PE. Restless legs syndrome induced by topiramate: two more cases. *J Neurol*. 2009 Apr;**256** (4):662–3. PubMed PMID: 19444538.

76. Okada M, Kaneko S, Hirano T, Mizuno K, Kondo T, Otani K, et al. Effects of zonisamide on dopaminergic system. *Epilepsy Res*. 1995 Nov;**22**(3):193–205. PubMed PMID: 8991786.

77. Silverdale MA, Nicholson SL, Crossman AR, Brotchie JM. Topiramate reduces levodopa-induced dyskinesia in the MPTP-lesioned marmoset model of Parkinson's disease. *Mov Disord*. 2005 Apr;**20**(4):403–9. PubMed PMID: 15593312.

78. Johnson BA. Topiramate-induced neuromodulation of cortico-mesolimbic dopamine function: a new vista for the treatment of comorbid alcohol and nicotine dependence? *Addict Behav*. 2004 Sep;**29**(7):1465–79. PubMed PMID: 15345276.

79. Garcia-Borreguero D, Ferini-Strambi L, Kohnen R, O'Keeffe S, Trenkwalder C, Hogl B, et al. European guidelines on management of restless legs syndrome: report of a joint task force by the European Federation of Neurological Societies, the European Neurological Society and the European Sleep Research Society. *Eur J Neurol*. 2012 Nov;**19**(11):1385–96. PubMed PMID: 22937989.

80. Trenkwalder C, Hening WA, Montagna P, Oertel WH, Allen RP, Walters AS, et al. Treatment of restless legs syndrome: an evidence-based review and implications for clinical practice. *Mov Disord*. 2008 Dec 15;**23**(16):2267–302. PubMed PMID: 18925578.

81. Trenkwalder C, Benes H, Grote L, Garcia-Borreguero D, Hogl B, Hopp M, et al. Prolonged release oxycodone-naloxone for treatment of severe restless legs syndrome after failure of previous treatment: a double-blind, randomised, placebo-controlled trial with an open-label extension. *Lancet Neurol*. 2013 Dec;**12**(12):1141–50. PubMed PMID: 24140442.

82. Vetrugno R, La Morgia C, D'Angelo R, Loi D, Provini F, Plazzi G, et al. Augmentation of restless legs syndrome with long-term tramadol treatment. *Mov Disord*. 2007 Feb 15;**22**(3):424–7. PubMed PMID: 17230457.

83. Earley CJ, Allen RP. Restless legs syndrome augmentation associated with tramadol. *Sleep Med*. 2006 Oct;**7**(7):592–3. PubMed PMID: 16926116.

84. Garcia-Borreguero D, Kohnen R, Silber MH, Winkelman JW, Earley CJ, Hogl B, et al. The long-term treatment of restless legs syndrome/Willis-Ekbom disease: evidence-based guidelines and clinical consensus best practice guidance: a report from the International Restless Legs Syndrome Study Group. *Sleep Med*. 2013 Jul;**14**(7):675–84. PubMed PMID: 23859128.

85. Terao T, Terao M, Yoshimura R, Abe K. Restless legs syndrome induced by lithium. *Biol Psychiatry*. 1991 Dec 1;**30**(11):1167–70. PubMed PMID: 1777530.

86. Heiman EM, Christie M. Lithium-aggravated nocturnal myoclonus and restless legs syndrome. *Am J Psychiatry*. 1986 Sep;**143**(9):1191–2. PubMed PMID: 3752305.

87. LaRochelle JS, Karp BI. Restless legs syndrome due to interferon-alpha. *Mov Disord*. 2004 Jun;**19**(6):730–1. PubMed PMID: 15197722.

88. Inal S, Golbas C, Onec K, Okyay GU, Derici UB. Methoxy polyethylene glycol-epoetin beta (CERA) induced restless legs syndrome. *Ther Apher Dial*. 2012 Aug;**16**(4):378–9. PubMed PMID: 22817128.

89. Tan EK, Ho SC, Koh L, Pavanni R. An urge to move with L-thyroxine: clinical, biochemical, and polysomnographic correlation. *Mov Disord*. 2004 Nov;**19**(11):1365–7. PubMed PMID: 15378680.

90. Santamaria J, Iranzo A, Tolosa E. Development of restless legs syndrome after dopaminergic treatment in a patient with periodic leg movements in sleep. *Sleep Med*. 2003 Mar;**4**(2):153–5. PubMed PMID: 14592347.

91. Garcia-Borreguero D, Williams AM. Dopaminergic augmentation of restless legs syndrome. *Sleep Medicine Rev*. 2010 Oct;**14**(5):339–46. PubMed PMID: 20219397.

92. Garcia-Borreguero D, Hogl B, Ferini-Strambi L, Winkelman J, Hill-Zabala C, Asgharian A, et al. Systematic evaluation of augmentation during treatment with ropinirole in restless legs syndrome (Willis-Ekbom disease): results from a prospective, multicenter study over 66 weeks. *Mov Disord*. 2012 Feb;**27**(2):277–83. PubMed PMID: 22328464.

93. Allen RP, Ondo WG, Ball E, Calloway MO, Manjunath R, Higbie RL, et al. Restless legs syndrome (RLS) augmentation associated with dopamine agonist and levodopa usage in a community sample. *Sleep Med*. 2011 May;**12**(5):431–9. PubMed PMID: 21493132.

94. Chokroverty S. Long-term management issues in restless legs syndrome. *Mov Disord*. 2011 Jul;**26** (8):1378–85. PubMed PMID: 21538518.

95. Winkelman JW, Johnston L. Augmentation and tolerance with long-term pramipexole treatment of restless legs syndrome (RLS). *Sleep Med*. 2004 Jan;**5**(1):9–14. PubMed PMID: 14725821.

96. Benes H, Heinrich CR, Ueberall MA, Kohnen R. Long-term safety and efficacy of cabergoline for the treatment of idiopathic restless legs syndrome: results from an open-label 6-month clinical trial. *Sleep*. 2004 Jun 15;**27**(4):674–82. PubMed PMID: 15283002.

97. Trenkwalder C, Benes H, Grote L, Happe S, Hogl B, Mathis J, et al. Cabergoline compared to levodopa in the treatment of patients with severe restless legs syndrome: results from a multi-center, randomized, active controlled trial. *Mov Disord*. 2007 Apr 15;**22** (5):696–703. PubMed PMID: 17274039.

98. Benes H, Garcia-Borreguero D, Ferini-Strambi L, Schollmayer E, Fichtner A, Kohnen R. Augmentation in the treatment of restless legs syndrome with transdermal rotigotine. *Sleep Med*. 2012 Jun;**13**(6):589–97. PubMed PMID: 22503658.

99. Hogl B, Garcia-Borreguero D, Kohnen R, Ferini-Strambi L, Hadjigeorgiou G, Hornyak M, et al. Progressive development of augmentation during long-term treatment with levodopa in restless legs syndrome: results of a prospective multi-center study. *J Neurol*. 2010 Feb;**257**(2):230–7. PubMed PMID: 19756826. Pubmed Central PMCID: 3085743.

100. Ondo W, Romanyshyn J, Vuong KD, Lai D. Long-term treatment of restless legs syndrome with dopamine agonists. *Arch Neurol*. 2004 Sep;**61**(9):1393–7. PubMed PMID: 15364685.

101. Garcia-Borreguero D, Allen RP, Kohnen R, Hogl B, Trenkwalder C, Oertel W, et al. Diagnostic standards for dopaminergic augmentation of restless legs syndrome: report from a World Association of Sleep Medicine-International Restless Legs Syndrome Study Group consensus conference at the Max Planck Institute. *Sleep Med*. 2007 Aug;**8**(5):520–30. PubMed PMID: 17544323.

102. Guilleminault C, Cetel M, Philip P. Dopaminergic treatment of restless legs and rebound phenomenon. *Neurology*. 1993 Feb;**43**(2):445. PubMed PMID: 8094897.

103. Walters AS, Hening W, Rubinstein M, Chokroverty S. A clinical and polysomnographic comparison of neuroleptic-induced akathisia and the idiopathic restless legs syndrome. *Sleep*. 1991 Aug;**14**(4):339–45. PubMed PMID: 1682986. Epub 1991/08/01. eng.

104. Paulus W, Trenkwalder C. Less is more: pathophysiology of dopaminergic-therapy-related augmentation in restless legs syndrome. *Lancet Neurol*. 2006 Oct;**5**(10):878–86. PubMed PMID: 16987735.

# Chapter 10

# Medication-induced tremors

Peter A. LeWitt

Tremor, a regular to-and-fro movement generated by the uniform repeated activations of lower motor units, is a characteristic manifestation of several neurological disorders. It arises as muscle entrainments enacted by neural oscillations, and for the most part is generated by circuitry in the brain. A low-amplitude tremor also can be detected as a normal physiological finding. Other causes for tremulous movements in limbs include the repetitive oscillations imparted by cardiac pulses. The differential diagnosis of tremor also includes the effects of a wide range of medications. Some of these drugs frequently cause tremors as a dose-related outcome, while for others, it is an unusual occurrence. For the most part, the mechanisms by which drugs produce tremors are not known. Nor is the similarity or difference of drug-induced tremor to essential tremor, a disorder that is often hereditary and which originates in the brain through a cortical-bulbar-cerebellar-thalamic-cortical loop [1]. Since there are several distinct neural structures that have been implicated in the creation of essential tremor, there also might be several sites at which tremorgenic drugs might be able to generate oscillations in motor output pathways.

Of the many hundreds of drugs in current medical practice, only a small number are known to produce tremor. Some reports of drug-induced tremor may represent unique circumstances. Examples of this include tremor that developed in several acquired immunodeficiency syndrome (AIDS) patients treated with trimethoprim-sulfamethoxazole [2], [3], or in a few patients after they received an injection of calcitonin [4]. While drug-induced tremor might arise from specific pharmacological actions on brain neuronal systems, another mechanism by which drugs might induce tremor is through enhancement of the mild tremor normally present (physiological tremor). The characteristic resting tremor of Parkinson's disease (PD) can be duplicated by the actions of drugs depleting presynaptic release of dopamine or blocking dopamine receptors. More commonly, tremor induced by drugs is evident during postural maintenance of the arms or during a targeted action such as handwriting. Drugs leading to this type of tremor include sympathomimetic compounds that duplicate the actions of adrenergic or noradrenergic neurotransmitters.

This chapter will provide a review of drug-induced tremor, updating previous compendia that have appeared in the medical literature over several decades [5], Pinder 1984, [6], [7]. As some reports of drug-induced tremor arise from a single case or provide only limited documentation, the verity of such claims may be questionable. Authors reporting a new cause of tremor need to take pains at excluding alternative explanations or considerations of coincidence (such as a patient exhibiting tremor thought to be due to a drug but in actuality related to adrenaline released from an unsuspected myocardial infarction). FDA-approved product information for a drug can list tremor as a possible adverse effect using relatively uncritical reporting criteria.

## Drug-induced Parkinsonian tremor

Pharmacological disruption of striatal dopaminergic neurotransmission can duplicate virtually all of the clinical features of PD [8], [9]. This includes resting tremor in the limbs and lips at 4–8 Hz and which can be unilateral, bilateral, symmetrical, or asymmetrical. This form of tremor tends to be more prevalent in women than men and often arises at an older age than typical PD. A coarse, flapping tremor or a tremor

*Medication-Induced Movement Disorders*, ed. Joseph H. Friedman. Published by Cambridge University Press.
© Cambridge University Press 2015.

initiated during action has also been described from the use of dopamine blocking medications [10], [11]. Tremor caused by dopamine blocking medications can evolve shortly after the start of the drug or at weeks to months later. Though this group of drugs reduces dopaminergic neurotransmission as a dose-related and reversible effect, the resting tremor and other Parkinsonian features have been known to persist for varying periods of time long afterwards (in some instances, up to several weeks).

Drugs responsible for inducing resting tremor and other clinical features of PD include a large number of compounds mostly targeted to the D-2 dopamine receptor family (which includes the D-3 dopamine receptor). These drugs, which form the mainstay of pharmacological treatment for schizophrenia and other psychoses, have been classified as "typical" and "atypical" neuroleptics. The drugs regarded as "typical" neuroleptics have been in use since the late 1950s, beginning with chlorpromazine. Among the later generation of compounds with similar psychiatric uses were fluphenazine, perphenazine, pimozide, mesoridazine, promazine, trifluoperazine, loxapine, sulpiride, and haloperidol, among many others used worldwide. A later generation of neuroleptics were modeled after the improved side effect profile of clozapine and received the term "atypical" because of their reduced propensity to produce extrapyramidal side effects such as Parkinsonism or acute dystonic reactions. Most researchers consider the only genuinely "atypical" neuroleptic to be clozapine, a drug that does not cause tardive dyskinesia or Parkinsonism (and which uniquely can block PD tremor [12]). Quetiapine, although not capable of diminishing Parkinsonian tremor, has a pharmacological profile that is closest to the actions of clozapine with respect to extrapyramidal reactions. In recent years, a number of antipsychotic drugs that have been promoted in marketing as "atypical" neuroleptics— among them olanzapine, risperidone, ziprasidone, and aripiprazole—are widely known to behave otherwise and commonly induce Parkinsonian side effects like resting tremor. One of the older neuroleptic drugs, thioridazine (now discontinued) possessed an additional anticholinergic property which would simultaneously provide some symptomatic effects against Parkinsonian resting tremor.

Two drugs in common use also can produce typical neuroleptic drug side effects such as tremor. These include the antinausea drug prochlorperazine and a drug used to enhance gastric motility, metoclopramide. Each of these drugs can enter the brain to antagonize striatal D-2 dopamine receptors and so can induce features of Parkinsonism. Another pharmacological way that dopaminergic neurotransmission can be disrupted is by depletion of presynaptic vesicular dopamine stores as occurs with reserpine (an antihypertensive drug no longer used in Western medicine) and tetrabenazine [13]. Each of these ways to diminish striatal dopaminergic neurotransmission can induce the full spectrum of Parkinsonian features, including resting tremor.

Drug-induced tremor caused by dopamine depletion or receptor blockade can respond to anticholinergic drugs or amantadine, and tends to be rapidly reversible. Some drug formulations, such as depot injections, can deliver drugs for long periods of time and as a result, tremor can persist long after discontinuation of therapy. Another outcome of neuroleptic drug use is a rare condition termed "tardive tremor." Tardive tremor arises when the long-term use of a neuroleptic medication induces a persisting resting tremor. This condition is akin to the phenomena of other tardive movement disorders such as dyskinesia or dystonia [14], [15]. There has been little further reporting of this condition, which potentially can be confused with the unmasking or simultaneous development of PD. One distinguishing feature of tardive tremor is that, unlike the tremor of PD, it is dampened by the reinstitution of a dopamine blocking or depleting drug.

A rare movement disorder termed "orthostatic tremor" also has been reported to occur as an outcome from use of dopamine blocking medications. Orthostatic tremor most commonly is a disorder of unknown etiology that develops spontaneously in otherwise healthy individuals. While localization of its origin in the brain or spinal cord is not well understood, it lies presumably within the central nervous system. It is characterized by a tremor that affects the legs and lower trunk exclusively during upright posture. Patients described as developing drug-induced orthostatic tremor during exposure to metoclopramide, sulpiride, and thiethylperazine experienced full remission in three of four reported cases and marked improvement in the fourth case [16].

# Tremor induced by anticonvulsant drugs

Drugs with anticonvulsant properties are widely used, in some instances for other approved or off-label indications in psychiatry and other fields of medicine. The use of these drugs as mood stabilizers for bipolar disorder may occur in patients previously treated with lithium salts, also a drug that commonly leads to drug-induced action tremor. Tremor is not produced by most of the anticonvulsant class drugs, however. Several of them, such as primidone, phenobarbital, and clonazepam, can be useful for treating essential tremor. However, among drugs often utilized for seizure control (and migraine prophylaxis), valproate is the one most likely to induce action tremor [17], [18]. An action tremor of the limbs is produced in up to one-quarter of all patients treated with conventional doses of valproate, and an even greater fraction of them will show the induction of tremor on sensitive recordings [19]. The tremor can be in the range of typical physiological tremor or up to 15 Hz and can also be associated with titubation of head, neck, and trunk [18]. In addition to action and postural tremor of the limbs, sometimes a resting tremor can be produced. Tremors caused by valproate can be suppressed by coadministration of other drugs including acetazolamide [20], amantadine, or propranolol [18]. In one report, a markedly asymmetrical tremor was described in a valproate-treated patient [21].

Other drugs with anticonvulsant properties also can produce relatively mild tremor in small fractions of patients receiving conventional doses. Among these are gabapentin, tiagabine, carbamazepine and related derivatives such as oxazepine, and lamotrigine. Reporting of tremor in placebo-controlled clinical trials has the potential for confounding by the not infrequent incidence of essential tremor and the target population of anticonvulsant therapy which commonly includes patients with injury to the nervous system (which can be another source of tremor). The properties of the various anticonvulsants vary substantially and so no clear mechanism of tremor induction can be gleaned from their pharmacological actions. In fact, the anticonvulsants topiramate and primidone can confer suppression of action and postural tremor in many patients affected with essential tremor.

## Tremor induced by lithium salts

One of the most common sources of drug-induced tremor is lithium, generally formulated as lithium carbonate and administered today primarily for bipolar disorder. The tremor produced by lithium affects up to a third or more of patients receiving conventional doses (particularly in men and older patients)

[22]; sometimes, the tremor is a dose-limiting side effect. Over time, the intensity of tremor can lessen [23] and the dosing can be adjusted in its timing and quantities to minimize the problems it can cause. The tremor can be both action and postural in affecting the limbs [24] and has shown a higher frequency (8–12 cycles per second) than in essential tremor [25]. In some instances, chronic use of lithium has resulted in enduring tremor even after discontinuation of the drug [26].

## Tremor induced by antidepressant medications

Among drugs developed for treatment of depression, the idiosyncratic and dose-related generation of tremor has become well recognized as a side effect. These drugs can also exacerbate physiological tremor as well as preexisting with PD and essential tremor. Up to half of all patients treated with a member of this drug class experience a postural or action tremor. Some studies have suggested that tremor due to these drugs may have an origin in increased noradrenergic activity in the brain, and find that drugs with beta-receptor blocking properties can attenuate them [27]. Postural tremor rather than action or resting tremor has been emphasized as a predominant clinical feature in many of the reports describing the older class of antidepressant medications (such as amitriptyline, nortriptyline, and imipramine). The second generation of antidepressant medications, which includes compounds classified as selective serotonin reuptake inhibitors and selective serotonin-norepinephrine reuptake inhibitors, also are prone to causing dose-related tremor in many treated patients. Generally, the severity is no more than mild and its clinical manifestations resemble those of essential tremor, although its frequency may be greater in some cases. Persistence of the tremors has been described for several months after discontinuation of fluoxetine in one report [28].

## Tremor induced by stimulant drugs

Drugs with sympathomimetic properties are well known to cause tremors either as a feature of excessive medication or even in therapeutic dosage. Since physiological tremor may also be driven in part by endogenous catecholamine actions similar to the effects of drugs like amphetamine, the mechanisms of tremor may be similar. Conventional therapy with the various drugs used for attention deficit disorder and hyperactivity syndrome does not generally lead to problematic occurrence of tremor in children or adults. Withdrawal of stimulant-class drugs for those individuals who were taking them in excess can result in markedly tremulous states.

Short- and longer-acting beta-adrenergic receptor agonists and various xanthine-structure compounds are routinely used in asthma therapeutics. These drugs share a structural similarity to caffeine, which also increases physiological tremor for some individuals (although not to the extent that popular myth sometimes implies [29]. Postural and action tremors are regularly encountered as dose-related effects of these drugs [30], possibly enhanced in some instances by a patient's endogenous release of epinephrine and norepinephrine due to the stress of breathing difficulty. Whether these effects originate in the central nervous system or skeletal muscle (or both) is not fully understood. Hypokalemia may also be a risk factor for tremor [31]. The synergistic role of a substituted xanthine (aminophylline) in exacerbating action tremor has been demonstrated in essential tremor patients treated with this drug [32]. Another commonly-used class of drugs for obstructive pulmonary disease, beta-adrenergic receptor agonists, also are routinely observed to produce enhancement of physiological or essential tremor. Since the use of beta-adrenergic receptor blocking medications is contraindicated in their management, this side effect needs to be balanced by the effectiveness of the drug in each patient using them. With beta-2-adrenergic receptor agonists, up to 4% of treated asthma patients report the side effect of tremor. Fortunately, tolerance to repeated use of beta-2-adrenergic agonists rarely is a reason for discontinuation of this form of treatment [31].

## Tremor induced by cardiac arrhythmics

Medication that can suppress cardiac arrhythmia is associated with a relatively high incidence of drug-induced tremor. Among these, amiodarone probably is the greatest offender [33], [34]. This drug has a dose-dependent induction of action and postural tremor similar to typical features of essential tremor and affecting up to one-half of treated patients [35], [36]. It has also been reported to cause a unilateral rest tremor [37]. Other antiarrhythmic drugs capable of

generating tremor include mexiletine [38], [39], and procainamide [40].

## Tremor induced by calcium channel blocking drugs

Flunarizine and a closely related compound cinnarizine act as selective calcium channel entry blockers and also have properties of antagonism at dopamine receptors. Not surprisingly, these drugs can induce resting tremor and other features of Parkinsonism at conventional doses [41], [42]. The resting tremors (which can include the so-called "rabbit syndrome," a tremor of the lip region) can remit rapidly with lowering or discontinuation of the drug, but can last for weeks afterwards. Other drugs acting on calcium channel entry do not cause tremor, and so the additional property of flunarizine and cinnarizine on D-2 dopamine receptors may be the key feature associated with the induction of tremor by these drugs.

## Additional drugs reported to cause tremor

Like adrenaline and noradrenaline, other sympathomimetic compounds can produce tremor (possibly through peripheral effects as well as central nervous system actions). Among these are compounds such as phenylpropylamine [43], ephedrine, and pseudoephedrine [44]. Action tremor can accompany the peak effects of this medication. Only pseudoephedrine is currently marketed in the US; it can be associated with a mild tremulous side effect in almost half of patients receiving it. Although pindolol is classified as a beta blocking drug (and so might be expected to behave like propranolol in suppressing action tremor), it has been observed to induce tremor based on its intrinsic sympathomimetic actions [28].

Tremor has been reported with the use of the antiviral drug acyclovir in several reports [45], [46]. Another antiviral therapy, vidarabine, has been found to cause action tremors in some treated patients [47]. This drug can cause sometimes severe generalized tremor [48]. Tremors and other features of neurological impairment (amidst multiple metabolic and postsurgical complications) can be observed in patients who are receiving cyclosporine-A for immunosuppression [49].

# References

1. Elble RJ. What is essential tremor? *Curr Neurol Neurosci Rep* 2013; **13**:353. DOI 10.1007/s11910-013-0353-4.

2. Borucki MJ, Matzke DS, Pollard RB. Tremor induced by trimethoprim-sulfamethoxazole in patients with the acquired immunodeficiency syndrome (AIDS). *Ann Intern Med* 1988; **109**: 77–78.

3. Patterson RG, Couchenour RI. Trimethoprim-sulfamethoxazole-induced tremor in an immunocompetent patient. *Pharmacotherapy* 1999; **19**: 1456–1458.

4. Conget JI, Vendrell J, Halperin I, Esmatjes E. Widespread tremor after injection of sodium calcitonin. *Br Med J* 1989; **298**: 189.

5. Brimblecombe RW, Pinder RM. *Tremors and Tremorogenic Agents*. Bristol (UK): Scientechnica, 1972.

6. LeWitt PA. Tremor induced or enhanced by pharmacological means. In: Findley L, Koller WC (eds), *Handbook of Tremor Disorders*, New York: Marcel Dekker., Chap 34, pp 473–481, 1995.

7. Morgan JC, Sethi KD. Drug-induced tremors. *Lancet Neurology* 2005; **4**:866–876.

8. Micheli F, Cerosimo MG. Drug-induced parkinsonism. *Handbook of Clinical Neurology*. 2007; **84**:399–416.

9. Shin H-W, Chung SJ. Drug-induced parkinsonism. *J Clin Neurol* 2012; **8**: 15–21.

10. Boshes RA, Oepen G, Handren M. Flapping tremor produced by high-potency neuroleptics. *J Clin Psychopharmacol* 1991: **11**: 76–77.

11. Friedman JH. "Rubral" tremor induced by a neuroleptic drug. *Mov Disord* 1992; **42**: 407–410.

12. Thomas AA, Friedman JH. Current use of clozapine in Parkinson disease and related disorders. *Clin Neuropharmacol* 2010; **33**:14–16.

13. Calne DB, Webster RA. Tremor induced by tetrabenazine. *Br J Pharmacol* 1969; **37**: 468–475.

14. Stacy M, Jankovic J. Tardive tremor. *Mov Disord* 1992; **7**: 71–76.

15. Shprecher D. Sensory trick with metoclopramide-associated tardive tremor. *Br Med J Case Rep* 2012 pii: bcr1120115/156. Doi: 10.1136/bcr-11-2011-5156.

16. Alonso-Navarro H, Orti-Pareja M, Jiménez-Jiménez FJ et al. [Orthostatic tremor induced by pharmaceuticals]. *Rev Neurol [in Spanish]* 2004; **39**: 834–836.

17. Hyman NM, Dennis PD, Sinclair KG. Tremor due to sodium valproate. *Neurology* 1979; **29;** 1177–1180.

18. Karas BJ, Wilder BJ, Hammond EJ, Bauman AW. Valproate tremors. *Neurology* 1982; **32**: 428–432.

19. Rinnerthaler M, Luef G, Mueller J, et al. Computerized tremor analysis of valproate induced tremor: a comparative study of controlled-release versus conventional valproate. *Epilepsia* 2005; **46**: 320–323.

20. Lancman ME, Asconape JJ, Walker F. Acetazolamine appears effective in the management of valproate-induced tremor. *Mov Disord* 1994; **9**:369.

21. Kakisaka Y, Ito S, Ohara T et al. Asymmetric drug-induced tremor: Rare feature of a common event. *Pediatric Neurology* 2013; **48**: 479–480.

22. Bech P, Thomsen J, Prytz S et al. The profile and severity of lithium-induced side-effects in mentally healthy subjects. *Neuropsychobiology* 1979; **5**: 160–166.

23. Vestergaard P, Poulstrup I, Shou M. Prospective studies on a lithium cohort. 3. Tremor, weight gain, diarrhea, psychological complaints. *Acta Psychiatr Scand* 1988; **78**: 434–441.

24. Tyrer P, Lee I, Trotter C. Physiologic characteristics of tremor after chronic lithium therapy. *Br J Psychiatr* 1981; **139**: 851–853.

25. Gelenberg AJ, Jefferson JW. Lithium tremor. *J Clin Psychiatr* 1995; **56**: 283–287.

26. Donaldson IM, Cunningham J. Persisting neurological sequelae of lithium carbonate therapy. *Arch Neurol* 1983; **40**: 747–751.

27. Kronfol Z, Greden JF, Zis AP. Imipramine-induced tremor: effects of a beta-adrenergic blocking agent. *J Clin Psychiatr* 1983; **44**:225–226.

28. Serrano-Duenas M. Fluoxetine-induced tremor: clinical features in 21 patients. *Parkinsonism Relat Disord* 2002; **8**: 325–327.

29. Koller W, Cone S, Herbster G. Caffeine and tremor. *Neurology* 1987;**37**):169–172.

30. Seddon P, Bara A, Ducharme FM, Lasserson TJ. Oral xanthines as maintenance treatment for asthma in children. *Cochrane Database Syst Rev* 2006; (**1**): CD002885.

31. Cazzola M, Matera MG. Tremor and β(2)-adrenergic agents: is it a real clinical problem? *Pulm Pharmacol Ther* 2012; **25**:4–10.

32. Buss DC, Marshall RW, Milligan N, et al. The effect of intravenous aminophylline on essential tremor. *Br J Clin Pharmacol* 1997; **43**:119–121.

33. Palakurthy PR, Iyer V, Meckler RJ. Unusual neurotoxicity associated with amiodarone therapy. *Ann Intern Med* 1987; **147**: 881–884.

34. Hilleman D, Miller MA, Parker R et al. Optimal management of amiodarone therapy: efficacy and side effects. *Pharmacotherapy* 1998; **18**:138S–145S.

35. Charness ME, Morady F, Scheinman MM. Frequent neurologic toxicity associated with amiodarone therapy. *Neurology* 1984; **34**: 669–671.

36. Coulter DM, Edwards IR, Savage RI. Survey of neurological problems with amiodarone in the New Zealand Intensive Medicines Monitoring Programme. *N Z Med J* 1990; **103**: 98–100.

37. Werner EG, Olanow CW. Parkinsonism and amiodarone therapy. *Ann Neurol* 1989; **25**:630–632.

38. Peyrieux JC, Boissel JP, Leizorovicz A. Relationship between plasma mexiletine levels at steady-state. Presence of ventricular arrhythmias and side effects. *Fundam Clin Pharmacol* 1987; **1**:45–47.

39. Manolis AS, Deering TF, Cameron J, Estes NA. Mexetiline: pharmacology and therapeutic use. *Clin Cardiol* 1990; **13**:349–359.

40. Rubenstein A, Cabili S. Tremor induced by procainamide. *Am J Cardiol* 1986; **57**:340–341.

41. Marti-Masso JF, Pozo JJ. Cinnizarine-induced parkinsonism: ten years later. *Mov Disord* 1998; **13**: 453–456.

42. Micheli F, Fernandez-Pardal M, Gatto M et al. Flunarizine- and cinnarizine-induced extrapyramidal reactions. *Neurology* 1987; **37**:881–884.

43. Dietz AJ. Amphetamine-like reactions to phenylpropylamine. *JAMA* 1981; **245**:439–442.

44. Supiyaphun P, Chochaipanichnon I, Kerekhanjanarong V, Saengpaniel S. A comparative study of the side effects between pseudoephedrine in loratidine plus pseudoephedrine sulfate repetabs and loratidine + pseudoephedrine sulfate in treatment of allergic rhinitis in Thai patients. *J Med Assoc Thai* 2002; **85**: 722–727.

45. Wade JC, Meyers JD. Neurologic symptoms associated with parenteral acyclovir treatment after marrow transplantation. *Ann Intern Med* 1983; **98**: 921–925.

46. Rashiq S, Briewa L, Mooney M, et al. Distinguishing acyclovir neurotoxicity from encephalomyelitis. *J Intern Med* 1993; **234**: 507–511.

47. Nadel AM. Vidarabine therapy for herpes simplex encephalitis. The development of an unusual tremor during treatment. *Arch Neurol* 1981; **38**: 384–385.

48. Buedge DR, Chow AW, Sacks SL. Neurotoxic effects during vidarabine therapy for herpes zoster. *Can Med Assoc J* 1985; **132**: 392–395.

49. Kahan DB, Flechner SM, Lorber MI et al. Complications of cyclosporine-prednisone immunosuppression in 402 renal allograft recipients exclusively followed at a single center for one to five years. *Transplantation* 1987; **43**:197–204.

50. Amery WK, Heykants J. Essential tremor and flunarizine. *Cephalalgia* 1988; **8**:227.

51. Capella D, Laporte JR, Castel JM et al. Parkinsonism, tremor, and depression induced by cinnarizine and flunarizine. *Brit Med J* 1988; **297**: 722–723.

52. Koller W, Orebaugh C, Lawson L, Potempa K. Pindolol-induced tremor. *Clin Neuropharmacol* 1987; **10**:449–452.

53. Topaktas S, Onur R, Dalkara T. Calcium channel blockers and essential tremor. *Eur Neurol* 1987; **27**:114–119.

# L-dopa dyskinesias

Juan Ramirez-Castaneda and Joseph Jankovic

## Introduction

Since its introduction in the late 1960s, levodopa (L-dopa), a dopamine (DA) precursor, has been the most widely used drug for the symptomatic therapy of Parkinson's disease (PD) and has remained the most efficacious treatment of motor manifestations of the disease. However, chronic L-dopa therapy is complicated by the development of long-term adverse effects, particularly motor fluctuations and dyskinesias, that can be disabling, difficult to treat, and may limit its utility.[1, 2] Levodopa-induced dyskinesia (LID) is typically manifested by "peak-dose dyskinesia," coinciding with the "on" response following L-dopa administration, also termed "IDI" (improvement-dyskinesia-improvement) response. This is in contrast to diphasic dyskinesia, which typically appears at the beginning of the medication effect prior to the attainment of a full "on" response and which may reappear as the medication effect starts to wear off, also termed "DID" (dyskinesia-improvement-dyskinesia) response. Chorea, stereotypy, and ballism are the most frequent forms of LIDs, especially in the IDI form. Other LIDs include off-dystonia, which is typically manifest when the dopaminergic benefit is wearing off or the patient is in an "off" state, such as early morning dystonia.[3] LIDs tend to first appear when patients still respond well to L-dopa but begin to experience motor fluctuations, such as the wearing off response.[4] The latency from the onset of L-dopa therapy to the onset of motor fluctuations and dyskinesia correlates with the age at onset of PD (the younger the patient, the shorter the latency), dosage, and duration of L-dopa therapy.[5] There are, however, many other clinical, pharmacologic, and genetic factors that influence the risk and severity of motor fluctuations and LIDs. These factors will be discussed later along with LID phenomenology, molecular and pharmacologic mechanisms, and medical and surgical therapies.

## Assessment of LIDs

LIDs are commonly assessed by a variety of clinical rating scales and home diaries, such as the Hauser diary.[6-9] Based on a comprehensive review of dyskinesia scales, including the Unified Dyskinesia Rating Scale (UDysRS) and other scales, only the Abnormal Involuntary Movement Scale (AIMS) and the Rush Dyskinesia Rating Scale (RDRS) fulfill criteria for "recommended" use in PD populations, "albeit weakly."[9] In a randomized placebo-controlled trial of amantadine, assessing dyskinesia at baseline and at 4 and 8 weeks using the following scales: UDysRS, RDRS, AIMS, Lang-Fahn Activities of Daily Living Dyskinesia Rating Scale (LF), 26-Item Parkinson's Disease Dyskinesia scale (PDD-26), patient diaries, dyskinesia items from the Movement Disorder Society–sponsored revision of the Unified Parkinson's Disease Rating Scale (MDS-UPDRS), and Clinical Global Impression (severity and change: CGI-S, CGI-C), only the UDysRS was considered superior to other scales for detecting treatment effects.[10] In addition, a screening questionnaire, the 9-item Wearing Off Questionnaire (WOQ9), has been developed as a tool to aid in the diagnosis of the wearing off phenomenon.[11] These scales are generally preferable to patient-based measures or portable, computer-based instruments that typically utilize triaxial accelerometers and other electronic or mechanical devices.[12] These tools are used not only in the clinics but also in assessing dyskinesia in clinical trials.

*Medication-Induced Movement Disorders*, ed. Joseph H. Friedman. Published by Cambridge University Press.
© Cambridge University Press 2015.

# Risk factors associated with the development of LIDs

The frequency of dyskinesia varies according to the population studied, instruments used to measure dyskinesia, duration and dosage of treatment, and a variety of other factors. Patients with young-onset PD have a higher prevalence of LIDs than those with late-onset PD.[13] The incidence of LIDs has been estimated at 91% at 5 years in individuals with PD onset before the age of 40 years.[14] Blanchet and colleagues[15] found that 56% of patients develop dyskinesia after a mean of 2.9 years. Dyskinetic patients were significantly younger at disease onset, but their mean latency to dyskinesia induction after levodopa initiation was no different from that of older dyskinetic individuals. The 5-year risk of dyskinesia has been estimated to be 50% for PD onset at 40–59 years, 26% with onset ages 60–69 years, and 16% age 70 or older.[16] In another study,[17] 70% of patients with PD onset between 40 and 49 years developed dyskinesia after 5 years of therapy, compared to 42% of patients with PD onset between 50 and 59 years. After 5 years of therapy, the risks become similarly high across all ages of onset between 40 and 79 years. The severity of PD is also considered a risk factor, as this may reflect a greater degree of striatal dopaminergic denervation. This is supported by numerous reports showing that LIDs are more frequent in animals and humans with severe PD than those with mild PD.[15, 18] Furthermore, LIDs are more likely to start on the side more severely affected by PD and may follow a somatotopic order corresponding to the topography of denervation of the caudate and putamen.[19] The DID dyskinesias predominantly affect the legs, starting typically in the foot on the most affected side and then spreading as an "ascending wave" to the contralateral side, the trunk, upper limbs, and head. In some cases dystonic movements transition to choreic movements or other hyperkinesias. In some cases dyskinesias may coexist with parkinsonian features such as tremor or hypomimia, and some patients are dyskinetic on one side of their body and bradykinetic (with or without rest tremor) on the other side, or in other anatomical sites distant from the dyskinetic limb. Some patients, particularly those with multiple system atrophy, may have orofacial stereotypic dyskinesia while the rest of the body exhibits bradykinesia and rigidity.

There is evidence that young-onset patients, about a third of whom have *PRKN* mutation (PARK2),

develop LIDs with less severe denervation than older patients.[20, 21] Shorter treatment duration and lower doses of L-dopa are needed to produce LIDs in severely parkinsonian primates than in primates with moderate parkinsonism.[18] On the other hand, pathological studies show a similar extent of degeneration of the substantia nigra pars compacta (SNc) in PD patients with and without LIDs.[22] Although LIDs almost never occur in individuals with normal nigrostriatal innervation, such as those wrongly treated with levodopa for essential tremor, nonparkinsonian monkeys can develop LIDs under circumstances of continuous, high-dose L-dopa exposure.[23]

Functional imaging studies such as PET and DaT scan studies provide support for the hypothesis that the severity of denervation correlates with the risk of developing LIDs.[24–27] The status of the presynaptic DA nigrostriatal pathway using DaTscan was studied in 14 patients with PD who developed early and severe LIDs despite using low doses of L-dopa and in ten patients without this complication, despite the use of high L-dopa doses.[28] Patients were matched for age at onset, duration, and severity of PD. The pattern of response to L-dopa and the uptake of (123I)N-w-fluoropropyl-2β-carbomethoxy-3β-(4-iodophenyl) nortropane, a DA transporter (DAT) ligand, were similar in both groups, suggesting that the extent of denervation alone is not sufficient to explain the emergence of LIDs.

The rate of progression of PD may also be a risk factor for LIDs, as suggested by the finding that primates with rapidly induced parkinsonism are more likely to develop LIDs than those with slowly induced parkinsonism.[29] Duration of L-dopa treatment is also considered a risk factor for LIDs as this motor complication is more frequent in PD patients with long-term L-dopa treatment than in recently treated patients.[15] The occurrence of LIDs is higher and at earlier onset than previously thought. In the past, reviews examining mainly retrospective data have estimated median LIDs frequency of less than 10% at 1 year of treatment, increasing to 40% after 5 years of L-dopa therapy.[30] A large randomized trial designed to examine the impact of L-dopa on PD progression (the ELLDOPA trial) found that 16.5% of patients treated with L-dopa 600 mg/day developed LIDs after only 9 months of therapy.[31] Several studies have found that LIDs may appear within a few weeks after beginning L-dopa treatment, especially in the young-onset patients, independent of the degree of denervation.[14, 15, 18, 20, 21, 32, 33]

The total daily dose of L-dopa is also a risk factor for the development of LIDs, particularly when high doses of L-dopa are used and in early phases of the disease.[15] As noted above, in the ELLDOPA trial 16.5% of patients treated with 600 mg/day of L-dopa for 40 weeks developed LIDs, in contrast to 2.3% of patients taking 300 mg/day and 3.3% of those taking 150 mg/day.[31] Several other studies have shown that low doses of L-dopa can cause LIDs in animals with severe parkinsonism and in patients with young-onset parkinsonism.[14, 18, 20, 21]

Many studies have found that early use of a DA agonist delays the onset of L-dopa related motor fluctuations and dyskinesias.[33–35] For example, LIDs were found in 45% of patients within 5 years receiving L-dopa compared to only 20% in those on ropinirole.[34] At 10 years, there was 72.8% prevalence of LIDs in the group initially treated with L-dopa, compared to 52.4% in the ropinirole group.[35] However, a long-term observational study suggested that although the frequency of LIDs was higher with early use of L-dopa after 5 years, the frequency of LIDs was similar after 10 years, regardless of the initial anti-PD medication used.[36]

A number of genetic polymorphisms have been implicated as potential markers for increased risk of LIDs. DRD2 polymorphism may increase the risk of LIDs in men.[37] The polymorphism DRD2Taq1A has been associated with an increased risk for developing motor fluctuations.[38] DRD3p.S9G has been associated with the presence of diphasic dyskinesia, but not peak-dose dyskinesia.[39] Conversely, one study found no association between genetic polymorphisms in DRD2, DRD3, and DRD4 and LIDs risk, but instead showed that 40-bp VNTR of the DAT gene was a predictor for LIDs.[40] This study also found that the possession of a single common allele of the brain-derived neurotropic factor (BDNF) gene doubles the risk for developing LIDs, and possessing two alleles quadruples the risk. Certain monogenic forms of PD, such as PARK2, have been known to be associated with a higher frequency of LIDs.[20]

## Dopamine receptors and molecular mechanisms of LID

Several lines of evidence have provided support for the notion that L-dopa-induced motor complications in PD are associated with nonphysiological, discontinuous, or pulsatile stimulation of striatal DA receptors and that the motor fluctuations can be prevented or ameliorated by more continuous stimulation of striatal DA receptors.[2, 41] In the normal basal ganglia system, nigral dopaminergic cells produce and release DA continuously, maintaining a relatively constant striatal concentration of this neurotransmitter and continuous activation of DA receptors.[42] Central to this concept are observations indicating that DA neurons in the SNc fire tonically at a nearly constant rate,[43] that striatal DA is maintained at a fairly constant concentration,[44] and that there is continuous activation of striatal DA receptors. In the striatum that has been denervated as a result of PD-related nigral degeneration, several pathological adaptive changes occur both at the presynaptic and postsynaptic sites.[45, 46] The maladaptive presynaptic changes mainly involve the regulation of DA release. Furthermore, the buffering capacity of the normal striatum is lost when exogenous L-dopa is administered, thus resulting in marked shortening of the striatal half-life and more pulsatile stimulation of the postsynaptic DA receptors.[42]

While the mechanisms involved in LID occurrence are still unclear, DA receptors are thought to play a central role.[47–49] The DA receptors belong to the superfamily of G protein-coupled receptors with five distinct subtypes of DA receptor that mediate the actions of DA, three of which (D2R, D3R, and D4R) belong to the D2R-like family and two of which (D1R and D5R) belong to the D1R-like family.[50] DA effects in the striatum are mediated principally through the D1R and D2R subtypes which are segregated to the direct and indirect pathways of striatal projection neurons, respectively.[51] D3R subtype is predominantly distributed in the limbic areas.[52] In normal dorsal striatum D3R expression is very low.[53] In the dorsal striatum, the GABAergic medium spiny neurons (MSNs) represent approximately 95% of all neurons. MSNs are present in the 1) "direct pathway" (direct projections from the putamen to the globus pallidus pars internalis and the substantia nigra pars reticulata) containing the D1R coexpressed with the peptide substance P and dynorphin which provide a direct inhibitory effect on basal ganglia output neurons; and 2) "indirect pathway" (connecting the putamen with the globus pallidus pars internalis/substantia nigra pars reticulata via the globus pallidus pars externalis and subthalamic nucleus) bearing the D2R and enkephalin peptides which also provide an inhibitory effect.[54] These two pathways have opposing effects on movements:

activation of the *direct striatonigral pathway* disinhibits thalamocortical neurons and facilitates motor activity, whereas activation of the *indirect striatopallidal pathway* enhances inhibition on thalamocortical neurons and reduces motor activity.[55]

Animal models have been very useful in the study of LIDs.[56] The behavioral sensitization model rendered by Di Chiara's team,[57, 58] using the unilateral 6-hydroxydopamine (6-OHDA)-lesioned rat model, demonstrated that repeated exposure to drugs acting as direct or indirect stimulants of central dopamine transmission resulted in sensitization to their behavioral stimulant properties. These results indicate that priming results in an increased responsiveness of postsynaptic DA receptor mechanisms in the caudate nucleus, possibly due to an increased affinity of the D1 receptor for its agonist. Priming, however, is not an absolute requirement for the expression of D1-dependent supersensitivity.[58] Another model studied the development of abnormal involuntary movements in the L-dopa-treated 6-OHDA-lesioned rat, demonstrating that chronic treatment with L-dopa but not with bromocriptine, a D2 receptor agonist, induced abnormal involuntary movements and that only D1 receptor stimulation (not D2) induced these involuntary movements.[59, 60]

In physiological conditions, cortical glutamate activates striatal output GABAergic neurons through a powerful excitatory influence via both ionotropic (NMDA and AMPA) and metabotropic receptors. Depletion of nigrostriatal DA leads to glutamatergic overactivity, which has been postulated to contribute to loss of dopaminergic neurons, progression of PD, and the appearance of LID.[61, 62] NMDA glutamate receptors consist of ligand-gated cation channels (permeable to $Na^+$ and $Ca^{2+}$) that are known to be expressed at both synaptic and extrasynaptic sites. They are made up of two obligatory NR1 subunits and up to two of four NR2 (NR2A-NR2D) subunits that confer distinct pharmacological and kinetic properties to the receptor.[63] After chronic L-dopa therapy, the glutamatergic signaling from the cortex to the striatum undergoes further adaptive changes. In particular, chronic L-dopa treatment has been found to profoundly modify NR1/NR2B NMDA receptor binding in the putamen of brains of PD patients experiencing motor complications.[64] NMDA receptor blockade ameliorates the dyskinetic complications of long-term L-dopa therapy in both experimental parkinsonism[65] and human PD patients[66] without diminishing the beneficial effects of L-dopa on parkinsonian signs. Although NMDA receptor structure modifications are considered important elements in the pathological cascade leading to the development of LIDs, the precise mechanisms regulating NMDA receptor subcellular trafficking and function have not been clearly elucidated.[42] Gardoni et al. demonstrated that NR2B subcellular redistribution from synaptic to extrasynaptic sites represents a key element in the complex modification of glutamatergic synapse in LIDs.[67] It is uncertain whether NMDA receptor structure modifications represent the primary molecular trigger leading to the development of dyskinetic behavior or represent compensatory mechanisms designed to counteract the modifications in glutamatergic signaling induced by dopaminergic denervation.

At the postsynaptic level, interactions between the D1 receptor and NMDA receptors appear to be particularly relevant in the development of LID.[68] An important mechanism of these interactions is the ability of DA, through D1 receptor activation, to potentiate NMDA glutamate receptor function. In striatal neurons, D1 receptor activation leads to rapid trafficking of NMDA receptor subunits, enhanced coclustering of these subunits, and increased surface expression.[69] D1 receptor activation can potentiate striatal NMDA subunit function by directly promoting the surface insertion of the receptor complexes. Modification of these pathways may be a useful therapeutic target for PD and LIDs.

Among adenosine receptors, A2A receptors appear to play the most important role in the control of motor behavior and in the modulation of DA-mediated responses. Blockade of the adenosine A2A receptor in striatopallidal neurons reduces postsynaptic effects of DA depletion, and in turn lessens the motor deficits of PD. A2A antagonists therefore might partially improve not only the symptoms of PD but also favorably alter its course, by slowing the underlying neurodegeneration and reducing the maladaptive neuroplasticity that complicates standard DA replacement treatments.[70, 71] Similarly to glutamate receptors, A2A-receptor activity is increased in the parkinsonian state.[72, 73]

# Synaptic plasticity and gene expression

Some investigators have hypothesized that neural plasticity may play a role in the development of LIDs.[74]

Drugs that change striatal DA neurotransmission can have long-term effects on striatal physiology and behavior, which may alter gene expression. Dopaminergic drugs rapidly cause changes in gene expression in striatal neurons[75–77] and these changes may be responsible for the alterations in striatal physiology. L-dopa applied in a pulsatile and nonphysiological manner can perturb the normal physiological mechanism that mediates motor control, and eventually result in remodeling of neuronal contacts and pathways, producing long-lasting, near-permanent changes.[78] Neural plasticity can lead to positive, adaptive responses but also to maladaptive responses that might underlie pathological conditions. LIDs can be regarded as maladaptive, negative consequences of neural plasticity.

LIDs can develop independently of the level of denervation and receptor supersensitivity.[79] Physiological changes in corticostriatal plasticity associated with DA denervation and L-dopa treatment differ depending on whether or not the animal has developed LID. This effect is in part due to disruption of protein phosphatase activity in the postsynaptic neurons.[80]

There are two major ways by which neural plasticity can be expressed: functional changes such as an increase in transmitter release, receptor regulation, and synaptic plasticity; and anatomical modifications such as axonal regeneration, sprouting, synaptogenesis, and neurogenesis.[74] In striatal neurons, the stimulation of D1 receptors (coupled to $G_s/G_{olf}$) and D2 receptors (coupled to $G_i/G_o$) that follow L-dopa therapy respectively activate and inhibit adenylyl cyclase, triggering opposite effects on the intracellular levels of cAMP.[81] Intracellular cAMP levels are known to modulate the activity of the cAMP-dependent protein kinase A (PKA).[82] PKA interacts with cAMP-regulated phosphoprotein 32 kDa (DARPP-32), the DA signal amplifier. DARPP-32, in turn, acts as a potent inhibitor of protein phosphatase-1 (PP-1) that regulates the functional activity of many physiological effectors, including NMDA and AMPA glutamate receptors.[81, 82] The D1 receptor signaling cascade (DA/PKA/DARPP-32/PP-1 cascade), involved in the activation of indirect pathway striatofugal neurons, seems to play a pivotal role in LID genesis.

D1 receptor activation appears to be necessary for striatal gene induction by cocaine or L-dopa.[83, 84] This induction occurs selectively in the 40%–50% of striatal neurons whose DA receptors are predominantly of the D1 type and project to the substantia nigra pars reticulata.[85, 86] Increased cAMP can activate PKA, which phosphorylates the transcription factor cAMP response element-binding protein (CREB). D1 receptor stimulation of striatal cells also appears to cause changes in CREB phosphorylation and *c-fos* expression by increasing intracellular calcium, entering through either voltage-sensitive calcium channels or NMDA receptors.[87, 88]

Using a differential display PCR a large number of genes have been identified that can be rapidly induced by D1 receptor stimulation in unilateral D1 receptor stimulated 6-OHDA-lesioned rats.[89] Some genes were expressed at near-maximal levels within 30 minutes, whereas others showed no substantial induction until 2 hours or more after stimulation. The 6-OHDA-lesioned striatum displayed increased DA responsiveness compared with the unlesioned striatum, and this could be increased further by D1 stimulation.[58, 90] Very similar sets of genes are induced by distinct drug classes including psychostimulants, antipsychotics, and dopaminergic medications despite quite different mechanisms of action.[89] The common induction of CREB in striatal neurons by these drugs may account for the observed similar program of gene induction.[91] Other transcription factors may also be involved.[92] Several of the identified genes (MKP-1, CREM, CHOP) may act as homeostatic responses to activation of signal transduction pathways. This diverse set of induced genes may be involved in several processes of neuronal adaptation, including alteration in sensitivity to neurotransmitters and changes in membrane properties.

Taking advantage of a primate brain bank to study LID, Aubert et al. reported changes affecting D1 and D2 receptors within the striatum of normal, parkinsonian, nondyskinetic levodopa-treated parkinsonian, and dyskinetic, levodopa-treated parkinsonian monkeys.[93] There was a linear relationship between D1 receptor sensitivity and LID severity, whereas the relationship with D1 receptor expression levels was less direct. Moreover, the striata of dyskinetic animals showed higher levels of cyclin-dependent kinase 5 (Cdk5) and of the DARPP-32. This data further suggests that LIDs result from increased dopamine D1 receptor-mediated transmission at the level of the direct pathway.

In addition to these biochemical alterations, D1 receptor availability to the ligands is pathologically increased in LIDs. Not only is D1 receptor expression increased, but D1 receptor subcellular distribution is also modified.[49] D1 receptors are more abundant at the plasma membrane compared with control animals,[94, 95] which suggests that LIDs are associated with deficiencies in D1 receptor desensitization and trafficking.[94] The protein machinery involved in this homologous desensitization process is impaired due to blockage of receptor internalization related to downregulation of GPCR and arrestins relative to D1 receptor levels in the striatum of dyskinetic monkeys[96] and rats.[97] Although impaired, D1 receptors retain their ability to internalize after stimulation by D1 receptor agonists.[95] Moreover, this phenomenon is not limited to D1 receptors, as both NMDA and AMPA receptors are recruited at the membrane in dyskinetic monkeys.[98, 99]

The involvement of D3 receptors has also been studied in LIDs. There is evidence of increased level of expression in the dorsal motor-related striatum in experimental mouse,[100] rat,[101] and monkey[53] models of LID. The D1 and D3 receptors have been suggested to directly interact through intramembrane D1-D3 receptor cross-talk.[102, 103] Therefore, the coactivation of both receptors by their natural ligand DA has been found to anchor D1 receptor at the plasma membrane.[49]

There may be other signaling cascades involved in striatal plasticity, such as the extracellular signal-regulated kinase (ERK) signaling cascade.[104] Ionotropic and metabotropic glutamate receptors are able to switch in the small GTPases of the Ras family, which in turn activate this cascade. Sustained activation of these biochemical pathways leads to synaptic rearrangement requiring de novo gene expression and protein synthesis. In striatal cells glutamate and DA receptors interact and provide a route for ERK activation.[105] It has been shown that aberrant supersensitivity of D1R leads to ERK hyperactivation in response to L-dopa, and the degree of ERK activation correlates with LID severity in the unilaterally 6-OHDA-lesioned rodent and the MPTP-treated primate.[96, 106]

The exact role of D2 receptors in LID is not yet fully understood. However, it has been shown that D2 agonists induce behavioral sensitization[58, 107] and LID in primed animals.[47, 48] The role of the D2 receptors in LID requires further investigation.[49]

There are two classic forms of synaptic plasticity at corticostriatal synapses which are opposite forms of long-term neuroplasticity: long-term potentiation (LTP) and long-term depression (LTD) which can be fully abolished after the genetic disruption of DARPP-32,[108] suggesting that the stimulation of the DA/PKA/DARPP-32/PP-1 cascade is required for the induction of these two opposite forms of neuroplasticity in the striatum. LTP and LTD represent long-lasting, activity-dependent changes in the efficacy of synaptic transmission. At striatal synapses, these two forms of plasticity are thought to underlie both motor learning and striatal-dependent cognitive tasks.[109] The requirement of DA for the induction of striatal LTP and LTD makes these two forms of synaptic plasticity unique. DA influences the physiological process of the striatum through several mechanisms, including the modulation of various voltage-gated currents. The induction of synaptic plasticity in the striatum requires interaction between DA and other neurotransmitters, including glutamate, primarily ionotropic (NMDA and AMPA) and metabotropic, receptors, as well as acetylcholine, nitric oxide, and endogenous cannabinoids. DA, functioning at DA receptors, crucially influences both the induction and the reversal of neuroplasticity at corticostriatal synapses.[110]

Normally, in striatal projecting GABAergic neurons, individual brief pulses of low-frequency stimulation (LFS) produce an excitatory postsynaptic potential (EPSP), a response that is stable to repetitive stimulation. LTP is considered to be the long-term increase of the amplitude of the EPSP that follows a burst of high-frequency stimulation of corticostriatal fibers. This long-term increase of the efficacy of synaptic transmission is widely considered to be a cellular model of learning and in the striatum strongly depends upon the activation of D1 receptors by DA arising from the substantia nigra.[111] LTP follows positive feedback rules that drive neuronal circuits toward maximal action potential firing frequency ranges, thus leading to synaptic saturation. Thus, the ability to forget or "ignore" irrelevant synaptic signals is critically important to render neurons able to encode subsequent plastic changes. The key mechanism that underlies synaptic forgetting is the "depotentiation," a form of plasticity that is considered to be the abolishment of the synaptic potentiation induced by several minutes of LFS.[42]

Several studies have been performed to characterize the modification of the main forms of striatal neuronal plasticity in experimental models of PD showing that the development of LID involves an aberrant form of plasticity at the corticostriatal synapse. In the 6-OHDA model of PD obtained by lesioning the nigrostriatal dopaminergic pathway with a local intracerebral injection of the neurotoxin 6-OHDA, LTP is lost. Nevertheless, in animals sustaining unilateral 6-OHDA lesions of the substantia nigra, corticostriatal LTP can be restored by chronic treatment with the DA precursor L-dopa.[80] Interestingly, the ability to "forget" irrelevant synaptic signals named "depotentiation" is selectively lost only in the dyskinetic animals chronically treated with L-dopa, whereas animals that do not develop involuntary movements maintain the physiological reversal of synaptic strength after LFS.[80] Such a loss of bidirectional plasticity at corticostriatal synapses may cause a pathological storage of nonessential motor information that would normally be erased, leading to the development or the expression of abnormal motor patterns. Moreover, the lack of "depotentiation" that probably represents the electrophysiological correlate of the abnormal motor patterns within the basal ganglia is attributable to changes occurring along the DA/PKA/DARPP-32/PP-1 cascade, because D1 agonists and adenylate cyclase activators can prevent LFS-induced "depotentiation".[80] It is worthwhile to note that LTP-like plasticity is deficient in PD patients and is restored by L-dopa in nondyskinetic but not in dyskinetic patients.[112] In line with this hypothesis, it has been suggested that D1 receptor blockade improves LID.[113]

Although preclinical and clinical findings suggest pulsatile stimulation of striatal postsynaptic receptors as a key pathogenic mechanism underlying LIDs, recent studies indicate that L-dopa-induced plasticity may also affect presynaptic mechanisms involving L-dopa or DA uptake, conversion, and metabolism in the brain.[114, 115] These studies also raise the possibility that individual differences in the susceptibility to dyskinesia may reflect a variation in the magnitude and kinetics of central changes in L-dopa and DA levels following peripheral drug administration. PET studies in PD patients have shown that rapid fluctuations in central DA levels are at the heart of both motor fluctuations and dyskinesias.[24, 116] The pathophysiological importance of central pharmacokinetic mechanisms is further supported by the observation that the incidence of dyskinesia is lower in patients on treatment with direct DA agonists instead of L-dopa.[34] Unlike L-dopa, the DA agonists have a long half-life, which prevents the occurrence of rapid and transient fluctuations in central levels of DA receptor

occupancy. Unfortunately these drugs do not provide an alternative to L-dopa in the more advanced stages of PD, as they are less effective than the DA precursor in ameliorating PD motor symptoms.[117]

# Therapeutic consideration in the management of LIDs

Treatment strategies of recently diagnosed PD patients or those with advanced disease should be tailored for each individual. For example, because of the higher risk of LIDs in young-onset patients, most parkinson specialists prefer delaying L-dopa therapy unless the PD symptoms interfere with the patient's functioning at home or at work (Figure 11.1). Although there are currently no drugs approved by the Food and Drugs Administration (FDA) for the treatment of LID, several novel anti-LID drugs are currently being investigated in preclinical and clinical trials.[118]

## 1. Glutamate receptor antagonists

Abnormalities in the thalamo- and cortico-striatal glutamatergic transmission have long been implicated in the pathogenesis of LIDs. The thalamostriatal system consists of multiple neural systems that originate from a wide variety of thalamic nuclei and terminate in functionally segregated striatal territories where ionotropic (NMDA and AMPA) and metabotropic receptors are densely present. Moreover, abnormal phosphorylation and synaptic redistribution of several NMDA subunit receptors seem to play an important role in the expression of LIDs, and have been found in the dyskinetic state.[119] An increase in the binding of these receptors has been reported in patients with LIDs,[120] leading to a state of hypersensitivity to glutamatergic action in the dopaminergic neurons in the substantia nigra.[121] Subsequently, glutamate-mediated neurodegeneration ensues, facilitating the expression of LIDs after L-dopa treatment.

Despite existing data at the preclinical level showing the antidyskinetic effect of several NMDA modulators, the results from clinical trials using NMDA antagonists for the treatment of LIDs have been disappointing. Therefore, none of the agents with anti-NMDA activity has been approved by the FDA for the treatment of LIDs.[122] The story is different, however, for amantadine.

Amantadine, a low-affinity, noncompetitive NMDA receptor antagonist has been considered the most effective drug used in reduction of dyskinesia

**Management of Motor Complications in Parkinson's Disease**

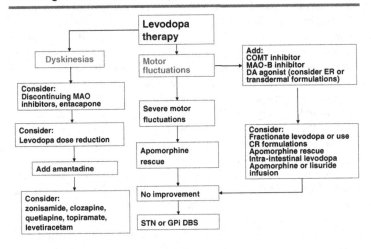

**Figure 11.1** Management of motor complications in Parkinson's disease

without worsening of motor performance. Luginger et al.[128] studied the effect of amantadine in patients with LIDs in a 5-week, double-blind crossover trial. Dyskinesia severity assessed following oral L-dopa challenges and by self-scoring dyskinesia diaries was reduced by approximately 50% after amantadine treatment compared with baseline or placebo. Similarly, dyskinesia assessments on the Unified Parkinson's Disease Rating Scale (UPDRS) part IV also revealed significant improvement after treatment with amantadine. The magnitude of the L-dopa motor response to oral challenges was not different after amantadine or placebo treatment, and there was no significant reduction of daily off time when patients received active treatment.[123] Another double-blind, placebo-controlled, crossover study of 18 advanced PD patients attempted to determine the effects of amantadine on LIDs and motor fluctuations in PD.[129] In the 14 patients completing this trial, amantadine significantly reduced dyskinesia severity by 60% compared to placebo, without altering the antiparkinsonian effect of L-dopa. Motor fluctuations occurring with patients' regular oral L-dopa regimen also improved according to UPDRS and patient-kept diaries[124] There have been a few more double-blind, placebo-controlled studies showing improvement of dyskinesia after amantadine administration. Snow et al.[130] showed a 24% reduction without any influence on the severity of "on" period parkinsonism. On the other hand Da Silva-Junior et al.[125] demonstrated that the duration of LIDs was reduced by amantadine

despite the fact that the dyskinesia scores were not changed, and that amantadine significantly decreased UPDRS scores, showing that this substance can improve the subjective experience of dyskinesias.

Most of these efficacy studies had active treatment periods of only 2 to 4 weeks and data on the long-term antidyskinetic effect of amantadine are limited and contradictory. A double-blind study was designed to assess the duration of the antidyskinetic effect of amantadine on LID over a period of 12 months. Forty patients treated for 7.5 (S.D. 2.2) years with levodopa 729.3 (S.D. 199.4) mg/day and DA agonists, having peak-dose or diphasic dyskinesia with or without pain, were assessed. Twenty patients received amantadine (300 mg) and 20 received a placebo. After 15 days of amantadine treatment there was a reduction by 45% in the total dyskinesia scores; however, all patients receiving amantadine were withdrawn in 3–8 months, inducing a rebound with increase of dyskinesia by 10%–20% in 11 patients.[126] One year after completion of an acute, double-blind, placebo-controlled, crossover study, 17 of the original 18 patients returned for reevaluation (13 remained on amantadine) of motor symptoms and duration of antidyskinetic effect of amantadine in advanced PD. Results showed that one year after initiation of amantadine cotherapy, its antidyskinetic effect was similar in magnitude (56% reduction in dyskinesia compared with 60% 1 year earlier). Motor complications occurring with the patients' regular oral L-dopa regimen also remained improved according to the UPDRS part

IV scores.[127] A randomized placebo-controlled parallel group study was performed to assess the long-term antidyskinetic effect of amantadine in 32 PD patients on stable amantadine therapy for LID over at least one year.[128] The mean duration of amantadine treatment in all patients was 4.8 (2.9) years. Patients were switched in a double-blind manner to amantadine or placebo and followed for 3 weeks. In order to determine whether early treatment with amantadine would delay the development of LIDs, patients with the clinical diagnosis of PD with no history of anti-PD drugs at first visit and subsequently treated with L-dopa for at least 5 years were divided in two groups. Group A received amantadine prior to L-dopa use while group B did not. Amantadine treatment prior to the use of L-dopa did not delay onset of LID nor reduce the incidence of LID.[129] Dyskinesia duration and intensity assessed in these intervals showed a significant increase of UPDRS part IV scores in patients treated with placebo compared with no significant change in patients staying on amantadine. In the AMANDYSK trial, 57 amantadine-treated patients were randomly switched to placebo and the washout of amantadine was associated with marked worsening of LIDs in a median time of 7 days.[130]

Currently, there are two ongoing multicenter, randomized, double-blind, placebo-controlled study to evaluate the tolerability and efficacy of each of three dose levels of extended-release formulations of amantadine (Adamas and Osmotica formulations), dosed once daily for the treatment of LIDs in subjects with PD. The use of this medication is expected to improve safety and tolerability of amantadine via the stabilization of its plasma concentrations throughout the day.[131]

Other agents that block NMDA receptors (remacemide[132] and riluzole,[133] both noncompetitive NMDA receptor antagonists) have not been proven to be of benefit for the management of LIDs in PD patients. However, another antagonist, dextromethorphan, was given to PD patients with motor fluctuations in a double-blind, placebo-controlled, crossover study, showing that average and maximum dyskinesia scores improved by >50%, without compromising the antiparkinsonian response magnitude or duration of L-dopa.[134] There is an ongoing clinical trial to evaluate the efficacy, safety, and tolerability of the use of a new compound containing 45mg dextromethorphan and 10mg quinidine (a potent inhibitor of CYP2D6 which in turn metabolizes

dextromethorphan rapidly and extensively) compared with placebo for the treatment of LIDs in PD patients.[135]

The effect of memantine on cardinal symptoms of PD on patients with LIDs was studied in a crossover design by randomizing subjects to memantine or placebo. Results showed that memantine may improve parkinsonian symptoms independently of dopaminergic drugs but without improvement of LIDs.[136] A randomized, double-blind study giving memantine versus placebo analyzed motor and dyskinesia scores and their axial subscores, demonstrating that memantine treatment was associated with lower axial motor symptoms and dyskinesia scores.[137] Varanese et al.[143] described the effects of memantine in 3 patients with motor complications and their follow-up evaluations at 1–5 years, suggesting that memantine may be a potentially effective drug with a low side effect profile for the treatment of LIDs in PD, particularly when other alternative agents such as amantadine are contraindicated. Unexpectedly, Vidal et al.[138] reported improvement of LIDs in 2 cases of individuals diagnosed with PD dementia who were started on memantine, given for cognitive improvement, but whose most impressive clinical outcome was the unanticipated improvement in dyskinesias. During the last few years, a number of studies have tested selective NMDA antagonists in the treatment of LIDs, though without robust effect.[139–141]

A number of preclinical studies have highlighted the involvement of metabotropic glutamate receptors (mGluRs) in the pathophysiology of LIDs.[142] Antagonists of mGluR5 reduce overactivity of NMDA receptors and resulting overexcitability, both important factors in the expression of LIDs. The effect of the mGluR5 antagonist [(2-methyl-1,3-thiazol-4-yl)ethynyl]pyridine (MTEP) was analyzed in an experimental model of PD with LID in 6-OHDA-lesioned rats, demonstrating that mGluR5 antagonists may be useful for the symptomatic treatment of LIDs.[143] Other mGluR5 inhibitors, such as AFQ056 (mavoglurant) and ADX48621 (dipraglurant) are currently in clinical trials in the treatment of LIDs.[144, 145]

A model of MPTP-induced PD monkeys treated with L-dopa was used to investigate the acute effects of the novel mGluR5 antagonist AFQ056 (mavoglurant) on motor behavior and dyskinesias, showing LIDs reduction without affecting the beneficial motor effects of L-dopa.[146] Berg et al.[152] assessed the efficacy, safety, and tolerability of AFQ056 in PD patients with

LIDs in two randomized, double-blind, placebo-controlled studies with moderate to severe LID (study 1) and severe LID (study 2) on stable dopaminergic therapy to those randomized to placebo. A double-blind, placebo-controlled study of patients with PD and moderate to severe LIDs who were receiving stable L-dopa/antiparkinsonian treatment and were not currently receiving amantadine, were randomized to receive either different doses of AFQ056 or placebo.[147] Patients randomized to AFQ056 200 mg daily administered in 2 doses had a significant improvement in dyskinesia at week 12 compared to those randomized to placebo in a dose-response relationship. The most common adverse events were dizziness, hallucinations, fatigue, nasopharyngitis, diarrhea, and insomnia. Currently, there is an ongoing, open-label study to generate long-term safety, tolerability, and efficacy data for AFQ056 in patients who have participated in and completed any AFQ056 phase II study in PD-LID.[148]

Dipraglurant (ADX48621), a novel mGluR5 negative allosteric modulator, was evaluated for the safety, tolerability, and antidyskinetic profile in PD patients with LID.[149] Seventy-six patients with moderate to severe LID were randomized in a double-blind placebo-controlled study. Dipraglurant significantly reduced dyskinesia without affecting L-dopa efficacy. There were no significant changes in safety monitoring parameters. Furthermore, dipraglurant increased daily "on" time without dyskinesia in weeks 1, 2, 3, and 4 and reduced daily "off" time at week 4.

There is evidence regarding the contribution of AMPA receptors to the pathogenesis of parkinsonian signs and LIDs. Konitsiotis et al.[156] compared the ability of an AMPA agonist (CX516) and a noncompetitive AMPA antagonist (LY300164) to alter parkinsonian symptoms and LID in MPTP-lesioned monkeys. CX516 alone, and when combined with low-dose L-dopa, did not affect motor activity but did induce dyskinesia. Moreover, following injection of the higher doses of L-dopa, it increased LID by up to 52%. LY300164 (talampanel) potentiated the motor activating effects of L-dopa and at the same time decreased LID by up to 40%.[150] Several clinical studies have evaluated the effects of talampanel in PD and LID; however, no data have been published.[122]

Perampanel, a novel, noncompetitive, selective AMPA-receptor antagonist demonstrated evidence of efficacy in reducing motor symptoms in animal models of PD. One study assessed the safety and efficacy of different doses of perampanel versus placebo for treatment of "wearing off" motor fluctuations in patients with PD.[151] There were no significant changes in dyskinesia or cognitive function when perampanel was compared to placebo. Two multicenter randomized, double-blind, placebo-controlled, parallel group phase III studies assessed the efficacy and safety of adjunctive perampanel in patients with PD and motor fluctuations. In neither of these studies was perampanel superior to placebo in improving motor symptoms or LIDs.[152] Another study aimed to assess the efficacy and tolerability of perampanel in L-dopa-treated patients with moderately severe PD and motor fluctuations using an active comparator study design.[153] Although perampanel was generally well tolerated, it was not superior to placebo on any efficacy end point measures including duration and severity of dyskinesias.

# 2. Alpha2-adrenergic receptor antagonists

Studies in the MPTP-lesioned primate model of PD have demonstrated that alpha2-adrenergic receptor antagonists can alleviate LID.[154–157] Fipamezole is an alpha2-antagonist which has a high affinity at human alpha(2A), alpha(2B), and alpha(2C) receptors. It also has a moderate affinity at histamine H1 and H3 receptors and serotonin (5-HT) transporter. In the MPTP-lesioned marmoset, fipamezole significantly reduced LID without compromising the antiparkinsonian action of L-dopa.[154] The duration of action of the combination of L-dopa and fipamezole was 66% greater than that of L-dopa alone.

A proof-of-concept study in 10 PD patients with LIDs showed beneficial effects at single doses of 60 and 90 mg of fipamezole in a double-blind, randomized, placebo-controlled, dose-escalating 28-day study conducted at 25 centers in the United States and seven centers in India.[155] There was no statistically significant difference in suppressing LID between fipamezole and placebo. However, because of inhomogeneity recognized between U.S. and Indian study populations, a prespecified subgroup analysis of the U.S. population showed that fipamezole at 90 mg reduced LIDs. Fipamezole was associated with an acceptable profile of adverse effects, including mild, transient elevation of blood pressure.

A study of the selective and potent alpha2-adrenergic receptor antagonist, idazoxan, showed that the drug reduces LIDs in the MPTP-lesioned marmoset model of PD.[162] Furthermore, the coadministration of idazoxan with L-dopa more than doubled its duration of action as an antiparkinsonian drug compared to that seen with L-dopa alone. However, idazoxan as a monotherapy displayed no antiparkinsonian effect. Another experimental study in MPTP-lesioned monkeys demonstrated that idazoxan alone increased locomotor activity and improved the disability score with virtually no dyskinesias in 50% of the animals.[156] In combination with L-dopa, idazoxan did not impair the antiparkinsonian response but significantly reduced dyskinesias in all animals up to 65% and delayed their onset. A pilot, randomized, placebo-controlled study in PD patients with LID assessed the effects of single oral doses of idazoxan on motor parkinsonian disability and LID. The severity of LID improved after 20 mg idazoxan pretreatment, while there was no concomitant deterioration in the antiparkinsonian response to L-dopa.[157] However, the same dosage in another trial proved to be ineffective and caused adverse effects.[158] An in vivo microdialysis analysis in 6-OHDA-lesioned rats with LIDs showed that the decrease of L-dopa-derived extracellular DA levels in the lesioned striatum in dyskinetic rats significantly contributed to the antidyskinetic effect of idazoxan.[159]

## 3. Adenosine A$_{2A}$-receptor antagonists

Preladenant is one of the most selective A2A-receptor antagonists, with a robust in vivo activity.[167] In 6-OHDA-lesioned rats, daily administration of preladenant showed inhibition of L-dopa-induced behavioral sensitization, which suggested that this drug had the potential to reduce the risk of LIDs. Subsequently, the effects of preladenant in MPTP-lesioned primate models of PD with LID were investigated showing evidence of improvement of motor ability without induction of LIDs.[160] Hauser et al.[161] aimed to assess the efficacy and safety of preladenant in patients with PD and motor fluctuations who were receiving L-dopa and other antiparkinsonian drugs. This phase 2, randomized, placebo-controlled, double-blind trial enrolled 253 patients at 44 sites in 15 countries. At week 12, the mean daily off time (primary outcome measure) was significantly reduced compared to placebo in patients on 5 mg and 10 mg of preladenant. The most common adverse events were worsening of parkinsonism, somnolence, dyskinesia, nausea, constipation, and insomnia. Although the use of

preladenant twice daily was clinically useful to reduce off time, it failed to significantly improve LID. The 36-week, open-label phase, follow-up study of preladenant 5 mg twice a day as an L-dopa adjunct in 140 subjects with fluctuating PD reported treatment-emergent adverse events by ≥15% of subjects, including dyskinesia (33%) and constipation (19%). Preladenant treatment also provided "off" time reductions and "on" time increases, but at the expense of increased dyskinesia rates.[162]

## 4. Nicotinic acetylcholine-receptor agonists

Nicotinic receptors have been implicated in the expression of LID in PD, although solid scientific support is lacking. Nicotine and nicotinic agonists increase dopamine release from mesolimbic and nigrostriatal neurons in vitro and in vivo. There is ample evidence from in vitro experiments on synaptosome preparations for the facilitation of basal dopamine release by presynaptic nicotinic receptors on striatal dopaminergic terminals causing excitation of dopaminergic SNc neurons as well as a modulatory influence.[163]

Nicotine, a nonspecific agonist of nicotinic receptors, is very effective in preventing the occurrence of LIDs and reducing established LIDs in several parkinsonian animal models. However, preclinical results are limited and should be interpreted with caution.[122]

## 5. Other pharmacological treatments

Clozapine was the first "atypical" antipsychotic, and appears to be free of extrapyramidal side effects despite its D2 receptor blocking action. It has effects on a large number of neurotransmitter systems so that interpretation of its modes of action is open to much speculation. In addition to having antitremor activity in PD, it has been reported in a double-blind, placebo-controlled trial of 50 subjects, to reduce dyskinesias, reduce on time with dyskinesias without increasing off time.[164] The mean dose used was 39 mg/d. Prospective, open-label studies have also supported the beneficial effect of clozapine on dyskinesias, without reducing on time or worsening motor function, with one study using only 30 mg/d,[165] whereas another used doses that were generally between 100 and 200 mg/d, with one subject on 400 mg/d.[166] The higher doses produced marked somnolence, offsetting the benefit.

**Table 11.1** Pharmacological compounds used for the management of LID

1. Glutamate receptor antagonists

   a. NMDA antagonists

      i. amantadine

      ii. extended-release formulation of amantadine (ADS-5102)

      iii. remacemide

      iv. riluzole

      v. dextromethorphan (+/- quinidine)

      iv. memantine

   b. mGluR antagonists

      i. mavoglurant (AFQ056)

      ii. dipraglurant (ADX48621)

   c. AMPA antagonists

      i. AMPA agonist (CX516)

      ii. talampanel (LY300164)

      iii. perampanel

2. Alpha2-adrenergic-receptor antagonists

   a. fipamezole

   b. idazoxan

3. Adenosine$A_{2A}$-receptor antagonists

   a. preladenant

   b. istradefylline

   c. tozadenant (SYN115)

4. Nicotinic acetylcholine-receptor agonists

   a. nicotine

   b. SIB-1508Y

5. Other potential pharmacological treatments

   a. partial dopamine agonists (aripiprazole, pardoprunox, aplindore)

   b. monoamine oxidase-B inhibitors (selegiline, rasagiline, safinamide)

   c. 5-HT agonists (tandospirone, sarizotane, piclozotan, neurolixis, anpirtoline)

   d. anticonvulsants (valproate, gabapentin, zonisamide, levetiracetam, topiramate)

   e. cannabidiol extract

   f. clozapine

   g. nalbuphine (µ receptor antagonist)

   h. pridopidine (dopamine stabilizer)

Other treatment options that have been studied include partial dopamine agonists (aripiprazole,[167] pardoprunox[168, 169]), monoamine oxidase-B inhibitors (selegiline,[170] rasagiline,[171] safinamide[172]), cannabidiol

extract,[173] 5-HT agonists, and anticonvulsants.[118] However, their use remains limited, as the great majority have failed to confirm safety, tolerability, or effectiveness. Numerous ongoing studies, involving dopaminergic and nondopaminergic pathways, are attempting to provide further information about these parameters, constituting innovative steps toward novel therapeutic approaches toward this disabling complication of L-dopa.

# Neurosurgical treatment of LIDs

It is beyond the scope of this chapter to comprehensively review the effects of neurosurgical interventions in the treatment of LIDs in PD. Both pallidotomy and pallidal deep brain stimulation (DBS) are probably the most effective neurosurgical treatment, because they significantly improve all of the LIDs, including off-period dystonia, without reduction of L-dopa dosage. Subthalamic (STN) DBS has no direct therapeutic effects on LID, but can substantially improve this iatrogenic symptom as a result of decreased L-dopa dosage.[174] Pallidotomy and globus pallidus internus (GPi) DBS or subthalamotomy and STN DBS have assumed a pivotal role in surgical treatment of PD. Interventions in either the STN or the GPi seem to be similar in controlling most of the other motor aspects of PD; nonetheless, GPi surgery seems to induce a more particular and direct effect on dyskinesia, while the antidyskinetic effect of STN interventions is mostly dependent on a reduction of dopaminergic drug dosages.[175]

The first double-blind, crossover study evaluating the results of GPi versus STN DBS in PD showed that both procedures significantly reduced dyskinesia (by 58% with STN DBS and 66% with GPi DBS).[176] Furthermore, the average medication dosage, measured in L-dopa equivalents, was decreased significantly more with STN DBS. Another study with a longer follow-up, mean 48.5 months, showed 64% mean improvement in LID after this period of observation.[177] Eleven PD patients undergoing GPi DBS were followed for 5 years showing that, despite a decline on the motor benefit for the off-period scores after 3 years, the improvement in LID was sustained.[178]

Long-term studies of bilateral STN DBS in patients with advanced PD have demonstrated the sustained efficacy of this therapy over time. A 5-year prospective study of 49 consecutive patients treated with STN DBS noted improvement of LIDs with dyskinesia disability and duration at 5 years being improved by 58% and 71%, respectively, in comparison with baseline.[179] Similar benefits with respect to dyskinesia were observed in a 5-year follow-up of 37 PD patients treated with stimulation of the STN.[180] Finally, a comprehensive metaanalysis of 921 patients who underwent STN DBS between 1993 and 2004 noted an average reduction in LID following surgery of 69.1%.[181]

In conclusion, although STN and GPi procedures have different mechanisms of action, both are effective treatment strategies to control LIDs. GPi interventions may have a more immediate effect, independent of reduction of L-dopa daily dosage; although the tendency is to adopt STN DBS, as this procedure also brings marginally better improvements in off-period motor scores than GPI DBS.[182]

# References

1. Obeso JA, Olanow CW, Nutt JG. Levodopa motor complications in Parkinson's disease. *Trends in neurosciences* 2000;**23**:S2–7.

2. Olanow CW. The scientific basis for the current treatment of Parkinson's disease. *Annual review of medicine* 2004;**55**:41–60.

3. Voon V, Fernagut PO, Wickens J, et al. Chronic dopaminergic stimulation in Parkinson's disease: from dyskinesias to impulse control disorders. *Lancet neurology* 2009;**8**:1140–1149.

4. Nutt JG, Chung KA, Holford NH. Dyskinesia and the antiparkinsonian response always temporally coincide: a retrospective study. *Neurology* 2010;**74**:1191–1197.

5. Fahn S, Jankovic J, Hallett M. *Principles and practice of movement disorders*, 2nd ed. Edinburgh; New York: Elsevier/Saunders, 2011.

6. Hauser RA, Friedlander J, Zesiewicz TA, et al. A home diary to assess functional status in patients with Parkinson's disease with motor fluctuations and dyskinesia. *Clinical neuropharmacology* 2000;**23**:75–81.

7. Fabbrini G, Brotchie JM, Grandas F, Nomoto M, Goetz CG. Levodopa-induced dyskinesias. *Movement disorders: official journal of the Movement Disorder Society* 2007;**22**:1379–1389;quiz 1523.

8. Reimer J, Grabowski M, Lindvall O, Hagell P. Use and interpretation of on/off diaries in Parkinson's disease. *Journal of neurology, neurosurgery, and psychiatry* 2004;**75**:396–400.

9. Colosimo C, Martinez-Martin P, Fabbrini G, et al. Task force report on scales to assess dyskinesia in Parkinson's disease: critique and recommendations. *Movement disorders: official journal of the Movement Disorder Society* 2010;**25**:1131–1142.

10. Goetz CG, Stebbins GT, Chung KA, et al. Which dyskinesia scale best detects treatment response? *Movement disorders: official journal of the Movement Disorder Society* 2013;**28**:341–346.

11. Stacy MA, Murphy JM, Greeley DR, et al. The sensitivity and specificity of the 9-item Wearing-off Questionnaire. *Parkinsonism & related disorders* 2008;**14**:205–212.

12. Katzenschlager R, Schrag A, Evans A, et al. Quantifying the impact of dyskinesias in PD: the PDYS-26: a patient-based outcome measure. *Neurology* 2007;**69**:555–563.

13. Jankovic J. Motor fluctuations and dyskinesias in Parkinson's disease: clinical manifestations. *Movement disorders: official journal of the Movement Disorder Society* 2005;**20** Suppl 11:S11–16.

14. Schrag A, Ben-Shlomo Y, Brown R, Marsden CD, Quinn N. Young-onset Parkinson's disease revisited-clinical features, natural history, and mortality. *Movement disorders: official journal of the Movement Disorder Society* 1998;**13**:885–894.

15. Blanchet PJ, Allard P, Gregoire L, Tardif F, Bedard PJ. Risk factors for peak dose dyskinesia in 100 levodopa-treated parkinsonian patients. *The Canadian journal of neurological sciences. Le journal canadien des sciences neurologiques* 1996;**23**:189–193.

16. Kumar N, Van Gerpen JA, Bower JH, Ahlskog JE. Levodopa-dyskinesia incidence by age of Parkinson's disease onset. *Movement disorders: official journal of the Movement Disorder Society* 2005;**20**:342–344.

17. Ku S, Glass GA. Age of Parkinson's disease onset as a predictor for the development of dyskinesia. *Movement disorders: official journal of the Movement Disorder Society* 2010;**25**:1177–1182.

18. Di Monte DA, McCormack A, Petzinger G, Janson AM, Quik M, Langston WJ. Relationship among nigrostriatal denervation, parkinsonism, and dyskinesias in the MPTP primate model. *Movement disorders: official journal of the Movement Disorder Society* 2000;**15**:459–466.

19. Vidailhet M, Bonnet AM, Marconi R, Gouider-Khouja N, Agid Y. Do parkinsonian symptoms and levodopa-induced dyskinesias start in the foot? *Neurology* 1994;**44**:1613–1616.

20. Khan NL, Graham E, Critchley P, et al. Parkin disease: a phenotypic study of a large case series. *Brain: a journal of neurology* 2003;**126**:1279–1292.

21. Scherfler C, Khan NL, Pavese N, et al. Striatal and cortical pre- and postsynaptic dopaminergic dysfunction in sporadic parkin-linked parkinsonism. *Brain: a journal of neurology* 2004;**127**:1332–1342.

22. Calon F, Morissette M, Rajput AH, Hornykiewicz O, Bedard PJ, Di Paolo T. Changes of GABA receptors and dopamine turnover in the postmortem brains of parkinsonians with levodopa-induced motor complications. *Movement disorders: official journal of the Movement Disorder Society* 2003;**18**:241–253.

23. Togasaki DM, Tan L, Protell P, Di Monte DA, Quik M, Langston JW. Levodopa induces dyskinesias in normal squirrel monkeys. *Annals of neurology* 2001;**50**:254–257.

24. de la Fuente-Fernandez R, Schulzer M, Mak E, Calne DB, Stoessl AJ. Presynaptic mechanisms of motor fluctuations in Parkinson's disease: a probabilistic model. *Brain: a journal of neurology* 2004;**127**:888–899.

25. Linazasoro G, Antonini A, Maguire RP, Leenders KL. Pharmacological and PET studies in patients with Parkinson's disease and a short duration-motor response: implications in the pathophysiology of motor complications. *Journal of neural transmission* 2004;**111**:497–509.

26. Troiano AR, de la Fuente-Fernandez R, Sossi V, et al. PET demonstrates reduced dopamine transporter expression in PD with dyskinesias. *Neurology* 2009;**72**:1211–1216.

27. Hong JY, Oh JS, Lee I, et al. Presynaptic dopamine depletion predicts levodopa-induced dyskinesia in de novo Parkinson disease. *Neurology* 2014;**82**:1597–1604.

28. Linazasoro G, Van Blercom N, Bergaretxe A, Inaki FM, Laborda E, Ruiz Ortega JA. Levodopa-induced dyskinesias in Parkinson disease are independent of the extent of striatal dopaminergic denervation: a pharmacological and SPECT study. *Clinical neuropharmacology* 2009;**32**:326–329.

29. Schneider JS, Gonczi H, Decamp E. Development of levodopa-induced dyskinesias in parkinsonian monkeys may depend upon rate of symptom onset and/or duration of symptoms. *Brain research* 2003;**990**:38–44.

30. Ahlskog JE, Muenter MD. Frequency of levodopa-related dyskinesias and motor fluctuations as estimated from the cumulative literature. *Movement disorders: official journal of the Movement Disorder Society* 2001;**16**:448–458.

31. Fahn S, Oakes D, Shoulson I, et al. Levodopa and the progression of Parkinson's disease. *The New England journal of medicine* 2004;**351**:2498–2508.

32. Khan NL, Valente EM, Bentivoglio AR, et al. Clinical and subclinical dopaminergic dysfunction in PARK6-linked parkinsonism: an 18F-dopa PET study. *Annals of neurology* 2002;**52**:849–853.

33. Dekker M, Bonifati V, van Swieten J, et al. Clinical features and neuroimaging of PARK7-linked parkinsonism. *Movement disorders: official journal of the Movement Disorder Society* 2003;**18**:751–757.

34. Rascol O, Brooks DJ, Korczyn AD, De Deyn PP, Clarke CE, Lang AE. A five-year study of the incidence of dyskinesia in patients with early Parkinson's disease who were treated with ropinirole or levodopa. 056 Study Group. *The New England journal of medicine* 2000;**342**:1484–1491.

35. Hauser RA, Rascol O, Korczyn AD, et al. Ten-year follow-up of Parkinson's disease patients randomized to initial therapy with ropinirole or levodopa. *Movement disorders: official journal of the Movement Disorder Society* 2007;**22**:2409–2417.

36. Lopez IC, Ruiz PJ, Del Pozo SV, Bernardos VS. Motor complications in Parkinson's disease: ten year follow-up study. *Movement disorders: official journal of the Movement Disorder Society* 2010;**25**:2735–2739.

37. Zappia M, Annesi G, Nicoletti G, et al. Sex differences in clinical and genetic determinants of levodopa peak-dose dyskinesias in Parkinson disease: an exploratory study. *Archives of neurology* 2005;**62**:601–605.

38. Wang J, Liu ZL, Chen B. Association study of dopamine D2, D3 receptor gene polymorphisms with motor fluctuations in PD. *Neurology* 2001;**56**:1757–1759.

39. Lee JY, Cho J, Lee EK, Park SS, Jeon BS. Differential genetic susceptibility in diphasic and peak-dose dyskinesias in Parkinson's disease. *Movement disorders: official journal of the Movement Disorder Society* 2011;**26**:73–79.

40. Foltynie T, Cheeran B, Williams-Gray CH, et al. BDNF val66met influences time to onset of levodopa induced dyskinesia in Parkinson's disease. *Journal of neurology, neurosurgery, and psychiatry* 2009;**80**:141–144.

41. Obeso JA, Grandas F, Herrero MT, Horowski R. The role of pulsatile versus continuous dopamine receptor stimulation for functional recovery in Parkinson's disease. *The European journal of neuroscience* 1994;**6**:889–897.

42. Calabresi P, Di Filippo M, Ghiglieri V, Picconi B. Molecular mechanisms underlying levodopa-induced dyskinesia. *Movement disorders: official journal of the Movement Disorder Society* 2008;**23** Suppl 3:S570–579.

43. Grace AA. Phasic versus tonic dopamine release and the modulation of dopamine system responsivity: a hypothesis for the etiology of schizophrenia. *Neuroscience* 1991;**41**:1–24.

44. Venton BJ, Zhang H, Garris PA, Phillips PE, Sulzer D, Wightman RM. Real-time decoding of dopamine concentration changes in the caudate-putamen during tonic and phasic firing. *Journal of neurochemistry* 2003;**87**:1284–1295.

45. Zigmond MJ, Abercrombie ED, Berger TW, Grace AA, Stricker EM. Compensations after lesions of central dopaminergic neurons: some clinical and basic implications. *Trends in neurosciences* 1990;**13**:290–296.

46. Lewitt PA, Mouradian MM. Predicting the development of levodopa-induced dyskinesias: A presynaptic mechanism? *Neurology* 2014;**82**:1574–1575.

47. Bezard E, Brotchie JM, Gross CE. Pathophysiology of levodopa-induced dyskinesia: potential for new therapies. *Nature reviews Neuroscience* 2001;**2**:577–588.

48. Jenner P. Molecular mechanisms of L-DOPA-induced dyskinesia. *Nature reviews Neuroscience* 2008;**9**:665–677.

49. Berthet A, Bezard E. Dopamine receptors and L-dopa-induced dyskinesia. *Parkinsonism & related disorders* 2009;**15** Suppl 4:S8–12.

50. Missale C, Nash SR, Robinson SW, Jaber M, Caron MG. Dopamine receptors: from structure to function. *Physiological reviews* 1998;**78**:189–225.

51. Le Moine C, Bloch B. D1 and D2 dopamine receptor gene expression in the rat striatum: sensitive cRNA probes demonstrate prominent segregation of D1 and D2 mRNAs in distinct neuronal populations of the dorsal and ventral striatum. *The Journal of comparative neurology* 1995;**355**:418–426.

52. Landwehrmeyer B, Mengod G, Palacios JM. Differential visualization of dopamine D2 and D3 receptor sites in rat brain. A comparative study using in situ hybridization histochemistry and ligand binding autoradiography. *The European journal of neuroscience* 1993;**5**:145–153.

53. Bezard E, Ferry S, Mach U, et al. Attenuation of levodopa-induced dyskinesia by normalizing dopamine D3 receptor function. *Nature medicine* 2003;**9**:762–767.

54. Gerfen CR, Engber TM, Mahan LC, et al. D1 and D2 dopamine receptor-regulated gene expression of striatonigral and striatopallidal neurons. *Science* 1990;**250**:1429–1432.

55. Alexander GE, Crutcher MD. Functional architecture of basal ganglia circuits: neural substrates of parallel processing. *Trends in neurosciences* 1990;**13**:266–271.

56. Le W, Sayana P, Jankovic J. Animal models of Parkinson's disease: a gateway to therapeutics? *Neurotherapeutics: the journal of the American Society for Experimental NeuroTherapeutics* 2014;**11**:92–110.

57. Di Chiara G, Morelli M, Barone P, Pontieri F. Priming as a model of behavioural sensitization. *Developmental pharmacology and therapeutics* 1992;**18**:223–227.

58. Morelli M, Fenu S, Garau L, Di Chiara G. Time and dose dependence of the 'priming' of the expression of dopamine receptor supersensitivity. *European journal of pharmacology* 1989;**162**:329–335.

59. Cenci MA, Lee CS, Bjorklund A. L-DOPA-induced dyskinesia in the rat is associated with striatal overexpression of prodynorphin- and glutamic acid decarboxylase mRNA. *The European journal of neuroscience* 1998;**10**:2694–2706.

60. Lundblad M, Andersson M, Winkler C, Kirik D, Wierup N, Cenci MA. Pharmacological validation of behavioural measures of akinesia and dyskinesia in a rat model of Parkinson's disease. *The European journal of neuroscience* 2002;**15**:120–132.

61. Picconi B, Centonze D, Rossi S, Bernardi G, Calabresi P. Therapeutic doses of L-dopa reverse hypersensitivity of corticostriatal D2-dopamine receptors and glutamatergic overactivity in experimental parkinsonism. *Brain: a journal of neurology* 2004;**127**:1661–1669.

62. Gasparini F, Di Paolo T, Gomez-Mancilla B. Metabotropic glutamate receptors for Parkinson's disease therapy. *Parkinson's disease* 2013;**2013**:196028.

63. van Zundert B, Yoshii A, Constantine-Paton M. Receptor compartmentalization and trafficking at glutamate synapses: a developmental proposal. *Trends in neurosciences* 2004;**27**:428–437.

64. Hurley MJ, Jackson MJ, Smith LA, Rose S, Jenner P. Immunoautoradiographic analysis of NMDA receptor subunits and associated postsynaptic density proteins in the brain of dyskinetic MPTP-treated common marmosets. *The European journal of neuroscience* 2005;**21**:3240–3250.

65. Bibbiani F, Oh JD, Kielaite A, Collins MA, Smith C, Chase TN. Combined blockade of AMPA and NMDA glutamate receptors reduces levodopa-induced motor complications in animal models of PD. *Experimental neurology* 2005;**196**:422–429.

66. Del Dotto P, Pavese N, Gambaccini G, et al. Intravenous amantadine improves levadopa-induced dyskinesias: an acute double-blind placebo-controlled study. *Movement disorders: official journal of the Movement Disorder Society* 2001;**16**:515–520.

67. Gardoni F, Picconi B, Ghiglieri V, et al. A critical interaction between NR2B and MAGUK in L-DOPA induced dyskinesia. *The Journal of neuroscience: the official journal of the Society for Neuroscience* 2006;**26**:2914–2922.

68. Missale C, Fiorentini C, Busi C, Collo G, Spano PF. The NMDA/D1 receptor complex as a new target in drug development. *Current topics in medicinal chemistry* 2006;**6**:801–808.

69. Hallett PJ, Spoelgen R, Hyman BT, Standaert DG, Dunah AW. Dopamine D1 activation potentiates striatal NMDA receptors by tyrosine phosphorylation-dependent subunit trafficking. *The Journal of neuroscience: the official journal of the Society for Neuroscience* 2006;**26**:4690–4700.

70. Schwarzschild MA, Agnati L, Fuxe K, Chen JF, Morelli M. Targeting adenosine A2A receptors in Parkinson's disease. *Trends in neurosciences* 2006;**29**:647–654.

71. Xiao D, Bastia E, Xu YH, et al. Forebrain adenosine A2A receptors contribute to L-3,4-dihydroxyphenylalanine-induced dyskinesia in

hemiparkinsonian mice. *The Journal of neuroscience: the official journal of the Society for Neuroscience* 2006;**26**:13548–13555.

72. Calon F, Dridi M, Hornykiewicz O, Bedard PJ, Rajput AH, Di Paolo T. Increased adenosine A2A receptors in the brain of Parkinson's disease patients with dyskinesias. *Brain: a journal of neurology* 2004;**127**:1075–1084.

73. Carta AR, Pinna A, Cauli O, Morelli M. Differential regulation of GAD67, enkephalin and dynorphin mRNAs by chronic-intermittent L-dopa and A2A receptor blockade plus L-dopa in dopamine-denervated rats. *Synapse* 2002;**44**:166–174.

74. Linazasoro G. New ideas on the origin of L-dopa-induced dyskinesias: age, genes and neural plasticity. *Trends in pharmacological sciences* 2005;**26**:391–397.

75. Robertson HA, Peterson MR, Murphy K, Robertson GS. D1-dopamine receptor agonists selectively activate striatal c-fos independent of rotational behaviour. *Brain research* 1989;**503**:346–349.

76. Dragunow M, Robertson GS, Faull RL, Robertson HA, Jansen K. D2 dopamine receptor antagonists induce fos and related proteins in rat striatal neurons. *Neuroscience* 1990;**37**:287–294.

77. Graybiel AM, Moratalla R, Robertson HA. Amphetamine and cocaine induce drug-specific activation of the c-fos gene in striosome-matrix compartments and limbic subdivisions of the striatum. *Proceedings of the National Academy of Sciences of the United States of America* 1990;**87**:6912–6916.

78. Calon F, Hadj Tahar A, Blanchet PJ, et al. Dopamine-receptor stimulation: biobehavioral and biochemical consequences. *Trends in neurosciences* 2000;**23**:S92–100.

79. Dunnett S. L-DOPA, dyskinesia and striatal plasticity. *Nature neuroscience* 2003;**6**:437–438.

80. Picconi B, Centonze D, Hakansson K, et al. Loss of bidirectional striatal synaptic plasticity in L-DOPA-induced dyskinesia. *Nature neuroscience* 2003;**6**:501–506.

81. Greengard P, Allen PB, Nairn AC. Beyond the dopamine receptor: the DARPP-32/protein phosphatase-1 cascade. *Neuron* 1999;**23**:435–447.

82. Walaas SI, Hemmings HC, Jr., Greengard P, Nairn AC. Beyond the dopamine receptor: regulation and roles of serine/threonine protein phosphatases. *Frontiers in neuroanatomy* 2011;**5**:50.

83. Morelli M, Cozzolino A, Pinna A, Fenu S, Carta A, Di Chiara G. L-dopa stimulates c-fos expression in dopamine denervated striatum by combined activation of D-1 and D-2 receptors. *Brain research* 1993;**623**:334–336.

84. Steiner H, Gerfen CR. Dynorphin opioid inhibition of cocaine-induced, D1 dopamine receptor-mediated immediate-early gene expression in the striatum. *The Journal of comparative neurology* 1995;**353**:200–212.

85. Gerfen CR, Keefe KA, Gauda EB. D1 and D2 dopamine receptor function in the striatum: coactivation of D1- and D2-dopamine receptors on separate populations of neurons results in potentiated immediate early gene response in D1-containing neurons. *The Journal of neuroscience: the official journal of the Society for Neuroscience* 1995;**15**:8167–8176.

86. Robertson GS, Vincent SR, Fibiger HC. Striatonigral projection neurons contain D1 dopamine receptor-activated c-fos. *Brain research* 1990;**523**:288–290.

87. Keefe KA, Gerfen CR. D1 dopamine receptor-mediated induction of zif268 and c-fos in the dopamine-depleted striatum: differential regulation and independence from NMDA receptors. *The Journal of comparative neurology* 1996;**367**:165–176.

88. Konradi C, Leveque JC, Hyman SE. Amphetamine and dopamine-induced immediate early gene expression in striatal neurons depends on postsynaptic NMDA receptors and calcium. *The Journal of neuroscience: the official journal of the Society for Neuroscience* 1996;**16**:4231–4239.

89. Berke JD, Paletzki RF, Aronson GJ, Hyman SE, Gerfen CR. A complex program of striatal gene expression induced by dopaminergic stimulation. *The Journal of neuroscience: the official journal of the Society for Neuroscience* 1998;**18**:5301–5310.

90. Juncos JL, Engber TM, Raisman R, et al. Continuous and intermittent levodopa differentially affect basal ganglia function. *Annals of neurology* 1989;**25**:473–478.

91. Konradi C, Heckers S. Haloperidol-induced Fos expression in striatum is dependent upon transcription factor cyclic AMP response element binding protein. *Neuroscience* 1995;**65**:1051–1061.

92. Huang KX, Walters JR. Dopaminergic regulation of AP-1 transcription factor DNA binding activity in rat striatum. *Neuroscience* 1996;**75**:757–775.

93. Aubert I, Guigoni C, Hakansson K, et al. Increased D1 dopamine receptor signaling in levodopa-induced dyskinesia. *Annals of neurology* 2005;**57**:17–26.

94. Guigoni C, Doudnikoff E, Li Q, Bloch B, Bezard E. Altered D(1) dopamine receptor trafficking in parkinsonian and dyskinetic non-human primates. *Neurobiology of disease* 2007;**26**:452–463.

95. Berthet A, Porras G, Doudnikoff E, et al. Pharmacological analysis demonstrates dramatic alteration of D1 dopamine receptor neuronal distribution in the rat analog of L-DOPA-induced dyskinesia. *The Journal of neuroscience: the*

official journal of the Society for Neuroscience 2009;**29**:4829–4835.

96. Bezard E, Gross CE, Qin L, Gurevich VV, Benovic JL, Gurevich EV. L-DOPA reverses the MPTP-induced elevation of the arrestin2 and GRK6 expression and enhanced ERK activation in monkey brain. *Neurobiology of disease* 2005;**18**:323–335.

97. Ahmed MR, Bychkov E, Gurevich VV, Benovic JL, Gurevich EV. Altered expression and subcellular distribution of GRK subtypes in the dopamine-depleted rat basal ganglia is not normalized by l-DOPA treatment. *Journal of neurochemistry* 2008;**104**:1622–1636.

98. Hallett PJ, Dunah AW, Ravenscroft P, et al. Alterations of striatal NMDA receptor subunits associated with the development of dyskinesia in the MPTP-lesioned primate model of Parkinson's disease. *Neuropharmacology* 2005;**48**:503–516.

99. Silverdale MA, Kobylecki C, Hallett PJ, et al. Synaptic recruitment of AMPA glutamate receptor subunits in levodopa-induced dyskinesia in the MPTP-lesioned nonhuman primate. *Synapse* 2010;**64**:177–180.

100. Gross CE, Ravenscroft P, Dovero S, Jaber M, Bioulac B, Bezard E. Pattern of levodopa-induced striatal changes is different in normal and MPTP-lesioned mice. *Journal of neurochemistry* 2003;**84**:1246–1255.

101. Bordet R, Ridray S, Carboni S, Diaz J, Sokoloff P, Schwartz JC. Induction of dopamine D3 receptor expression as a mechanism of behavioral sensitization to levodopa. *Proceedings of the National Academy of Sciences of the United States of America* 1997;**94**:3363–3367.

102. Fiorentini C, Busi C, Gorruso E, Gotti C, Spano P, Missale C. Reciprocal regulation of dopamine D1 and D3 receptor function and trafficking by heterodimerization. *Molecular pharmacology* 2008;**74**:59–69.

103. Marcellino D, Ferre S, Casado V, et al. Identification of dopamine D1-D3 receptor heteromers. Indications for a role of synergistic D1-D3 receptor interactions in the striatum. *The Journal of biological chemistry* 2008;**283**:26016–26025.

104. Brambilla R. Targeting Ras/ERK signaling in the striatum: will it help? *Molecular psychiatry* 2003;**8**:366–368.

105. Valjent E, Pascoli V, Svenningsson P, et al. Regulation of a protein phosphatase cascade allows convergent dopamine and glutamate signals to activate ERK in the striatum. *Proceedings of the National Academy of Sciences of the United States of America* 2005;**102**:491–496.

106. Westin JE, Vercammen L, Strome EM, Konradi C, Cenci MA. Spatiotemporal pattern of striatal ERK1/2 phosphorylation in a rat model of L-DOPA-induced

dyskinesia and the role of dopamine D1 receptors. *Biological psychiatry* 2007;**62**:800–810.

107. Morelli M, Di Chiara G. Agonist-induced homologous and heterologous sensitization to D-1- and D-2-dependent contraversive turning. *European journal of pharmacology* 1987;**141**:101–107.

108. Calabresi P, Gubellini P, Centonze D, et al. Dopamine and cAMP-regulated phosphoprotein 32 kDa controls both striatal long-term depression and long-term potentiation, opposing forms of synaptic plasticity. *The Journal of neuroscience: the official journal of the Society for Neuroscience* 2000;**20**:8443–8451.

109. Calabresi P, Picconi B, Parnetti L, Di Filippo M. A convergent model for cognitive dysfunctions in Parkinson's disease: the critical dopamine-acetylcholine synaptic balance. *Lancet neurology* 2006;**5**:974–983.

110. Calabresi P, Picconi B, Tozzi A, Di Filippo M. Dopamine-mediated regulation of corticostriatal synaptic plasticity. *Trends in neurosciences* 2007;**30**:211–219.

111. Centonze D, Grande C, Saulle E, et al. Distinct roles of D1 and D5 dopamine receptors in motor activity and striatal synaptic plasticity. *The Journal of neuroscience: the official journal of the Society for Neuroscience* 2003;**23**:8506–8512.

112. Morgante F, Espay AJ, Gunraj C, Lang AE, Chen R. Motor cortex plasticity in Parkinson's disease and levodopa-induced dyskinesias. *Brain: a journal of neurology* 2006;**129**:1059–1069.

113. Grondin R, Doan VD, Gregoire L, Bedard PJ. D1 receptor blockade improves L-dopa-induced dyskinesia but worsens parkinsonism in MPTP monkeys. *Neurology* 1999;**52**:771–776.

114. Meissner W, Ravenscroft P, Reese R, et al. Increased slow oscillatory activity in substantia nigra pars reticulata triggers abnormal involuntary movements in the 6-OHDA-lesioned rat in the presence of excessive extracellular striatal dopamine. *Neurobiology of disease* 2006;**22**:586–598.

115. Carta M, Lindgren HS, Lundblad M, Stancampiano R, Fadda F, Cenci MA. Role of striatal L-DOPA in the production of dyskinesia in 6-hydroxydopamine lesioned rats. *Journal of neurochemistry* 2006;**96**:1718–1727.

116. de la Fuente-Fernandez R, Sossi V, Huang Z, et al. Levodopa-induced changes in synaptic dopamine levels increase with progression of Parkinson's disease: implications for dyskinesias. *Brain: a journal of neurology* 2004;**127**:2747–2754.

117. Cenci MA, Lundblad M. Post- versus presynaptic plasticity in L-DOPA-induced dyskinesia. *Journal of neurochemistry* 2006;**99**:381–392.

118. Poewe W, Mahlknecht P, Jankovic J. Emerging therapies for Parkinson's disease. *Current opinion in neurology* 2012;**25**:448–459.

119. Napolitano M, Picconi B, Centonze D, Bernardi G, Calabresi P, Gulino A. L-DOPA treatment of parkinsonian rats changes the expression of Src, Lyn and PKC kinases. *Neuroscience letters* 2006;**398**:211–214.

120. Smith Y, Raju D, Nanda B, Pare JF, Galvan A, Wichmann T. The thalamostriatal systems: anatomical and functional organization in normal and parkinsonian states. *Brain research bulletin* 2009;**78**:60–68.

121. Blandini F. An update on the potential role of excitotoxicity in the pathogenesis of Parkinson's disease. *Functional neurology* 2010;**25**:65–71.

122. Bargiotas P, Konitsiotis S. Levodopa-induced dyskinesias in Parkinson's disease: emerging treatments. *Neuropsychiatric disease and treatment* 2013;**9**:1605–1617.

123. Luginger E, Wenning GK, Bosch S, Poewe W. Beneficial effects of amantadine on L-dopa-induced dyskinesias in Parkinson's disease. *Movement disorders: official journal of the Movement Disorder Society* 2000;**15**:873–878.

124. Verhagen Metman L, Del Dotto P, van den Munckhof P, Fang J, Mouradian MM, Chase TN. Amantadine as treatment for dyskinesias and motor fluctuations in Parkinson's disease. *Neurology* 1998;**50**:1323–1326.

125. da Silva-Junior FP, Braga-Neto P, Sueli Monte F, de Bruin VM. Amantadine reduces the duration of levodopa-induced dyskinesia: a randomized, double-blind, placebo-controlled study. *Parkinsonism & related disorders* 2005;**11**:449–452.

126. Thomas A, Iacono D, Luciano AL, Armellino K, Di Iorio A, Onofrj M. Duration of amantadine benefit on dyskinesia of severe Parkinson's disease. *Journal of neurology, neurosurgery, and psychiatry* 2004;**75**:141–143.

127. Metman LV, Del Dotto P, LePoole K, Konitsiotis S, Fang J, Chase TN. Amantadine for levodopa-induced dyskinesias: a 1-year follow-up study. *Archives of neurology* 1999;**56**:1383–1386.

128. Wolf E, Seppi K, Katzenschlager R, et al. Long-term antidyskinetic efficacy of amantadine in Parkinson's disease. *Movement disorders: official journal of the Movement Disorder Society* 2010;**25**:1357–1363.

129. Jahangirvand AR, A. Early use of amantadine to prevent or delay onset of levodopa-induced dyskinesia in Parkinson's disease. *Movement disorders: official journal of the Movement Disorder Society* 2013;**28**:207.

130. Ory-Magne F CJ, Azulay JP, Bonnet AM, Brefel-Courbon C, Damier P, Dellapina E, Destée A, Durif F, Galitzky M, Lebouvier T, Meissner W, Thalamas C, Tison F, Salis A, Sommet A, Viallet F, Vidailhet M, Rascol O; NS-Park CIC Network. Withdrawing amantadine in dyskinetic patients with Parkinson disease: The AMANDYSK trial. *Neurology* 2014;**82**:300–307.

131. Pahwa RT, C. Hauser, R. Sethi, K. Isaacson, D. Truong, D. Struck, L. Stempien, M. Went, G. Randomized trial of extended release amantadine in Parkinson's disease patients with levodopa-induced dyskinesia (EASED study). *Movement disorders: official journal of the Movement Disorder Society* 2013;**28**:158.

132. Parkinson Study G. Evaluation of dyskinesias in a pilot, randomized, placebo-controlled trial of remacemide in advanced Parkinson disease. *Archives of neurology* 2001;**58**:1660–1668.

133. Bara-Jimenez W, Dimitrova TD, Sherzai A, Aksu M, Chase TN. Glutamate release inhibition ineffective in levodopa-induced motor complications. *Movement disorders: official journal of the Movement Disorder Society* 2006;**21**:1380–1383.

134. Verhagen Metman L, Del Dotto P, Natte R, van den Munckhof P, Chase TN. Dextromethorphan improves levodopa-induced dyskinesias in Parkinson's disease. *Neurology* 1998;**51**:203–206.

135. Pharmaceuticals A. Safety and Efficacy of AVP-923 in the Treatment of Levodopa-induced Dyskinesia in Parkinson's Disease Patients (LID in PD) [online]. Available at: http://clinicaltrials.gov/show/NCT01767129. Accessed April 30, 2014.

136. Merello M, Nouzeilles MI, Cammarota A, Leiguarda R. Effect of memantine (NMDA antagonist) on Parkinson's disease: a double-blind crossover randomized study. *Clinical neuropharmacology* 1999;**22**:273–276.

137. Moreau C, Delval A, Tiffreau V, et al. Memantine for axial signs in Parkinson's disease: a randomised, double-blind, placebo-controlled pilot study. *Journal of neurology, neurosurgery, and psychiatry* 2013;**84**:552–555.

138. Vidal EI, Fukushima FB, Valle AP, Villas Boas PJ. Unexpected improvement in levodopa-induced dyskinesia and on-off phenomena after introduction of memantine for treatment of Parkinson's disease dementia. *Journal of the American Geriatrics Society* 2013;**61**:170–172.

139. Nash JE, Ravenscroft P, McGuire S, Crossman AR, Menniti FS, Brotchie JM. The NR2B-selective NMDA receptor antagonist CP-101,606 exacerbates L-DOPA-induced dyskinesia and provides mild potentiation of anti-parkinsonian effects of L-DOPA in the MPTP-lesioned marmoset model of

Parkinson's disease. *Experimental neurology* 2004;**188**:471–479.

140. Nutt JG, Gunzler SA, Kirchhoff T, et al. Effects of a NR2B selective NMDA glutamate antagonist, CP-101,606, on dyskinesia and Parkinsonism. *Movement disorders: official journal of the Movement Disorder Society* 2008;**23**:1860–1866.

141. Ltd. NP. A Double-blind, Placebo Controlled, Crossover, Ascending Single Dose Safety Tolerability, Pharmacokinetic and Pharmacodynamic Study of Neu-120 in Patients With Advanced Phase Idiopathic Parkinson's Disease With Levodopa Induced Dyskinesia [online]. Available at: http://www.clinicaltrials.gov/ct2/show/NCT00607451?term=NCT00607451%26rank=1. Accessed April 30, 2014.

142. Picconi B, Calabresi P. Targeting metabotropic glutamate receptors as a new strategy against levodopa-induced dyskinesia in Parkinson's disease? *Movement disorders: official journal of the Movement Disorder Society* 2014;**29**:715–719.

143. Dekundy A, Pietraszek M, Schaefer D, Cenci MA, Danysz W. Effects of group I metabotropic glutamate receptors blockade in experimental models of Parkinson's disease. *Brain research bulletin* 2006;**69**:318–326.

144. Johnston TH, Fox SH, McIldowie MJ, Piggott MJ, Brotchie JM. Reduction of L-DOPA-induced dyskinesia by the selective metabotropic glutamate receptor 5 antagonist 3-[(2-methyl-1,3-thiazol-4-yl)ethynyl]pyridine in the 1-methyl-4-phenyl-1,2,3,6-tetrahydropyridine-lesioned macaque model of Parkinson's disease. *The Journal of pharmacology and experimental therapeutics* 2010;**333**:865–873.

145. Levandis G, Bazzini E, Armentero MT, Nappi G, Blandini F. Systemic administration of an mGluR5 antagonist, but not unilateral subthalamic lesion, counteracts l-DOPA-induced dyskinesias in a rodent model of Parkinson's disease. *Neurobiology of disease* 2008;**29**:161–168.

146. Gregoire L, Morin N, Ouattara B, et al. The acute antiparkinsonian and antidyskinetic effect of AFQ056, a novel metabotropic glutamate receptor type 5 antagonist, in L-Dopa-treated parkinsonian monkeys. *Parkinsonism & related disorders* 2011;**17**:270–276.

147. Stocchi F, Rascol O, Destee A, et al. AFQ056 in Parkinson patients with levodopa-induced dyskinesia: 13-week, randomized, dose-finding study. *Movement disorders: official journal of the Movement Disorder Society* 2013;**28**:1838–1846.

148. Pharmaceuticals N. An Open-label Treatment Study to Evaluate the Safety, Tolerability and Efficacy of AFQ056 in Parkinson's Patients With L-dopa Induced Dyskinesias [online].

Available at: http://www.clinicaltrials.gov/ct2/show/NCT01173731?term=NCT01173731%26rank=1. Accessed April 30, 2014.

149. Tison FD, Corvol J, Eggert K, Trenkwalder C, Lew, M, Isaacson S, Keywood C, Rascol O. Safety, tolerability and anti-dyskinetic efficacy of dipraglurant, a novel mGluR5 negative allosteric modulator (NAM) in Parkinson's disease (PD) patients with levodopa-induced dyskinesia (LID). *Neurology* 2013;**80**:004.

150. Konitsiotis S, Blanchet PJ, Verhagen L, Lamers E, Chase TN. AMPA receptor blockade improves levodopa-induced dyskinesia in MPTP monkeys. *Neurology* 2000;**54**:1589–1595.

151. Eggert K, Squillacote D, Barone P, et al. Safety and efficacy of perampanel in advanced Parkinson's disease: a randomized, placebo-controlled study. *Movement disorders: official journal of the Movement Disorder Society* 2010;**25**:896–905.

152. Lees A, Fahn S, Eggert KM, et al. Perampanel, an AMPA antagonist, found to have no benefit in reducing "off" time in Parkinson's disease. *Movement disorders: official journal of the Movement Disorder Society* 2012;**27**:284–288.

153. Rascol O, Barone P, Behari M, et al. Perampanel in Parkinson disease fluctuations: a double-blind randomized trial with placebo and entacapone. *Clinical neuropharmacology* 2012;**35**:15–20.

154. Savola JM, Hill M, Engstrom M, et al. Fipamezole (JP-1730) is a potent alpha2 adrenergic receptor antagonist that reduces levodopa-induced dyskinesia in the MPTP-lesioned primate model of Parkinson's disease. *Movement disorders: official journal of the Movement Disorder Society* 2003;**18**:872–883.

155. Lewitt PA, Hauser RA, Lu M, et al. Randomized clinical trial of fipamezole for dyskinesia in Parkinson disease (FJORD study). *Neurology* 2012;**79**:163–169.

156. Grondin R, Hadj Tahar A, Doan VD, Ladure P, Bedard PJ. Noradrenoceptor antagonism with idazoxan improves L-dopa-induced dyskinesias in MPTP monkeys. *Naunyn-Schmiedeberg's archives of pharmacology* 2000;**361**:181–186.

157. Rascol O, Arnulf I, Peyro-Saint Paul H, et al. Idazoxan, an alpha-2 antagonist, and L-DOPA-induced dyskinesias in patients with Parkinson's disease. *Movement disorders: official journal of the Movement Disorder Society* 2001;**16**:708–713.

158. Manson AJ, Iakovidou E, Lees AJ. Idazoxan is ineffective for levodopa-induced dyskinesias in Parkinson's disease. *Movement disorders: official journal of the Movement Disorder Society* 2000;**15**:336–337.

159. Buck K, Voehringer P, Ferger B. The alpha(2) adrenoceptor antagonist idazoxan alleviates L-DOPA-induced dyskinesia by reduction of striatal dopamine levels: an in vivo microdialysis study in 6-hydroxydopamine-lesioned rats. *Journal of neurochemistry* 2010;**112**:444–452.

160. Hodgson RA, Bedard PJ, Varty GB, et al. Preladenant, a selective A(2A) receptor antagonist, is active in primate models of movement disorders. *Experimental neurology* 2010;**225**:384–390.

161. Hauser RA, Cantillon M, Pourcher E, et al. Preladenant in patients with Parkinson's disease and motor fluctuations: a phase 2, double-blind, randomised trial. *Lancet neurology* 2011;**10**:221–229.

162. Factor SA, Wolski K, Togasaki DM, et al. Long-term safety and efficacy of preladenant in subjects with fluctuating Parkinson's disease. *Movement disorders: official journal of the Movement Disorder Society* 2013;**28**:817–820.

163. Jones IW, Bolam JP, Wonnacott S. Presynaptic localisation of the nicotinic acetylcholine receptor beta2 subunit immunoreactivity in rat nigrostriatal dopaminergic neurones. *The Journal of comparative neurology* 2001;**439**:235–247.

164. Durif F, Debilly B, Galitzky M, et al. Clozapine improves dyskinesias in Parkinson disease: a double-blind, placebo-controlled study. *Neurology* 2004;**62**:381–388.

165. Pierelli F, Adipietro A, Soldati G, Fattapposta F, Pozzessere G, Scoppetta C. Low dosage clozapine effects on L-dopa induced dyskinesias in parkinsonian patients. *Acta neurologica Scandinavica* 1998;**97**:295–299.

166. Bennett JP, Jr., Landow ER, Dietrich S, Schuh LA. Suppression of dyskinesias in advanced Parkinson's disease: moderate daily clozapine doses provide long-term dyskinesia reduction. *Movement disorders: official journal of the Movement Disorder Society* 1994;**9**:409–414.

167. Meco G, Stirpe P, Edito F, et al. Aripiprazole in L-dopa-induced dyskinesias: a one-year open-label pilot study. *Journal of neural transmission* 2009;**116**:881–884.

168. Rascol O, Bronzova J, Hauser RA, et al. Pardoprunox as adjunct therapy to levodopa in patients with Parkinson's disease experiencing motor fluctuations: results of a double-blind, randomized, placebo-controlled, trial. *Parkinsonism & related disorders* 2012;**18**:370–376.

169. Hauser RA, Bronzova J, Sampaio C, et al. Safety and tolerability of pardoprunox, a new partial dopamine agonist, in a randomized, controlled study of patients with advanced Parkinson's disease. *European neurology* 2009;**62**:40–48.

170. Waters CH, Sethi KD, Hauser RA, Molho E, Bertoni JM, Zydis Selegiline Study G. Zydis selegiline reduces off time in Parkinson's disease patients with motor fluctuations: a 3-month, randomized, placebo-controlled study. *Movement disorders: official journal of the Movement Disorder Society* 2004;**19**:426–432.

171. Rascol O, Brooks DJ, Melamed E, et al. Rasagiline as an adjunct to levodopa in patients with Parkinson's disease and motor fluctuations (LARGO, Lasting effect in Adjunct therapy with Rasagiline Given Once daily, study): a randomised, double-blind, parallel-group trial. *Lancet* 2005;**365**:947–954.

172. Stocchi F, Borgohain R, Onofrj M, et al. A randomized, double-blind, placebo-controlled trial of safinamide as add-on therapy in early Parkinson's disease patients. *Movement disorders: official journal of the Movement Disorder Society* 2012;**27**:106–112.

173. Carroll CB, Bain PG, Teare L, et al. Cannabis for dyskinesia in Parkinson disease: a randomized double-blind crossover study. *Neurology* 2004;**63**:1245–1250.

174. Sugiyama K, Yokoyama T, Namba H. [Neurosurgical treatment for dopamine-induced dyskinesias in Parkinson's disease patients]. *Nihon rinsho Japanese journal of clinical medicine* 2000;**58**:2115–2119.

175. Munhoz RP, Cerasa A, Okun MS. Surgical treatment of dyskinesia in Parkinson's disease. *Frontiers in neurology* 2014;**5**:65.

176. Deep-Brain Stimulation for Parkinson's Disease Study G. Deep-brain stimulation of the subthalamic nucleus or the pars interna of the globus pallidus in Parkinson's disease. *The New England journal of medicine* 2001;**345**:956–963.

177. Rodriguez-Oroz MC, Obeso JA, Lang AE, et al. Bilateral deep brain stimulation in Parkinson's disease: a multicentre study with 4 years follow-up. *Brain: a journal of neurology* 2005;**128**:2240–2249.

178. Volkmann J, Allert N, Voges J, Sturm V, Schnitzler A, Freund HJ. Long-term results of bilateral pallidal stimulation in Parkinson's disease. *Annals of neurology* 2004;**55**:871–875.

179. Krack P, Batir A, Van Blercom N, et al. Five-year follow-up of bilateral stimulation of the subthalamic nucleus in advanced Parkinson's disease. *The New England journal of medicine* 2003;**349**:1925–1934.

180. Schupbach WM, Chastan N, Welter ML, et al. Stimulation of the subthalamic nucleus in Parkinson's disease: a 5 year follow up. *Journal of neurology, neurosurgery, and psychiatry* 2005;**76**:1640–1644.

181.  Kleiner-Fisman G, Herzog J, Fisman DN, et al. Subthalamic nucleus deep brain stimulation: summary and meta-analysis of outcomes. *Movement disorders: official journal of the Movement Disorder Society* 2006;**21** Suppl 14:S290–304.

182.  Odekerken VJ, van Laar T, Staal MJ, et al. Subthalamic nucleus versus globus pallidus bilateral deep brain stimulation for advanced Parkinson's disease (NSTAPS study): a randomised controlled trial. *Lancet neurology* 2013;**12**:37–44.

# Chapter 12

# VPA, lithium, amiodarone, and other non-DA

Michael R. Silver and Stewart A. Factor

## Introduction

Considering that the characteristic motor features of Parkinson's disease (PD) are caused by a loss of dopamine in the brain, it stands to reason that medications which decrease dopamine's action would cause a parkinsonian condition. Drugs known to deplete dopamine, such as reserpine or tetrabenazine, certainly have this effect. However, the most common scenario in which drug-induced parkinsonism (DIP) arises is with postsynaptic dopamine receptor blocking agents such as antipsychotic or antiemetic medications. These drugs are covered elsewhere in this book.

Lesser known and often enigmatic is when parkinsonism is caused by medications that have no apparent action upon the dopamine system. Perhaps this is an indication that there is an occult antidopaminergic effect or that there is another lesser understood alternate mechanism that causes the clinical effect of parkinsonism. Such is the case with the medications we will discuss in this chapter. Most of the medications were designed for a specific purpose, such as blood pressure control in the case of the calcium channel blockers, but have caused a significant amount of morbidity in the form of DIP. DIP can also develop with exposure to naturally occurring substances used as therapeutic agents as well. For instance, lithium is a naturally occurring element that has been used since ancient times when its clinical effect became apparent, but there was no knowledge of pharmacology. Lithium probably exerts its psychiatric benefits through several mechanisms and may cause DIP through several as yet unknown mechanisms as well.

In this chapter, we will cover the nondopaminergic medications that induce parkinsonism. Table 12.1 summarizes such agents. Although antidepressants fall into this category, they will be covered elsewhere, with the exception of lithium.

The incidence and prevalence of DIP under these circumstances is difficult to quantify because DIP is often not recognized (1), and in some cases is extremely rare and unexpected. For example, while most physicians would know to attribute extrapyramidal side effects to neuroleptics, many may not know of the role that valproic acid has in causing parkinsonism. Furthermore, in situations where single or few cases have been reported it is hard to know for sure if there is a cause and effect relationship. A good example of this is the drug amlodipine which enjoys widespread use for hypertension and cardiac arrhythmias, and yet only two cases of parkinsonism have been reported. Nevertheless, several studies have attempted to examine the incidence of DIP. A French pharmacovigilance center tallied up all of its cases from 1993 to 2009. Parkinsonism was defined as having either resting tremor, rigidity, or akinesia (2). Dopamine antagonists constituted 54% of the DIP cases, antidepressants 8%, leaving a substantial percentage being due to a variety of nondopaminergic medications, suggesting that this type of DIP is of significant importance.

## Cardiac medications

### Antihypertensives

#### Calcium channel blockers: nondihydropyridine

The antihypertensive/antiarrhythmic medications diltiazem (3, 4) and verapamil (5, 6) are both widely used in the US, but were only implicated in causing DIP in a few case reports decades ago. On the other hand, two calcium channel blockers that are not

*Medication-Induced Movement Disorders*, ed. Joseph H. Friedman. Published by Cambridge University Press.
© Cambridge University Press 2015.

**Table 12.1** An overview of the classes of nonneuroleptic medications that cause parkinsonism

| Category of medications | Class of medications | Subclass | Drug names |
|---|---|---|---|
| Cardiac Medications | Antihypertensives | | |
| | | Calcium channel antagonists Nondihydropyridine | cinnarizine, flunarizine, diltiazem, verapamil |
| | | Calcium channel antagonists Dihydropyridines | amlodipine |
| | | ACE inhibitors | captopril |
| | Antiarrhythmics | | amiodarone, aprindine |
| | Antiischemics | | trimetazidine |
| Antiepileptic Drugs | | | valproic acid, phenytoin |
| Bipolar Agents | | | Lithium |
| Immunosuppressant | | | Cyclosporin |
| Antifungal | | | Amphotericin |
| Chemotherapeutic Agents | | | Vincristine, Cytosine arabinoside, Cyclophosphamide, Paclitaxel, 5-Fluorouracil, Methotrexate, Busulfan, etoposide, methotrexate, mitoxantrone, Adriamycin, gemcitabine, carboplatin |
| Miscellaneous | | | Procaine, propiverine, buformin, diazoxide, tacrine, cephaloridine, chloroquine, interferon, meperidine |

approved in the US, cinnarizine and its derivative flunarizine, are well known to cause parkinsonism. These are utilized for migraine prophylaxis, vestibular disorders, and as adjunctive treatment for epilepsy in southern Europe and South America (7). DIP caused by these two calcium channel blockers is characterized by the presence of a symmetric akinetic-rigid syndrome which may or may not be accompanied by rest or postural tremor. Other associated features include akathisia and dyskinesia (8). Risk factors for developing DIP from calcium channel blockers include female gender and age over 60 (7, 9–11).

In one prospective study, 93 out of 101 patients who were prescribed flunarizine or cinnarizine developed parkinsonism (9). Some studies (9, 11) indicated a good outcome after the drugs were discontinued with all or almost all patients recovering over the course of months. Garcia-Ruiz et al. found a difference in outcome based on the phenotype of their parkinsonism; the akinetic-rigid symptoms were mostly reversible, but tremor tended to persist long after the drug was removed (7). Conversely, Negrotti et al., had only 13 patients in their study, but found that all continued to have nonprogressive extrapyramidal side effects seven years after withdrawal of the offending medications (10).

Cinnarizine and flunarizine have antihistaminic, antiserotonergic, and antidopaminergic activity, so there are several theories as to why they cause parkinsonism. This could be a presynaptic process via loss of tyrosine hydroxylase (12) leading to dopamine depletion, by interfering with calcium-mediated neurotransmitter release (9), or it could be a postsynaptic process by blocking striatal dopamine receptors (9, 11).

### Calcium channel blockers: dihydropyridine

The class of dihydropyridine calcium channel blockers includes amlodipine and manidipine, both indicated for the treatment of hypertension. There are only two reported cases of amlodipine-induced parkinsonism. A 68-year-old woman developed tremor and parkinsonism upon initiating amlodipine, then improved within months of medication discontinuation (13). Another woman, 83 years old, developed tremor and parkinsonism within two months after starting amlodipine, which then resolved a month after stopping it (14). Manidipine has not been linked to "de novo" DIP, but rather worsening in two patients with preexisting PD (15). Amlodipine is widely used in parkinsonian patients with hypertension. Based on these reports we are left to ponder whether they are worsening motor features. Only a larger prospective examination of these agents in PD will address the issue of whether these drugs should be contraindicated in PD.

### ACE inhibitor (captopril)

One other medication that bears mention is the Angiotensin Converting Enzyme (ACE) inhibitor captopril. There are two case reports that implicate this medication in the induction of reversible tremor and parkinsonism (16, 17) or worsening of preexisting PD (18). Onset of parkinsonism and then resolution of symptoms took just days. This side effect is unexpected, since none of the other ACE inhibitors have been associated with DIP.

## Antiarrythmics

Amiodarone is a class III antiarrhythmic, typically prescribed for supraventricular tachycardia. It carries a variety of neurological side effects including neuropathy, ataxia, visual problems, fatigue, dizziness, and tremor (19). Neurological side effects tend to be dose-dependent and can be seen during the loading period or after long-term use. Tremor is the most common neurological symptom, with 30% of users exhibiting this complication (19). Most of the time, the tremor resembles essential tremor. It has a postural predilection and a frequency of 6 to 10 Hz (20). However, it can take on a distinctly parkinsonian character as well (21). Werner and Olanow reviewed the literature and described several cases of parkinsonism caused by amiodarone (22). Most cases did not resemble PD, but instead had nonspecific extrapyramidal syndromes featuring tremor, which interestingly included jaw tremor. Amiodarone can also cause a pure akinetic syndrome (23).

The amount of time from withdrawal to resolution of symptoms depends on the duration of exposure. Symptoms appearing with short courses of amiodarone only take days to improve, while longer courses may take several months (21). Tremor is a dose-dependent side effect and it can be reduced by lowering the dosage (20). Also, adding propranolol may be helpful in treating the postural component of tremor (20).

Aprindine is a lesser known antiarrhythmic medication which reportedly caused parkinsonism in a single case report (24). A 78-year-old man developed disorientation and parkinsonism after a month's use then recovered a few days after withdrawal. The mechanism by which amiodarone and aprindine cause parkinsonism is unknown, but they have been shown to block D1 and D2 receptors as part of in vivo and in vitro studies (25). In addition, amiodarone has been shown to interfere with mitochondrial function (26), which could explain its side effect profile. There have been two amiodarone-induced parkinsonian cases with pathological reports and they showed discrepant findings. LeMair presented a case whose pathology demonstrated depigmentation of the substantia nigra, without Lewy Bodies (27), whereas Ishida's case revealed a lack of Lewy Bodies, with normal pigmentation of the substantia nigra (28). The former case might suggest that amiodarone has a toxic effect on nigral neurons. Further study is needed.

## Antiischemic

Trimetazidine is an antiischemic medication that has been tied to parkinsonism. Two retrospective case series with 21 cases by Masmoudi (29) and 20 cases by Martí Massó (30) demonstrate this convincingly. Parkinsonism would develop over months to years and symptoms would generally improve weeks to months after withdrawal of the drug. This medication has the same piperazine core as the aforementioned calcium channel blockers, cinnarizine and flunarizine. Therefore, it is thought that the D2 receptor antagonism leads to the development of parkinsonism.

## Antiepileptics

### Valproic acid

Valproic acid (VPA) is well known to cause a reversible form of parkinsonism in pediatric populations (31–36). Features include marked bradykinesia and bradyphrenia which is sometimes associated with a reversible atrophic appearance of the brain called "pseudoatrophy." VPA-induced parkinsonism is also a well described clinical entity in adult populations (37). VPA is best known as a cause of nonparkinsonian postural hand tremor that has been estimated to occur in up to 45% of users and is not dose- or serum level–related (38). A smaller percentage of patients have been identified to develop actual parkinsonian features. In addition to causing de novo DIP, VPA was shown to worsen symptoms in those with preexisting parkinsonism (39). The studies that have examined the frequency of DIP from VPA have primarily looked at an exclusively epileptic patient population. There were disparate rates of parkinsonism described (39–43), with the highest estimates finding parkinsonism in 10% of those exposed. The incidence in the elderly treated for bipolar disorder remains unknown.

The diagnosis can sometimes be challenging in the elderly since this is the demographic in which one would expect to see PD, and normal aging is associated with mild parkinsonism. VPA-induced parkinsonism can present as an akinetic-rigid state or, as mixed postural/rest tremors, and it can look identical to PD with a unilateral bradykinesia and rest tremor. The parkinsonism that VPA causes is not a consequence of medication overdosage or toxicity, as low doses and therapeutic serum drug

concentrations can result in this complication. For instance, one patient from our own series was on a dose of only 250mg per day when she developed her symptoms (44). Further complicating the distinction between VPA-induced parkinsonism and PD is the fact that VPA-induced parkinsonism takes months to years to develop, so symptoms do not appear upon initiation of the offending agent as more typically seen with neuroleptics. Furthermore, symptoms typically require weeks to months to resolve after discontinuation of the VPA, so it takes time to assess for clinical improvement and clarify the diagnosis. The average duration in our series was seven months (44). Yet another confounding factor to distinguish between VPA-induced parkinsonism and PD is the fact that it is responsive to levodopa (44, 45) and one can even see levodopa-induced dyskinesia (44).

The mechanism by which VPA causes parkinsonism is unknown. Like other causes of DIP, it displays normal dopamine transporter density on SPECT scan (41), hence it does not appear to be toxic to presynaptic dopaminergic neurons. Based on the fact that this condition can be levodopa responsive, one would not expect a postsynaptic dopaminergic blockade to be the cause. Theories with regard to the mechanism of development of DIP include GABAergic effects, since VPA is known to increase GABAergic transmission (38), which is significant in the basal ganglia, including the substantia nigra. This may result in a net inhibition of dopaminergic activity (46). Other theories include the slow accumulation of a toxic metabolite of VPA in the substantia nigra (47), inhibition of mitochondrial metabolism (48), and inhibition of neurite outgrowth (49).

### Phenytoin

There are only two cases in the literature of parkinsonism associated with phenytoin. The first case described a 68-year-old man with seizures as a result of cranial injury who developed parkinsonism and tremors within one month of initiating the drug. Symptoms resolved over 6 months after switching to an alternative antiepileptic medication (50). The other case describes parkinsonism, tremor, and cerebellar ataxia within two weeks of phenytoin exposure, but his drug level was exceptionally high, at 40 mg/dL (51). Both patients had a history of severe cerebral trauma, so perhaps phenytoin requires the substrate of brain injury to cause parkinsonism.

# Bipolar medications

## Lithium

Lithium is known to cause a variety of movement disorders including tremor, parkinsonism, and chorea (52). Like VPA, lithium causes a postural and action high frequency tremor that is distinct from PD, similar to essential tremor, and is thought to be a form of enhanced physiologic tremor (53). In fact, it might be the most common form of drug-induced tremor seen (52), with an incidence as high 33%–65% (54). The variance among different estimates of incidence is the result of lithium frequently being prescribed with other tremor-producing medications. The tremor can occur even when the drug levels are therapeutic.

The notion that lithium can cause parkinsonism has been a controversial and complicated one. Certainly, when it does truly cause parkinsonism, it does so rarely. But patients who are prescribed lithium usually take it for bipolar disorder, often with neuroleptic drugs. Furthermore, much of the early literature on the matter probably overdiagnosed parkinsonism based on the physical exam findings of postural tremor and cogwheel phenomena without true rigidity. Cogwheeling is a nonspecific exam finding that does not necessarily indicate rigidity and is noted in patients with all types of postural tremor, probably as an extension of the tremor itself.

The first two papers on the matter examined randomly selected lithium users for "cogwheel rigidity" (55, 56), but it was not made clear if this represented true parkinsonism. In addition, in the first paper it was not clear if any were treated concomitantly with neuroleptics. Kane et al. then reported on 38 patients with therapeutic levels of lithium, two of whom had parkinsonian features, but both had been on neuroleptics in the year prior (57). It has been shown that neuroleptic-induced parkinsonism can last that long or even longer after neuroleptic discontinuation, complicating interpretation (1). Asnis evaluated the largest series of patients, 97, but again focused on cogwheeling instead of true parkinsonian signs (58).

The more solid evidence that lithium causes parkinsonism comes from more recent case reports, as summarized by Factor (52). Cogwheeling along with such parkinsonian traits as bradykinesia, rigidity, resting tremor, masked facies, and postural instability solidified the diagnosis of parkinsonism in these cases. All patients were on chronic lithium therapy, some with therapeutic, others with toxic serum levels. One can draw the conclusion based on these cases that the duration of lithium treatment, older age, and higher therapeutic levels of lithium appear to be risk factors for the development of parkinsonism. However, dopamine transporter SPECT scanning was not available for these cases, so it is possible some or all actually had PD.

Lithium's mechanism of action for improving bipolar disorder is unknown, and the same is true for inducing parkinsonism. Lithium affects many different neurotransmitters and modulates several biochemical pathways. For instance, lithium has been shown to block inositol phospholipid hydrolysis, part of a second-messenger system which has been theorized to explain lithium's benefit in affective disorder. This may be related to its upstream effect of blocking the stimulus-based release and the enhancement of reuptake of norepinephrine in animal models. Lithium also affects serotonin, GABA, glutamate, and several neuropeptides. Animal studies yield conflicting data for how lithium might cause parkinsonism, with lithium exerting contrasting effects on the dopaminergic system (52).

# Immunosuppressant therapy

## Cyclosporine

Causal relationships are difficult to determine when there are many medications given simultaneously. This especially becomes murky when it is against a background of an acute underlying illness. Such is the case when trying to attribute parkinsonism to an agent used in an organ transplant recipient. However, there are several convincing case reports of the calcineurin-inhibitor immunosuppressant agent cyclosporine (also referred to as cyclosporine A) causing a reversible form of parkinsonism (59–63). Cyclosporine is better known to cause action tremor (occurs in approximately 20%), and can also cause cerebellar ataxia, myoclonus, seizures, headache, cortical blindness, visual hallucinations, and encephalopathy (61, 63).

Cases of cyclosporine-induced parkinsonism varied in duration of exposure, ranging from days to years. The clinical syndrome includes rest tremor, bradykinesia, hypomimia, and rigidity. This could develop even with therapeutic serum levels of the drug. Generally resolution was fairly rapid, over days to weeks, upon stopping the medication. The parkinsonian symptoms in these cases sometimes responded to levodopa. Unfortunately, none of these cases included functional dopamine transporter imaging.

## Antifungal agents

### Amphotericin

Amphotericin B is prescribed for life-threatening fungal infections and frequently used alongside chemotherapeutic agents in immunosuppressed patients with leukemia. There are reports of amphotericin itself causing parkinsonism (64). Amphotericin may have some synergistic effects with the chemotherapeutic agent cytosine arabinoside (65, 66, 67) to cause parkinsonism. This parkinsonian syndrome is characterized by bradykinesia, rigidity, and resting tremor, which can resolve over days to months after discontinuation of the offending medication. Levodopa appears to be of no benefit.

## Chemotherapeutic agents

There are multiple case reports of different chemotherapeutic agents, most given in combinations, leading to parkinsonism. This is nicely summarized in a table by Chuang based on the experience of 17 patients (68). Many of these patients responded to levodopa. Among the implicated agents were cytosine arabinoside, cyclophosphamide, etoposide, methotrexate, mitoxantrone, 5-fluorouracil, Adriamycin, vincristine, CHOP (cyclophosphamide, doxorubicin, vincristine, and prednisolone), gemcitabine, carboplatin, paclitaxel, and busulfan. Not all cases were treated with levodopa, but of those cases treated, all responded, except for the case by Luque (66) in a patient taking cytosine arabinoside. This case was mentioned in the prior section, as the patient also received amphotericin.

## Miscellaneous

There are several medications that have been linked to parkinsonism in single cases or very small case series, but the true causality is unclear. These are listed in Table 12.2.

## How to distinguish DIP and PD

When the clinician is faced with a patient that is parkinsonian and on a medication known to cause these symptoms, the question will always be if this is a pure DIP, purely PD, or if this represents medication "unmasking" PD that would have eventually

**Table 12.2** Medications implicated in causing parkinsonism by single or few case reports

| Name of Medication and use | Number of cases with references |
| --- | --- |
| Procaine, an injectable anesthetic medication | 1 (69) |
| Propiverine, an anticholinergic medication | 1 (70),3(71) |
| Buformin, a biguanide diabetes medication | 1(24) |
| Diazoxide, an antihypoglycemic/antihypertensive agent | 6 had parkinsonism or mixed extrapyramidal syndromes (72) |
| Tacrine, a centrally acting acetylcholinesterase inhibitor | 1 case(73) |
| Cephaloridine, a cephalosporin antibiotic | 1(74) |
| Chloroquine, an antimalarial antibiotic | 1(75) |
| Interferon, immune modulating | 1(76),1(77) |
| Meperidine, an opiate | 1(78), 1(79) |

manifested itself in the future. This is a complex situation, as DIP from nearly all drugs can look identical to PD. Many of the DIP cases we have referenced in this chapter had PD that was worsened or unmasked by the offending medication. Only a long-term follow-up after the drug discontinuation will reveal the correct diagnosis. This was the case in our valproate-induced parkinsonism case series (44), where the patient who did not make a full recovery was followed for years and turned out to have PD. In our clinic the same scenario has played out with neuroleptics and cyclosporine and amiodarone as well. The problem is compounded when the patient cannot discontinue the causative agent, as is often the case.

There are several clues one could use to distinguish between PD and DIP caused by a nondopamine blocking agent. First, the time course is important. If symptoms started within a few months of starting the medication or increasing the medication, and the onset is fairly abrupt, then suspicion should be high for DIP, although this scenario does not always occur. Second, if the parkinsonism begins with bilateral symptoms, then one should be more suspicious for DIP since PD more commonly starts off with asymmetric features. Third, if the patient is young, then that would make DIP more likely since most PD has onset near or after the age of 60. The fourth point to consider is that DIP will sometimes present concurrently with other neurological symptoms. One may see akathisia, myoclonus, action tremor, or cognitive impairment mixed in with the parkinsonism. One would not expect PD to present with many of these features.

The dopamine transporter scan, [$^{123}$I] ioflupane SPECT scan, has served as a useful tool in generating an appropriate diagnosis in relation to DIP (80). An abnormal scan indicates presynaptic nigrostriatal neuronal loss and would suggest patients have degenerative parkinsonism, which may or may not be worsened by medications. Its use has been limited in the DIP reported in this chapter, but the scan has been shown to be normal in VPA-induced (41) and amiodarone-induced parkinsonism (81) in a limited number of cases. However, more research will be needed to precisely quantify the sensitivity and specificity of dopamine transporter imaging in DIP as there is the theoretical concern that some medications may interfere with ligand binding or alter neuronal metabolism, or cause nigral degeneration. It is not approved for this purpose.

Management of the DIP should first involve discontinuation or lowering the dose of the offending medication, if possible. Even if the patient has PD, the most prudent decision would be to stop the medication, since it may have aggravated the already present dopamine-depleted status. Improvement may take days or many months. As we have seen with valproate, this can even happen over the course of years (37). In the case of amiodarone, it seems to be dependent upon total duration of exposure (21). This seems to be more variable than neuroleptic-induced DIP, which generally resolves within a year (1).

In those patients who cannot stop the offending agent, treating DIP from nondopamine blocking agents with PD medications may or may not be effective. Levodopa has had some success in a few cases (11, 44, 45, 62, 68), but no prospective trials have been completed. It is difficult to comment on responsiveness in many of these cases because the offending agent was stopped concomitantly with initiating the levodopa. Anticholinergics, amantadine, and dopamine agonists would all be reasonable options to try but there is not enough experience to comment on their efficacy. Nevertheless, in situations where the causative agent cannot be stopped, it is reasonable to initiate a trial.

The mechanisms by which medications induce parkinsonism without reducing dopamine transmission remain a mystery. It challenges the simplistic dogma that parkinsonism comes from simply less dopamine in the system, and will require further study to elucidate this uncommon, fascinating, and underrecognized phenomenon.

## References

1. Esper CD, Factor SA. Failure of recognition of drug-induced parkinsonism in the elderly. *Mov Disord.* 2008;**23**(3):401–4.

2. Bondon-Guitton E, Perez-Lloret S, Bagheri H, Brefel C, Rascol O, Montastruc JL. Drug-induced parkinsonism: a review of 17 years' experience in a regional pharmacovigilance center in France. *Mov Disord.* 2011;**26**(12):2226–31.

3. Remblier C, Kassir A, Richard D, Perault MC, Guibert S. [Parkinson syndrome from diltiazem]. *Therapie.* 2001;**56**(1):57–9.

4. Dick RS, Barold SS. Diltiazem-induced parkinsonism. *Am J Med.* 1989;**87**(1):95–6.

5. Padrell MD, Navarro M, Faura CC, Horga JF. Verapamil-induced parkinsonism. *Am J Med.* 1995;**99**(4):436.

6. Garcia-Albea E, Jimenez-Jimenez FJ, Ayuso-Peralta L, Cabrera-Valdivia F, Vaquero A, Tejeiro J. Parkinsonism unmasked by verapamil. *Clin Neuropharmacol.* 1993;**16**(3):263–5.

7. Garcia-Ruiz PJ, Javier Jimenez-Jimenez F, Garcia de Yebenes J. Calcium channel blocker-induced parkinsonism: clinical features and comparisons with Parkinson's disease. *Parkinsonism Relat Disord.* 1998;**4**(4):211–4.

8. Teive HA, Troiano AR, Germiniani FM, Werneck LC. Flunarizine- and cinnarizine-induced parkinsonism: a historical and clinical analysis. *Parkinsonism Relat Disord.* 2004;**10**(4):243–5.

9. Micheli FE, Pardal MM, Giannaula R, Gatto M, Parera I, Paradiso G, et al. Movement disorders and depression due to flunarizine and cinnarizine. *Mov Disord.* 1989;**4**(2):139–46.

10. Negrotti A, Calzetti S. A long-term follow-up study of cinnarizine- and flunarizine-induced parkinsonism. *Mov Disord.* 1997;**12**(1):107–10.

11. Marti-Masso JF, Poza JJ. Cinnarizine-induced parkinsonism: ten years later. *Mov Disord.* 1998;**13**(3):453–6.

12. Takada M, Kono T, Kitai ST. Flunarizine induces a transient loss of tyrosine hydroxylase immunoreactivity in nigrostriatal neurons. *Brain Res.* 1992; **590** (1–2): 311–5.

13. Sempere AP, Duarte J, Cabezas C, Coria F, Claveria LE. Parkinsonism induced by amlodipine. *Mov Disord.* 1995;**10**(1):115–6.

14. Teive HA, Germiniani FM, Werneck LC. Parkinsonian syndrome induced by amlodipine: case report. *Mov Disord.* 2002;**17**(4):833–5.

15. Nakashima K, Shimoda M, Kuno N, Takahashi K. Temporary symptom worsening caused by manidipine hydrochloride in two patients with Parkinson's disease. *Mov Disord.* 1994;**9**(1):106–7.

16. Sandyk R. Parkinsonism induced by captopril. *Clin Neuropharmacol.* 1985;**8**(2):197–8.

17. Shimoda K, Hikasa C, Nishikawa S, Takahashi K. [A case report of captopril-induced parkinsonism]. *Rinsho Shinkeigaku.* 1987;**27**(3):366–8.

18. Chang YP, Shih PY. A case of Parkinson's disease worsened by captopril: an unexpected adverse effect. *Mov Disord.* 2009;**24**(5):790.

19. Hilleman D, Miller MA, Parker R, Doering P, Pieper JA. Optimal management of amiodarone therapy: efficacy and side effects. *Pharmacotherapy.* 1998; **18**(6 Pt 2): 138S–45S.

20. Charness ME, Morady F, Scheinman MM. Frequent neurologic toxicity associated with amiodarone therapy. *Neurology.* 1984;**34**(5):669–71.

21. Werner EG, Olanow CW. Parkinsonism and amiodarone therapy. *Ann Neurol.* 1989;**25**(6):630–2.

22. Berg A, Bellander BM, Wanecek M, Gamrin L, Elving A, Rooyackers O, et al. Intravenous glutamine supplementation to head trauma patients leaves cerebral glutamate concentration unaffected. *Intensive Care Med.* 2006;**32**(11):1741–6.

23. Malaterre HR, Renou C, Kallee K, Gauthier A. Akinesia and amiodarone therapy. *Int J Cardiol.* 1997;**59**(1):107–8.

24. Marti Masso JF, Carrera N, Urtasun M. Drug-induced parkinsonism: a growing list. *Mov Disord.* 1993;**8**(1):125.

25. Matsui A, Matsuo H, Takanaga H, Sasaki S, Maeda M, Sawada Y. Prediction of catalepsies induced by amiodarone, aprindine and procaine: similarity in conformation of diethylaminoethyl side chain. *J Pharmacol Exp Ther.* 1998;**287**(2):725–32.

26. Dotti MT, Federico A. Amiodarone-induced parkinsonism: a case report and pathogenetic discussion. *Mov Disord.* 1995;**10**(2):233–4.

27. Lemaire JF, Autret A, Biziere K, Romet-Lemone JL, Gray F. Amiodaron neuropathy: further arguments for human drug-induced neurolipidosis. *Eur Neurol.* 1982;**21**(1):65–8.

28. Ishida S, Sugino M, Hosokawa T, Sato T, Furutama D, Fukuda A, et al. Amiodarone-induced liver cirrhosis and parkinsonism: a case report. *Clin Neuropathol.* 2010;**29**(2):84–8.

29. Masmoudi K, Masson H, Gras V, Andrejak M. Extrapyramidal adverse drug reactions associated with trimetazidine: a series of 21 cases. *Fundam Clin Pharmacol.* 2012;**26**(2):198–203.

30. Marti Masso JF, Marti I, Carrera N, Poza JJ, Lopez de Munain A. *Trimetazidine induces parkinsonism, gait disorders and tremor. Therapie.* 2005;**60**(4):419–22.

31. Papazian O, Canizales E, Alfonso I, Archila R, Duchowny M, Aicardi J. Reversible dementia and apparent brain atrophy during valproate therapy. *Ann Neurol.* 1995;**38**(4):687–91.

32. Guerrini R, Belmonte A, Canapicchi R, Casalini C, Perucca E. Reversible pseudoatrophy of the brain and mental deterioration associated with valproate treatment. *Epilepsia.* 1998;**39**(1):27–32.

33. Galimberti CA, Diegoli M, Sartori I, Uggetti C, Brega A, Tartara A, et al. Brain pseudoatrophy and mental regression on valproate and a mitochondrial DNA mutation. *Neurology.* 2006;**67**(9):1715–7.

34. McLachlan RS. Pseudoatrophy of the brain with valproic acid monotherapy. *Can J Neurol Sci.* 1987;**14**(3):294–6.

35. Straussberg R, Kivity S, Weitz R, Harel L, Gadoth N. Reversible cortical atrophy and cognitive decline induced by valproic acid. *Eur J Paediatr Neurol.* 1998;**2**(4):213–8.

36. Yamanouchi H, Ota T, Imataka G, Nakagawa E, Eguchi M. Reversible altered consciousness with brain atrophy caused by valproic acid. *Pediatr Neurol.* 2003;**28**(5):382–4.

37. Mahmoud F, Tampi RR. Valproic acid-induced parkinsonism in the elderly: a comprehensive review of the literature. *Am J Geriatr Pharmacother.* 2011;**9**(6):405–12.

38. Perucca E. Pharmacological and therapeutic properties of valproate: a summary after 35 years of clinical experience. *CNS Drugs.* 2002;**16**(10):695–714.

39. Zadikoff C, Munhoz RP, Asante AN, Politzer N, Wennberg R, Carlen P, et al. Movement disorders in patients taking anticonvulsants. *J Neurol Neurosurg Psychiatry.* 2007;**78**(2):147–51.

40. van der Zwan A, Jr. [Transient Parkinson syndrome and tremor caused by the use of sodium valproate]. *Ned Tijdschr Geneeskd.* 1989;**133**(24):1230–2.

41. Easterford K, Clough P, Kellett M, Fallon K, Duncan S. Reversible parkinsonism with normal beta-CIT-SPECT in patients exposed to sodium valproate. *Neurology.* 2004;**62**(8):1435–7.

42. Jamora D, Lim SH, Pan A, Tan L, Tan EK. Valproate-induced Parkinsonism in epilepsy patients. *Mov Disord.* 2007;**22**(1):130–3.

43. Ristic AJ, Vojvodic N, Jankovic S, Sindelic A, Sokic D. The frequency of reversible parkinsonism and

cognitive decline associated with valproate treatment: a study of 364 patients with different types of epilepsy. *Epilepsia*. 2006;**47**(12):2183–5.

44. Silver M, Factor SA. Valproic acid-induced parkinsonism: levodopa responsiveness with dyskinesia. *Parkinsonism Relat Disord*. 2013;**19**(8):758–60.

45. Onofrj M, Thomas A, Paci C. Reversible parkinsonism induced by prolonged treatment with valproate. *J Neurol*. 1998;**245**(12):794–6.

46. Sasso E, Delsoldato S, Negrotti A, Mancia D. Reversible valproate-induced extrapyramidal disorders. *Epilepsia*. 1994;**35**(2):391–3.

47. Loscher W, Nau H. Distribution of valproic acid and its metabolites in various brain areas of dogs and rats after acute and prolonged treatment. *J Pharmacol Exp Ther*. 1983;**226**(3):845–54.

48. Armon C, Shin C, Miller P, Carwile S, Brown E, Edinger JD, et al. Reversible parkinsonism and cognitive impairment with chronic valproate use. *Neurology*. 1996;**47**(3):626–35.

49. Qian Y, Zheng Y, Tiffany-Castiglioni E. Valproate reversibly reduces neurite outgrowth by human SY5Y neuroblastoma cells. *Brain Res*. 2009;**1302**:21–33.

50. Goni M, Jimenez M, Feijoo M. Parkinsonism induced by phenytoin. *Clin Neuropharmacol*. 1985;**8**(4):383–4.

51. Ertan S, Ulu MO, Hanimoglu H, Tanriverdi T, Kafadar AM, Acar ZU, et al. Phenytoin-induced parkinsonism. *Singapore Med J*. 2006;**47**(11):981–3.

52. Factor S. Lithium-induced movement disorders. In: Sethi K, editor. *Drug-Induced Movement Disorders*. New York: Marcel Dekker, Inc.; 2004. p. 209–31.

53. Baek JH, Kinrys G, Nierenberg AA. Lithium tremor revisited: pathophysiology and treatment. *Acta Psychiatr Scand*. 2014;**129**(1):17–23.

54. Vestergaard P. Clinically important side effects of long-term lithium treatment: a review. *Acta Psychiatr Scand Suppl*. 1983;**305**:1–36.

55. Branchey MH, Charles J, Simpson GM. Extrapyramidal side effects in lithium maintenance therapy. *Am J Psychiatry*. 1976;**133**(4):444–5.

56. Shopsin B, Gershon S. Cogwheel rigidity related to lithium maintenance. *Am J Psychiatry*. 1975;**132**(5):536–8.

57. Kane J, Rifkin A, Quitkin F, Klein DF. Extrapyramidal side effects with lithium treatment. *Am J Psychiatry*. 1978;**135**(7):851–3.

58. Asnis GM, Asnis D, Dunner DL, Fieve RR. Cogwheel rigidity during chronic lithium therapy. *Am J Psychiatry*. 1979;**136**(9):1225–6.

59. Lima MA, Maradei S, Maranhao Filho P. Cyclosporine-induced parkinsonism. *J Neurol*. 2009;**256**(4):674–5.

60. Ling H, Bhidayasiri R. Reversible Parkinsonism after chronic cyclosporin treatment in renal transplantation. *Mov Disord*. 2009;**24**(12):1848–9.

61. Kim HC, Han SY, Park SB, Suh SJ. Parkinsonism during cyclosporine treatment in renal transplantation. *Nephrol Dial Transplant*. 2002;**17**(2):319–21.

62. Wasserstein PH, Honig LS. Parkinsonism during cyclosporine treatment. *Bone Marrow Transplant*. 1996;**18**(3):649–50.

63. Munhoz RP, Teive HA, Germiniani FM, Gerytch JC, Jr., Sa DS, Bittencourt MA, et al. Movement disorders secondary to long-term treatment with cyclosporine A. *Arq Neuropsiquiatr*. 2005;**63**(3A):592–6.

64. Fisher JF, Dewald J. Parkinsonism associated with intraventricular amphotericin B. *J Antimicrob Chemother*. 1983;**12**(1):97–9.

65. Mott SH, Packer RJ, Vezina LG, Kapur S, Dinndorf PA, Conry JA, et al. Encephalopathy with parkinsonian features in children following bone marrow transplantations and high-dose amphotericin B. *Ann Neurol*. 1995;**37**(6):810–4.

66. Luque FA, Selhorst JB, Petruska P. Parkinsonism induced by high-dose cytosine arabinoside. *Mov Disord*. 1987;**2**(3):219–22.

67. Manley TJ, Chusid MJ, Rand SD, Wells D, Margolis DA. Reversible parkinsonism in a child after bone marrow transplantation and lipid-based amphotericin B therapy. *Pediatr Infect Dis J*. 1998;**17**(5):433–4.

68. Chuang C, Constantino A, Balmaceda C, Eidelberg D, Frucht SJ. Chemotherapy-induced parkinsonism responsive to levodopa: an underrecognized entity. *Mov Disord*. 2003;**18**(3):328–31.

69. Gjerris F. Transitory procaine-induced Parkinsonism. *J Neurol Neurosurg Psychiatry*. 1971;**34**(1):20–2.

70. Matsuo H, Matsui A, Nasu R, Takanaga H, Inoue N, Hattori F, et al. Propiverine-induced Parkinsonism: a case report and a pharmacokinetic/pharmacodynamic study in mice. *Pharm Res*. 2000;**17**(5):565–71.

71. Sugiyama Y. [Parkinsonism induced by propiverine hydrochloride–report of 3 cases]. *Rinsho Shinkeigaku*. 1997;**37**(10):873–5.

72. Neary D, Thurston H, Pohl JE. Development of extrapyramidal symptoms in hypertensive patients treated with diazoxide. *Br Med J*. 1973;**3**(5878):474–5.

73. Ott BR, Lannon MC. Exacerbation of parkinsonism by tacrine. *Clin Neuropharmacol*. 1992;**15**(4):322–5.

74. Mintz U, Liberman UA, de Vries A. Parkinsonism syndrome due to cephaloridine. *JAMA*. 1971;**216**(7):1200.

75. Parmar RC, Valvi CV, Kamat JR, Vaswani RK. Chloroquine induced parkinsonism. *J Postgrad Med*. 2000;**46**(1):29–30.

76. Mizoi Y, Kaneko H, Oharazawa A, Kuroiwa H. [Parkinsonism in a patient receiving interferon alpha therapy for chronic hepatitis C]. *Rinsho Shinkeigaku.* 1997;**37**(1):54–6.

77. Sarasombath P, Sumida K, Kaku DA. Parkinsonism associated with interferon alpha therapy for chronic myelogenous leukemia. *Hawaii Med J.* 2002;**61**(3):48, 57.

78. Lieberman AN, Goldstein M. Reversible parkinsonism related to meperidine. *N Engl Med J.* 1985;**312**(8):509.

79. Olive JM, Masana L, Gonzalez J. Meperidine and reversible parkinsonism. *Mov Disord.* 1994;**9**(1):115–6.

80. Kagi G, Bhatia KP, Tolosa E. The role of DAT-SPECT in movement disorders. *J Neurol Neurosurg Psychiatry.* 2010;**81**(1):5–12.

81. Hambye AS, Vervaet A, Dethy S. FP-CIT SPECT in clinically inconclusive Parkinsonian syndrome during amiodarone treatment: a study with follow-up. *Nucl Med Commun.* 2010;**31**(6):583–9.

# Chapter 13

# Antidepressants and movement disorders

Gilles Fénelon

In a study performed in 18 countries from every continent, the 12-month prevalence estimate of major depressive episodes (according to the DSM-IV criteria) ranged from 2.2% to 10.4%. The midpoint across all countries was 5%. A substantial proportion of people who seek treatment for major depression have a chronic-recurrent course of illness, and the lifetime prevalence is 2–3 times that of 12 months prevalence.[1] Although the proportion of patients with depression who receive treatment may be less than one-half even in high-income countries, antidepressants are widely used. Moreover, other conditions than depression are treated with antidepressants, in the psychiatric field (e.g., obsessive-compulsive disorder, generalized anxiety disorder) or in nonpsychiatric conditions (e.g., chronic pain). All available antidepressants act via the monoamine neurotransmitters, serotonin and noradrenaline[2] (Table 13.1). The older medications, i.e., tricyclic antidepressants and monoamine oxidase inhibitors, have been supplanted in most cases by newer agents with fewer side effects, mainly selective serotonin reuptake inhibitors (SSRIs) and serotonin and noradrenaline reuptake inhibitors (SNRIs). Although not the most frequent adverse effects of antidepressants, movement disorders may occur during the course of treatment. The study of this topic is hampered by several limiting factors: a) the rarity of systematic prospective studies properly designed to detect movement disorders; b) the use of ill-defined terms, such as "extrapyramidal symptoms" in the older medical literature; c) finally, the fact that a number of patients receiving antidepressants also receive other psychoactive drugs that may also generate movement disorders (e.g., neuroleptics, lithium), so that the imputability may be difficult to establish.

## Tremor

### Antidepressants associated with tremor

Tricyclics, including amitriptyline, clomipramine, and imipramine have been identified as a cause of postural tremor in several controlled trials comparing the effects of these drugs with those of antidepressants of other pharmacological classes. In a systematic review and metaanalysis of 39 trials comparing efficacy and safety of amitriptyline to placebo, significantly more participants in the amitriptyline group suffered from tremor (OR 5.68, 95% CI 3.19 to 10.10, $P < 0.00001$, 10 RCTs, 1230 participants).[4] Tremor is also a common side effect of SSRIs, as shown by systematic reviews and metaanalyses.[5,6]

### Clinical features

Typical rest tremor of parkinsonism is not addressed in this section, which focuses on postural and action tremor. Drug-induced tremor involves upper limbs, with a frequency of 6 to 12 Hz.[7,8] In patients disclosing a tremor while receiving antidepressant drugs, some suggestive features may help orientate the diagnosis (Table 13.2). However, the responsibility of an antidepressant drug may be difficult to ascertain: a) patients under antidepressant treatment often receive other medications with tremorogenic properties, such as mood stabilizers (valproic acid, lithium), neuroleptics, or other nonpsychoactive drugs; b) many chronic conditions in the field of movement disorders (e.g., Parkinson's disease, dystonic syndromes) may display postural tremor and are associated with a high risk of depression and therefore of receiving antidepressant therapy.

*Medication-Induced Movement Disorders*, ed. Joseph H. Friedman. Published by Cambridge University Press.
© Cambridge University Press 2015.

**Table 13.1** Currently available antidepressant drugs (adapted from ref. 2)

| Type of drug | Mode of action | Examples |
|---|---|---|
| Tricyclics | Inhibition of noradrenaline and serotonin reuptake | Imipramine, desipramine, amitriptyline, clomipramine, amoxapine[a],... |
| Selective serotonin reuptake inhibitors SSRIs] | Inhibition of serotonin-selective reuptake | Fluoxetine, citalopram, escitalopram, sertraline, paroxetine |
| Noradrenaline reuptake inhibitors | Inhibition of noradrenaline-selective reuptake | Atomoxetine, reboxetine[b] |
| Serotonin and noradrenaline reuptake inhibitors [SNRIs] | Inhibition of noradrenaline and serotonin reuptake | Venlafaxine, duloxetine, desvenlafaxine |
| Monoamine oxidase inhibitors | Inhibition of monoamine oxidase A | Isocarboxazid, phenelzine |
| | Partially unknown or complex. Presumed antidepressant actions[3]<br>– mirtazapine: enhanced release of noradrenaline and 5-HT1A-mediated serotonergic transmission<br>– bupropion: enhanced release and inhibition of the reuptake of dopamine and noradrenaline<br>– trazodone: 5HT2 receptor antagonism, weak serotonin reuptake inhibition | mirtazapine, bupropion, trazodone |

a. Amoxapine, although usually classified as an antidepressant, has clinically relevant antidopaminergic properties with a profile close to that of atypical antipsychotics [Kapur et al. 1999].

b. Atomoxetine is currently approved in the United States to treat attention deficit–hyperactivity disorder. Reboxetine is not approved for any use in the USA and many countries due to a low benefit/risk ratio.

**Table 13.2** Diagnostic clues for antidepressant-induced tremor [after ref. 9 and 10].

Clear temporal relationship between tremor onset and drug initiation

Relationship between tremor severity and dose

Improvement or cessation of tremor when antidepressant is suspended

Exclusion of common medical or neurological causes of tremor (e.g., hyperthyroidism, essential tremor)

Relative symmetry of upper limb tremor, and absence of head (i.e., neck) tremor

Absence of worsening over time (if doses of antidepressants are stable)

## Pathogenesis

Little is known about the mechanisms of drug-induced tremors in general, and of antidepressant-induced tremors in particular. The current view is that tremorogenic drugs act through an enhancement of the oscillations of peripheral physiological tremor, through an increase in the gain of the muscle receptors and spinal reflex loops. However, an electrophysiological study of patients with postural hand tremor following amitriptyline administration suggested an enhancement of the centrally driven component of physiological tremor in spinal or supraspinal pathways.[11] It has been suggested that fluoxetine-induced tremors result from an increase of serotoninergic activation of the inferior olivary nucleus and/or the red nucleus, two structures which have been involved in the generation of tremors.[7]

## Parkinsonism

### Antidepressants associated with parkinsonism

Although occasionally mentioned,[12] the existence of parkinsonism associated with tricyclic use is questionable. Indeed, in a review of the literature describing the tricyclic-related "extrapyramidal" (i.e., movement disorder) side effects, Vandel et al. identified 30 case reports of such side effects, but none of them was called parkinsonism.[13] Another review on the same topic did not report parkinsonism as a side effect of tricyclic antidepressants.[14] Similarly, in a more recent systematic literature review, movement disorders ("extrapyramidal symptoms") were identified in 89 patients taking only one antidepressant, but none of them had parkinsonism.[15] However, in a study of 155 cases of drug-induced parkinsonism reported to a French pharmacovigilance center, tricyclics were involved in three (2%).[16] Conversely, imipramine was found to have a beneficial effect on parkinsonian signs, independently of an effect on mood, in two early controlled studies, which raise a number of methodological issues. [17,18] Interestingly, a metaanalysis using a database compiled from six clinical trials suggested that early Parkinson's disease patients treated with tricyclics, amitriptyline in particular, experienced a significant delay in the initiation of dopaminergic therapy, an effect not attributable to a symptomatic effect.[19] The evidence of a role of newer antidepressants in inducing or aggravating preexisting parkinsonism is stronger. In 1979, Meltzer et al. published the case of a 25-year severely depressed man who, four days after the onset of a treatment with fluoxetine, acutely developed torticollis and parkinsonism.[12] These symptoms cleared rapidly under treatment with trihexyphenidyl, despite continuous administration of fluoxetine. Since that report, many cases of parkinsonism induced by SSRIs have been reported.[16,20–22]

## Clinical features and risk factors

Although drug-induced parkinsonism is often said to be relatively symmetrical with no rest tremor, this is far from being the rule, and the clinical presentation may mimic that of Parkinson's disease.[23] Parkinsonism usually occurs within the first three months of treatment.[16] Subjects aged 65 years and older are more likely to develop parkinsonism under SSRIs.[22] Identified potential risk factors include in one study the presence of the A1 allele of the D2 dopamine receptor gene [DRD2] Taq1A polymorphism.[22] A facilitating role for CYP2D6 polymorphisms has also been postulated.[24]

## Do SSRIs worsen motor condition in patients with Parkinson's disease?

Depressive disorders as well as depressive symptoms are common in Parkinson's disease and are important factors affecting quality of life. Although their efficacy has been questioned, antidepressants are therefore widely used in patients with Parkinson's disease. In these patients, conflicting data as to whether SSRIs worsen parkinsonism have been reported. Although some individual case reports suggested a reversible motor worsening in some patients, several open-label prospective studies on small groups of patients (14 to 33 each at inclusion) found that the following SSRIs did not modify motor function: fluoxetine,[25] sertraline,[26] paroxetine,[27] citalopram, fluoxetine, fluvoxamine, and sertraline.[28] However, in one prospective study of 65 patients with Parkinson's disease and depression receiving paroxetine during at least three months, 13 patients stopped paroxetine because of adverse events, consisting in two cases in increased "off" time duration and exacerbation of tremor. Motor worsening resolved completely within 48 hours after discontinuation of the drug. [29] In a Dutch retrospective study of levodopa users from a prescription database, it was shown that the start of SSRIs was accompanied by a faster increase of antiparkinsonian drug treatment as compared with starters of tricyclic antidepressants and patients not receiving antidepressants.[30] In a systematic review and metaanalysis of five randomized controlled trials comparing SSRIs to placebos, the dropout rate was not significantly different in both groups of patients.[31] In one of these studies, one patient under citalopram dropped out because of increased bradykinesia, which resolved after treatment discontinuation.[32] Finally, in a recent placebo-controlled trial comparing the efficacy and the safety of paroxetine and of venlafaxine, there was no evidence of treatment-associated worsening of motor function (actually, mean motor scores slightly improved in all groups).[33] In summary, SSRIs seem to very rarely worsen motor function in patients with Parkinson's disease. If it happens, this effect is rapidly reversible after discontinuation of treatment. Nevertheless, most controlled studies were short (no more than four months), and the risk of treatment-related worsening of parkinsonism cannot be ruled out for long-term use.[34]

## Pathogenesis

Although the exact mechanism or SSRI-induced parkinsonism remains controversial, most authors believe it could involve inhibition of dopaminergic neurons by serotonin. This view derives from early studies showing that experimental manipulations aimed at decreasing central serotonergic function enhanced dopaminergic transmission.[35] Moreover, in one patient who developed parkinsonism on fluoxetine, it was found that serum prolactin levels increased while homovanillic acid levels decreased in the cerebrospinal fluid.[12] However, the picture seems to be much more complex. Midbrain raphe neurons emit 5-HT axons which arborize in virtually all components of basal ganglia, and it has been shown that they exert their influence at both ends of the nigrostriatal dopaminergic projection. The nature of this influence is not simple: several 5-HT receptor subtypes (including 5-HT$_{1A}$, 5-HT$_{1B}$, 5-HT$_{2A}$, 5-HT$_3$, and 5-HT$_4$) act to facilitate dopamine release, while the 5-HT2 C receptor mediates an inhibitory effect of 5-HT on dopamine release.[35] Finally, the relative rarity of parkinsonism on SSRIs, and the identification of risk factors, such as older age, female sex, and drug interaction through cytochrome P450 (CYPD2D6), suggest that the modulatory effect of serotonergic systems on dopaminergic systems is not a factor sufficient for parkinsonism to develop.[15,16]

## Akathisia and restless legs syndrome

### Akathisia

Sensu stricto, this term refers to the inability to remain seated, but encompasses more generally motor activity as a voluntary effort to relieve continuous uncomfortable sensations of restlessness. Frequently observed in patients treated with antipsychotics, it may also occur with antidepressants, with many observations following that of Zubenko et al. [36] Akathisia has been described following treatment with tricyclic drugs,[13] fluoxetine and other SSRIs, [37,38] and mianserin.[39] Interestingly, trazodone, an atypical antidepressant with serotoninergic antagonistic properties, improved neuroleptic-induced akathisia in a small controlled study.[40]

The antidepressant-induced akathisia has the same characteristics as those observed in patients with antipsychotics.[37] It has been suggested that, in some instances, antidepressants, including the SSRIs, could increase suicidal behavior by inducing akathisia with associated self-destructive impulses.[41] It may also be associated with violent behavior.[38]

### Restless legs syndrome

**Antidepressants as a risk factor for RLS, prevalence.** The prevalence of RLS in the general population has been found to be around 10%. The prevalence is higher in women than in men and it increases with age.[42] Current evidence is contradictory regarding the question of RLS as a side effect of antidepressants. [43] In a large study of almost 19,000 subjects performed in Europe, the prevalence of RLS was 5.5%. Users of SSRIs but not of other antidepressants were more likely to have RLS.[42] In one prospective study of patients treated for the first time with antidepressants, RLS was recorded as a side effect in 9%.[43] However, another community-based cross-sectional study found a prevalence of RLS of 10.6 and revealed no association between antidepressants and RLS.[44] In a retrospective chart review of 200 consecutive patients referred for sleep initiation insomnia, 45% of the patients had RLS and no significant association was found between the use of antidepressants and RLS.[45] Moreover, one retrospective chart review study found improvement of preexisting RLS by SSRIs in most patients.[46] Another study suggested that the association of RLS and antidepressant use may vary by gender and type of antidepressant: antidepressant was more strongly associated with RLS for men, but not for women, and further analyses revealed an association between RLS and fluoxetine for women, and associations between RLS and citalopram, paroxetine, and amitriptyline for men.[47] The discrepancy between these studies might have various causes[43]: a) in the study by Dimmitt et al.,[46] preexisting RLS did deteriorate in 12% of the patients, and RLS developed in 9% of the patients free of RLS prior to treatment, which is in keeping with the results of other studies; b) RLS typically occurs during the initial days of treatment, and cross-sectional studies of patients with long-standing antidepressant treatment may miss the association with RLS; c) finally, the association between the use of antidepressants and RLS should be interpreted cautiously, as several cross-sectional, population-based, and clinic-based studies reported significantly higher rates of depression symptoms in individuals with RLS than in controls.[48] A prospective study in a cohort of women followed up during six years also showed that subjects with preexisting RLS had an increased risk of developing clinical depression and clinically relevant depressive symptoms.[49] In cross-sectional studies investigating the relationship between antidepressants and RLS, analyses should therefore adjust for depression.[47]

**Antidepressants associated with restless legs syndrome.** Most antidepressants have been reported to provoke or deteriorate RLS: mianserin, mirtazapine, SSRIs, SNRIs, and tricyclic antidepressants. [43,47,50] Conversely, bupropion, an antidepressant devoid of serotonergic effect did not aggravate the symptoms of preexisting RLS in a controlled trial, and there was a trend suggesting a possible beneficial effect, yet to be confirmed.[51]

**Pathogenesis.** The pathogenesis of RLS is poorly understood. It is generally agreed that dopamine and iron availability in the brain modulate emergence of symptoms, while dopaminergic agonists, iron, but also opioid drugs, alleviate the symptoms. Genetic factors seem critical.[45,52] How SSRIs could aggravate or induce RLS in some subjects is unknown. However, a SPECT study showed that in a group of patients with RLS, the severity of symptoms increased as the availability of serotonin transporter decreased. The authors therefore suggested that an increase in serotonergic transmission might exacerbate RLS, possibly via modulations on striatal dopaminergic transmission and on the spinal motor and sensory neurons.[53]

# Periodic limb movements of sleep

Periodic limb movements [PLM] are characterized by brief 0.5–10 s stereotyped lower limb movements during sleep, which typically occur at 20–40 s intervals. PLM can result in electroencephalographic arousals or awakenings and contribute to insomnia, or excessive daytime sleepiness. PLM may be associated with restless legs syndrome. An association between the use of fluoxetine and/or myoclonic jerks during non-REM sleep was described in the 1990s.[54] PLM was described with the use of fluoxetine in depressed patients[55] and soon after with venlafaxine in normal volunteers.[56] In a large case-control study, Yang et al. found that in patients referred for polysomnography (mainly to rule out sleep apnea), the use of venlafaxine and SSRI, and the risk of PLM was increased.[57] An increased risk of PLM in subjects receiving SSRI has also been demonstrated in children.[58] The risk of PLM seems to be independent of the type of SSRI, although differences in severity might exist.[57,59] Other antidepressants involved include venlafaxine and mirtazapine.[60]

# Serotonin syndrome[1]

Serotonin syndrome is a potentially life-threatening adverse drug reaction caused by excessive activation of postsynaptic serotonin receptors, usually in the context of an SSRI treatment.[61–63] Its incidence is not known. Most severe cases result from the interaction of two or more drugs that enhance serotoninergic transmission, among which, in a recent series, were SSRIs, SNRIs, trazodone, mirtazapine, antiemetics (ondansetron), and opiates.[63] Attention has also been drawn on the potential risk of serotonin syndrome in patients with Parkinson's disease receiving both an antidepressant and an inhibitor of monoamine oxidase B.

The clinical features of serotonin syndrome are: 1) neuromuscular hyperactivity: myoclonus, tremor, hyperreflexia, rigidity (predominant in lower limbs); 2) autonomic dysfunction: diaphoresis, fever, tachycardia, tachypnea, mydriasis, hypertension; and 3) altered mental status: agitation, confusion. [61–63] Several sets of clinical criteria have been put forward. The "Hunter serotonin toxicity criteria," more specific and sensitive than previous ones, are displayed in Table 13.3.[63,64] Some nonspecific laboratory findings may develop, including an elevated white blood cell count, elevated creatine phosphokinase, and metabolic acidosis. The serotonin syndrome shares clinical features with neuroleptic malignant syndrome, an idiosyncratic reaction with antipsychotic drugs. Patients with the latter condition usually have higher fever, more severe rigidity, and higher levels of creatine phosphokinase due to rhabdomyolysis. However, the diagnosis may be

**Table 13.3** The Hunter serotonin toxicity criteria (after ref. 63 and 64)

| Exposure to a serotonergic agent, plus one of the following: |
| --- |
| • Spontaneous clonus |
| • Inducible or ocular clonus and agitation or diaphoresis |
| • Inducible or ocular clonus and increased muscle tone and temperature > 38°C |
| • Tremor and hyperreflexia |

---

1 See also chapter 4.

difficult in patients receiving both antipsychotic and serotoninergic drugs.[65] Treatment of serotonin syndrome consists of removal of all serotonergic drugs, supportive measures, and administration of benzodiazepines and in some cases of serotonin antagonists such as cyproheptadine.[63] Most patients recover within a few days of initiating care.

# Other antidepressant-induced hyperkinesia

## Chorea

Chorea is not mentioned in a number of studies reviewing the antidepressant-induced movement disorders and focusing mainly on tricyclics and SSRIs, although the syndromic nature of "dyskinesia" or "dyskinesia-like movements" is imprecise and may include choreic movements.[66] Rare anecdotal reports of choreic syndrome have been published, involving trazodone,[67] and escitalopram in association with paliperidone, an atypical neuroleptic.[68] In one small but controlled study, fluoxetine did not aggravate chorea in patients with Huntington's disease.[69]

## Dystonia and dyskinesia

Dyskinesia is an ambiguous term that refers either to hyperkinetic movement disorders in general, or more specifically to some drug-induced movement disorders occurring with an acute course, or after long-term treatment. In the latter case, the abnormal movements are referred to as "tardive dyskinesia." Tardive dyskinesia consists in most cases in orofacial movements and/or choreic movements. Dystonia may be included in dyskinesia or described apart. Tardive dyskinesia and dystonia most often result from the use of dopamine receptor antagonist treatment. Dystonia and dyskinesia associated with antidepressants have been occasionally reported, but their incidences are unknown and seem to be much lower than that observed with neuroleptics.[15,21,65,70] In most cases, drugs implicated are SSRIs, with some cases of tardive dystonia involving SNRIs, trazodone, and amitriptyline.[13,71] Precise clinical data are lacking in most cases.

## Bruxism

Bruxism, defined as involuntary tooth grinding or tooth clenching, may occur during sleep or in wakefulness, and is frequent in the general adult population. Since the initial report by Ellison and Stanziani,[72] bruxism has been reported as a frequent adverse event of SSRIs and in rare cases following the use of SNRIs, i.e., duloxetine and venlafaxine.[70,73] SSRI-induced bruxism may resolve by reducing the antidepressant dose or by adding buspirone, a $5-HT1_A$ receptor agonist.[74]

## Myoclonus

Reversible action-myoclonus has been predominantly reported following the administration of tricyclics.[13,75] In a prospective study, Garvey and Tollefson found that, in 98 patients receiving cyclic antidepressant therapy, 39 developed myoclonus which was "clinically significant" in nine cases.[76] Cyclic antidepressant-induced myoclonus may be associated with EEG abnormalities and enlarged cortical somato-sensory evoked potentials, suggesting cortical hyperexcitability.[75] SSRIs may also induce myoclonus, outside the context of the serotonin syndrome. In a French pharmacovigilance database study, antidepressants, in most cases SSRIs, were involved in 15% of 423 reports of drug-induced myoclonus.[77]

## References

1. Kessler RC, Bromet EJ. The epidemiology of depression across cultures. *Annu Rev Public Health* 2013; **34**: 119–38.

2. Berton O, Nestler EJ. New approaches to andidepressant drug discovery: beyond monoamines. *Nat Rev Neurosci* 2006; **7**: 137–51.

3. Ciraulo DA, Shader RI, Greenblatt DJ. Clinical pharmacology and therapeutics of antidepressants. In: Ciraulo DA, Shader RI, eds, *Pharmacology of depression*, DOI 10.1007/978-1-60327-435-7_2, Springer Science +Business Media, LLC 2011

4. Leucht C, Huhn M, Leucht S. Amitriptyline versus placebo for major depressive disorder. *Cochrane Database Syst Rev* 2012; **12**: CD009138.

5. Edwards JG, Anderson I. Systematic review and guide to selection of selective serotonin reuptake inhibitors. *Drugs* 1999; **57**: 507–33.

6. Watanabe N, Omori IM, Nakagawa A, et al. Safety reporting and adverse-event profile of mirtazapine described in randomized controlled trials in comparison with other classes of antidepressants in the acute-phase treatment of adults with depression: systematic review and meta-analysis. *CNS Drugs* 2010; **24**: 35–53.

7. Serrano-Dueñas M. Fluoxetine-induced tremor: clinical features in 21 patients. *Parkinsonism Relat Disord* 2002; **8**: 325–7.

8. Zeuner KE, Deuschl G. An update on tremors. *Curr Opin Neurol* 2012; **25**: 475–482.

9. Morgan JC, Sethi KD. Drug-induced tremors. *Lancet* 2005; **4**: 866–76.

10. Burkhard PR. Acute and subacute drug-induced movement disorders. *Parkinsonism Relat Disord* 2014; **20S1**: S108–12.

11. Raethjen J, Lemke MR, Lindemann M, Wenzelburger R, Krack P, Deuschl G. Amitriptyline enhances the central component of physiological tremor. *J Neurol Neurosurg Psychiatry* 2001; **70**: 78–82.

12. Meltzer HY, Young M, Metz J, Fang VS, Schyve PM, Arora RC. Extrapyramidal side effects and increased serum prolactin following fluoxetine, a new antidepressant. *J Neural Transm* 1979; **45**: 165–75.

13. Vandel P, Bonin B, Leveque E, Sechter D, Bizouard P. Tricyclic antidepressant-induced extrapyramidal side effects. *Eur Neuropsychopharmacol* 1997; **7**: 207–12.

14. Gill HS, DeVane CL, Risch SC. Extrapyramidal symptoms associated with cyclic antidepressant treatment: a review of the literature and consolidating hypotheses. *J Clin Psychopharmacol* 1997; **17**: 377–89.

15. Madhusoodanan S, Alexeenko L, Sanders R, Brenner R. Extrapyramidal symptoms associated with antidepressants. A review of the literature and an analysis of spontaneous reports. *Ann Clin Psychiatry* 2010; **22**: 148–56.

16. Bondon-Guitton E, Perez-Lloret S, Bagheri H, Brefel C, Rascol O, Montatsruc JL. Drug-induced parkinsonism: a review of 17 years experience in a regional pharmacovigilance center in France. *Mov Disord* 2011; **26**: 2226–31.

17. Strang RR. Imipramine in treatment of parkinsonism: a double-blind placebo study. *Brit Med J* 1965; **2**: 33–34.

18. Laitinen L. Desipramine in treatment of Parkinson's disease. A placebo-controlled study. *Acta Neurol Scand* 1969; **45**: 109–13.

19. Paumier KL, Siderowf AD, Auinger P, et al. Tricyclic antidepressants delay the need for dopaminergic therapy in early Parkinson's disease. *Mov Disord* 2012; **27**: 880–7.

20. Leo RJ. Movement disorders associated with the serotonin selective reuptake inhibitors. *J Clin Psychiatry* 1996; **57**: 449–54.

21. Spigset O. Adverse reactions of selective serotonin reuptake inhibitors: reports from a spontaneous reporting system. *Drug Saf* 1999; **20**: 277–87.

22. Hedenmalm K, Güzey C, Dalh ML, Yue QY, Spigset O. Risk factors for extrapyramidal symptoms during treatment with selective serotonin reuptake inhibitors, including cytochrome P-450 enzyme, and serotonin and dopamine transporter and receptor polymorphisms. *J Clin Psychopharmacol* 2006; **26**: 192–7.

23. Montastruc JL, llau ME, Rascol O, Senard JM. Drug-induced parkinsonism: a review. *Fundam Clin Pharmacol* 1994; **8**: 293–306.

24. García-Parujuà P, de Ugarte L, Baca E. More data for the CYP2D6 hypothesis? The in vivo inhibition of CYP2D6 isoenzyme and extrapyramidal symptoms induced by antidepressants in the elderly. *J Clin Psychopharmacol* 2004; **24**: 111–2.

25. Montastruc J-L, Fabre N, Blin O, Senard J-M, Rascol O, Rascol A. Does fluoxetine aggravate Parkinson's disease? A pilot prospectice study. *Mov Disord* 1995; **10**: 355–7.

26. Hauser RA, Zesiewicz TA. Sertraline for the treatment of depression in Parkinson's disease. *Mov Disord* 1997; **12**: 756–759.

27. Ceravolo R, Nuti A, Piccinni A, et al. Paroxetine in Parkinson's disease: effects on motor and depressive symptoms. *Neurology* 2000; **55**: 1216–8.

28. Dell'Agnello G, Ceravolo R, Nuti A, et al. SSRIs do not worsen Parkinson's disease: evidence from an open-label, prospective study; *Clin Neuropharmacol* 2001; **24**: 221–7.

29. Tesi S, Antonini A, Canesi M, Zecchinelli A, Mariani CB, Pezzoli G. Tolerability of paroxetine in Parkinson's disease: a prospective study. *Mov Disord* 2000; **15**: 986–9.

30. van de Vijer DAMC, Roos RAC, Jansen PAF, Porsius AJ, de Boer A. Start of a selective serotonin reuptake inhibitor (SSRI) and increase of antparkinsonian drug treatment in patients on levodopa. *Br J Clin Pharmacol* 2002; **54**: 168–170.

31. Skapinakis P, Bakola E, Salanti G, Lewis G, Krytsis AP, Mavreas V. Efficacy and acceptability of selective serotonin reuptake inhibitors for the treatment of depression in Parkinson's disease: a systematic review and meta-analysis of randomized controlled trials. *BMC Neurol* 2010; **10**: 49.

32. Devos D, Dujardin K, Poirot I, et al. Comparison of desipramine and citalopram treatments for depression in Parkinson's disease: a double-blind, randomized, placebo-controlled study. *Mov Disord.* 2008; **23**: 850–7.

33. Richard IH, McDermott MP, Kurlan R. A randomized, double-blind, placebo-controlled trial of antidepressants in Parkinson disease. *Neurology* 2012; **78**: 1229–36.

34. Perez-Lloret S, Rascol O. Serotonin reuptake inhibitors for depression in PD. *Nat Rev Neurol* 2012; **8**: 365–6.

35. Esposito E, Di Matteo V, Di Giovanni G. Serotonin-dopamine interaction: an overview. *Progress Brain Res* 2008; **172**: 3–6.

36. Zubenko GS, Cohen BM, Lipinski JF Jr. Antidepressant-related akathisia. *J Clin Psychopharmacol* 1987; **7**: 254–7.

37. Lipinski JF Jr, Mallya G, Zimmerman P, Pope HG Jr. Fluoxetine-induced akathisia: clinical and theoretical implications. *J Clin Psychiatry* 1989; **50**: 339–42.

38. Lucire Y, Crotty C. Antidepressant-induced akathisia-related homicides associated with diminishing mutations in metabolizing genes of the CYP450 family. *Pharmacogenomics Pers Med* 2011; **4**: 65–81.

39. Markoula S, Konistiotis S, Chatzistafanidis D, Lagos G, Krytsis AP. Akathisia induced by mirtazapine after 20 years of continuous treatment. *Clin Neuropharmacol* 2010; **33**: 50–1.

40. Stryjer R, Rosenzcwaig S, Bar F, Ulman AM, Weizman A, Spivak B. Trazodone for the treatment of neuroleptic-induced acute akathisia: a placebo-controlled, double-blind, crossover study. *Clin Neuropharmacol* 2010; **33**: 219–22.

41. Hansen L. Fluoxetine dose-increment related akathisia in depression: implications for clinical care, recognition and management of selective serotonin reuptake inhibitor-induced akathisia. *J Psychopharmacol* 2003; **17**: 451–2.

42. Ohayon MM, Roth T. Prevalence of restless legs syndrome and periodic limb movement disorder in the general population. *J Psychosom Res* 2002; **53**: 547–554.

43. Rottach KG, Schaner BM, Kirch MH, et al. Restless legs syndrome as side effect of second generation antidepressants. *J Psychiatr Res* 2009; **43**: 70–5.

44. Högl B, Kiechl S, Willeit J, et al. Restless syndrome. A community-based study of prevalence, severity, and risk factors. *Neurology* 2005; **64**: 1920–24.

45. Brown LK, Decrick DL, Doggett JW, Guido PS. Antidepressant medication use and restless legs syndrome in patients presenting with insomnia. *Sleep Med* 2005; **6**: 443–50.

46. Dimmitt SB, Riley GJ. Selective serotonin receptor uptake inhibitors can reduce restless legs symptoms. *Arch Intern Med* 2000; **160**: 147.

47. Baughman KR, Bourguet CC, Ober SK. Gender differences in the association between antidepressant use and restless legs syndrome. *Mov Disord* 2009; **24**: 1054–9.

48. Picchietti D, Winkelmann JW. Restless legs syndrome, periodic limb movements in sleep, and depression. *Sleep* 2005; **28**: 891–98.

49. Li Y, Mirzaei F, Eilis J, et al. Prospective study of restless legs syndrome and risk of depression in women. *Am J Epidemiol* 2012; **176**: 279–88.

50. Page RL II, Ruscin JM, Bainbridge JL, Brieke AA. Restless legs syndrome induced by escitalopram: case report and review of the literature. *Pharmacotherapy* 2008; **28**: 271–80.

51. Bayard M, Bailey B, Acharya D, et al. Bupropion and restless legs syndrome: a randomized controlled trial. *J Am Board Fam Med* 2011; **24**: 422–8.

52. Freeman AA, Rye DB. The molecular basis of restless legs syndrome. *Curr Opin Neurobiol* 2013; **23**: 895–900.

53. Jhoo JH, Yoon I-Y, Kim YK, et al. Availability of brain serotonin transporters in patients with restless legs syndrome. *Neurology* 2010; **74**: 513–8.

54. Armitage R, Trived M, Rush JA. Fluoxetine and oculomotor activity during sleep in depressed patients. *Neuropsychopharmacol* 1995; **12**: 159–65.

55. Dorsey CM, Lukas SE, Cunningham SL. Fluoxetine-induced sleep disturbance in depressed patients. *Neuropsychopharmacol* 1996; **14**: 437–42.

56. Salin-Pascual RJ, Galicia-Polo L, Drucker-Colin R. Sleep changes after 4 consecutive days of venlafaxine administration in normal volunteers. *J Clin Psychiatry* 1997; **58**: 348–50.

57. Yang C, White DP, Winkelman JW. Antidepressants and periodic leg movements of sleep. *Biol Psychiatry* 2005; **58**: 510–4.

58. Vendrame M, Zarowski M, Loddenkemper T, Steinborn B, Kothare SV. Selective serotonin reuptake inhibitors and periodic limb movements of sleep. *Pediatr Neurol* 2011; **45**: 175–7.

59. Zhang B, Hao Y, Jia F, et al. Sertraline and periodic limb movements during sleep: an 8-week open-label study in depressed patients with insomnia. *Sleep Med* 2013; **14**: 1405–12.

60. Fulda S, Kloiber S, Dose T, et al. Mirtazapine provokes periodic leg movements during sleep in young healthy men. *Sleep* 2013; **36**: 661–9.

61. Lane R, Baldwin D. Selective serotonin reuptake inhibitor-induced serotonin syndrome: review. *J Clin Psychopharmacol* 1997; **17**: 208–21.

62. Talarico G, Tosto G, Pietracupa S, et al. Serotonin toxicity: a short review of the literature and two case reports involving citalopram. *Neurol Sci* 2011; **32**: 507–9.

63. Pedavally S, Fugate JE, Rabisntein AA. Serotonin syndrome in the intensive care unit: clinical presentations and precipitating medications. *Neurocrit Care* 2014; **21**: 108–113.

64. Dunkley EJC, Isbister GK, Sibbritt D, Dawson AH, Whyte IM. The Hunter serotonin toxicity criteria: simple and accurate diagnostic decision rules for serotonin toxicity. *Q J Med* 2003; **96**: 635–42.

65. Dosi R, Ambaliya A, Joshi H, Patell R. Serotonin syndrome versus neuroleptic malignant syndrome: a challenging clinical quandary. *BMJ Case Rep* 2014 pii: bcr2014204154.

66. Schillevoort I, van Puijenbroek EP, de Boer A, Roos RAC, Jansen PAF, Leufkens HGM. Extrapyramidal

syndromes associated with selective serotonin reuptake inhibitors: a case-control study using spontaneous reports. *Int Clin Psychopharmacol* 2002; **17**: 75–9.

67. Mcneill A. Chorea induced by low-dose trazodone. *Eur Neurol* 2006; **55**:101–102.

68. Hüther R, Gebhart C, Mirisch S, Bäuml J, Förstl H. Choreatic symptoms during and after treatment with paleperidone and escitalopram. *Pharmacopsychiatry* 2008; **41**: 203–4.

69. Como PG, Rubin AJ, O'Brien CF et al. A controlled trial study in nondepressed patients with Huntington's disease. *Mov Disord* 1997; **12**: 397–401.

70. Gerber PE, Lynd LD. Selective serotonin reuptake inhibitor-induced movement disorders. *Ann Pharmacother* 1998; **32**: 692–8.

71. Chen P-Y, Lin P-Y, Tien S-C, Chang Y-Y, Lee Y. Duloxetine-related tardive dystonia and tardive dyskinesia: a case report. *Gen Hosp Psychiatry* 2010; **32**: 646–9.

72. Ellison JM, Stanziani P. SSRI-associated nocturnal bruxism in four patients. *J Clin Psychiatry* 1993; **54**: 432–4.

73. Falisi G, Rastelli C, Panti F, Maglione H, Quezada Arcega R. Psychotropic drugs and bruxism. *Expert Opin Drug Saf* 2014; **13**: 1319–26.

74. Bostwick JM, Jaffee MS. Buspirone as an antidote to SSRI-induced bruxism in 4 cases. *J Clin Psychiatry* 1999; **60**: 857–60.

75. Jiménez-Jiménez FJ, Puertas I, de Toledo-Heras M. Drug-induced myoclonus. Frequency, mechanisms and management. *CNS Drugs* 2004; **18**: 93–104.

76. Garvey MJ, Tollefson GD. Occurrence of myoclonus in patients treated with cyclic antidepressants. *Arch Gen Psychiatry* 1987; **44**: 269–72.

77. Brefel-Courbon C, Gardette V, Ory F, Montastruc J-L. Drug-induced myoclonus: a French phamacovigilance database study. *Neurophysiol Clin* 2006; **36**: 333–6.

# Ataxia

Marina Sanchez Abraham and Oscar S. Gershanik

## Introduction

In this chapter we will review the different types of drugs that may cause cerebellar ataxia as part of their side effect profile. Ataxia as a drug-induced movement disorder occurs most often in the setting of acute intoxication with phenytoin (PHT) and carbamazepine (CBZ) as the two drugs most commonly implicated [1]. The frequent occurrence of ataxia due to drug exposure stems from the fact that the cerebellum is particularly susceptible to intoxication. Among all cerebellar cells, Purkinje neurons are especially susceptible to this form of injury. Cerebellar circuits are also a main target of drug exposure. However, figures on the prevalence and incidence of cerebellar involvement secondary to drug intoxication are still lacking for most drugs [2].

As is often the case with exposure to neuroleptics and the development of parkinsonism or tardive dyskinesia, the occurrence of ataxia in the setting of an epileptic patient treated either with PHT or CBZ is an expected event. However, it may not be the case with many other drugs that have been only occasionally reported as causing ataxia, and for that reason the treating physician may be unaware. Therefore, when faced with an unexpected event, such as the development of ataxia in a patient undergoing any pharmacological treatment, it may be useful to bear in mind the existence of certain instruments that may help in the ascertainment of the drug-induced nature of the phenomenon, such as the Adverse Drug Reaction (ADR) Probability Scale (Naranjo's Scale)[3].

## Definition of ataxia

Ataxia is both a neurologic symptom and a sign seen only in association with movement or with an attempt to maintain position against a deflecting force such as gravity. Ataxic movements are poorly organized and usually are due to dysfunction of the cerebellum or its numerous connections with other brain regions [4]. Limb and gait ataxia are quite common, but incoordination can also affect speech articulation, swallowing, vision, and truncal movements. The most common phenomenology in ataxia involves limb incoordination, unsteady and broad based gait, tremor, nystagmus, and scanning speech. Like all movement disorders, ataxia can be described in terms of its location, amplitude, frequency, modifying factors, course over time, and associated neurologic and nonneurologic symptoms. The differential diagnosis of ataxia includes a large number of neurologic disorders, so efficient evaluation requires a careful history and a thorough physical and neurologic examination to place ataxia in its appropriate context.

An appreciation of the broad differential diagnosis of movement disorders is also necessary when attempting to implicate a specific drug as causative. Classification and differential diagnosis of ataxic syndromes have an intrinsic complexity owing to the variability in phenotypic presentations and in etiologies, which include trauma, toxic and metabolic causes, neoplasms, immune mechanisms, drugs, and genetic diseases. Pure cerebellar symptoms are rarely observed, while the clinical picture of both genetic and sporadic ataxia syndromes is sometimes complicated by the presence of extracerebellar neurological or multisystem extraneural pathology [5]. Even when the suspected cause is attributable to drug exposure there should be a comprehensive evaluation both clinical and through the use of ancillary diagnostic methods, to rule out other etiologies, as well as a causality assessment. Drug-induced ataxia should

*Medication-Induced Movement Disorders*, ed. Joseph H. Friedman. Published by Cambridge University Press.
© Cambridge University Press 2015.

always be considered in the differential diagnosis in sporadic cases of this disorder.

# Drugs inducing ataxia

The drugs that have been most frequently held responsible for the development of drug-induced ataxia are antiepileptic drugs, and there is ample experience and a comprehensive body of literature, particularly related to PHT and CBZ. However, there are a growing number of published reports describing similar side effects with other AEDs besides the two most often cited in the literature. Similarly, other classes of drugs have been held responsible for the occurrence of drug-induced ataxia through anecdotal case reports or small series of patients. In Table 14.1 the case reports or reviews of drugs that produce ataxia published from 1990 through 2014 are cited. For PHT, due to the large number of published cases, a single review is cited.

## Antiepileptic drugs

### Phenytoin

Among the common movement disorders associated with PHT, cerebellar ataxia is the most frequently reported, followed by asterixis and myoclonus, although a variety of other movement disorders, including chorea, orofacial dyskinesias, tremor, tics, and dystonia, can occur. The classical signs of PHT intoxication are coarse nystagmus, limb and gait ataxia, and dysarthria, which are all signs of cerebellar dysfunction. In a review of 94 cases of PHT intoxication in a general hospital, ataxia was observed in 59/94 patients (63%), and of these, 18 patients had fallen, and nine of these had suffered injuries from their falls severe enough to require medical care. In the reported cases serum PHT levels ranged from 21.4–90 micrograms/ml, with a mean level 44.4 +/–12.5 micrograms/ml [6]. While the outcome in these patients is usually good, with the resolution of ataxia after the drug is metabolized to nontoxic levels, some patients develop chronic complications, such as a slight cognitive deficit or a peripheral neuropathy.

Although acute intoxication is quite frequent, cerebellar signs may develop after several years of chronic treatment. Complete recovery from cerebellar deficits is the usual outcome in these patients once the offending drug has been discontinued or tapered.

However, irreversible lesions may develop. Usually, patients who develop irreversible cerebellar deficits have been exposed to higher doses for longer periods of time [7, 8].

Computed tomography (CT) and brain magnetic resonance imaging (MRI) show cerebellar atrophy of variable degree in patients developing irreversible cerebellar signs following chronic treatment with PHT [2], with the vermian region predominantly affected [9]. In a case-controlled study, cerebellar atrophy was seen in patients with epilepsy exposed to PHT in the absence of seizures and preexisting cerebellar damage [10]. Cerebellar atrophy due to acute PHT intoxication is unusual, but a few cases have been reported [11], although it is controversial whether this effect is due to PHT itself, the underlying seizure disorder, or other causes.

Hospital admission is indicated in symptomatic cases until a declining serum PHT level is observed and ataxia resolves [6].

### Carbamazepine/Oxcarbazepine

Carbamazepine (CBZ) is also commonly implicated as a cause of ataxia. Typically, patients complain of dizziness and exhibit gaze-evoked nystagmus, action tremor, and ataxia of stance/gait. CBZ induces dose-dependent ataxic effects. In a study by Seymour [12], of 33 cases of intentional or accidental CBZ overdose, ataxia, nystagmus, or ophthalmoplegia were seen in 48% of adults with a mean overdose of 12 grams (range 1.6–45). It appears that the presence of cerebellar atrophy as seen on MRI predisposes CBZ-treated patients to ataxia at significantly lower serum levels compared to patients without cerebellar atrophy [13].

Oxcarbazepine (OXC) is the 10-keto analog of carbamazepine which blocks high-frequency voltage–dependent repetitive firing of sodium channels. Indirect comparisons between these AEDs, taking into account dose effect, showed that OXC may be associated with more frequent neurological adverse events than lacosamide (LCM) and eslicarbazepine acetate (ESL). Abnormal coordination/ataxia and diplopia were significantly more frequently observed in patients treated with OXC compared to patients treated with LCM and ESL. The study reveals that the number needed to harm (NNH) associated with OXC 1200 mg (95% IC) was 5 for ataxia/abnormal coordination [14].

**Table 14.1** Drugs inducing ataxia, evidence and references (1990–2014)

| Drug class | Drug (specific) | Evidence | Reference |
|---|---|---|---|
| Antiepileptic | Phenytoin | Review | (Awada et al., 2001) [56] |
| | Carbamazepine Oxcarbazepine | Retrospective review (n: 519) | (Zaccara et al., 2013) [14] |
| Other antiepileptics | Phenobarbital | Clinical review | (Factor et al., 2008) [1] |
| | Gabapentin | Case report | (Steinhoff et al., 1997) [15] |
| | Vigabatrin | Case report | (Sander et al., 1991) [16] |
| | Lamotrigine | Case report | (Fife et al., 2006) [17] |
| | Levetiracetam | Case report | (Chayasirisobhon et al., 2010) [18] |
| | Zonisamide | Systematic review | (Carmichael et al., 2013) [20] |
| | Rufinamide | Randomized controlled trial | (Brodie et al., 2009) [21] |
| | Lacosamide | Randomized controlled trial | (Ben-Menachem et al., 2007) [22] |
| Antineoplastics | 5-fluorouracil | Case report | (Pirzada et al., 2000) [57] (Noguerón et al., 1997) [58] (Barbieux et al., 1996) [59] |
| | Cytarabine (Ara-C) | Case report | (Friedman et al., 2001) [60] (Yeshurun et al., 2001) [61] (Hasle et al., 1990) [62] |
| | Capecitabine | Case report Case report Case report | (Gounaris et al., 2010) [34] (Lam et al., 2008) [33] (Renouf et al., 2006) [32] |
| | Methotrexate | Case report (n:2) Case report | (Masterson et al., 2008) [35] (Ferhanoglu et al., 2003) [63] |
| | Platinum (Cisplatin, Oxaliplatin, Paclitaxel) | Review (phase I) | (Kobrinsky et al., 2013) [64] |
| | Epothilone D | Review (phase II) | (Beer et al., 2007) [36] |
| Antiarrhythmic | Amiodarone | Case report Case report Case report Case report Case report Case report (n:5) | (Chaubey et al., 2013) [65] (Willis et al., 2009) [66] (Hindle et al., 2008) [37] (Krauser et al., 2005) [40] (Garreto et al., 1994) [67] (Arnaud et al., 1992) [68] |
| | Procainamide | Case report | |
| | Propafenone | Case report (n:3) | (Odeh et al., 2000) [42] |
| Antibiotic | Metronidazole | Systematic review | (Kuriyama et al., 2011) [69] |
| | Isoniazid | Case report (pediatric) | (Lewin et al., 1993) [46] |
| Other drugs | Lithium | Case report (n:3) Case report (n:6) | (Niethammer et al., 2007) [70] (Manto et al., 1996) [47] |
| | Calcineurin (Tacrolimus, cyclosporine) | Case report Case report Case report (pediatric) | (Yamaguchi et al., 2007) [49] (Kaczmarek et al., 2007) [71] (Kaleyias et al., 2006) [50] |
| | Bismuth | Case report Case report Case report | (Masannat et al., 2013) [52] (Gordon et al.,1995) [51] (Playford et al., 1990) [53] |
| | Statins | Case report | (Teive et al., 2012) [54] |

## Other AEDs

### Phenobarbital

Phenobarbital (PB) may induce transient ataxic signs at toxic levels, both acutely and after chronic exposure. The most common deficits are gaze-evoked nystagmus, kinetic tremor, and ataxia of stance and gait. Most patients will exhibit concomitant drowsiness. It is estimated that about 5% of epileptic patients treated with barbiturates show cerebellar deficits. Nevertheless, evidence of cellular toxicity and neuronal loss in adults is lacking. Experimental studies underline the vulnerability of the cerebellum during growth, but clinical implications are unclear [2].

### Gabapentin

The mechanism of action of gabapentin (GBT) is through the inhibition of calcium influx and the subsequent release of excitatory neurotransmitters. It is a well-tolerated drug when used for monotherapy or associated with other AEDs. However, movement disorders have been reported previously as rare side effects in individual patients. Steinhoff [15] reported two patients, who developed isolated severe ataxia on low-doses of GBT which resolved abruptly after discontinuation of the drug. One of the patients was receiving GBP as monotherapy and in the other patient, GBP was taken with CBZ. When GBP was stopped for one week, the ataxia disappeared.

### Vigabatrin

Vigabatrin (VGB) is a structural analog of gamma aminobutyric acid (GABA) which irreversibly inhibits the enzyme GABA transaminase. It has been used in refractory epilepsy and infantile spasms (IS) for more than 10 years. Use was restricted due to concern about its safety profile. VGB can induce mild ataxic posture in adults with poorly controlled epilepsy. Gait ataxia appears to be dose-related [16]. There is no data on ataxia as an ADR of VGB in children with epilepsy.

### Lamotrigine

Lamotrigine (LTG) acts by blocking the voltage-dependent sodium channels and thus blocks the release of glutamate through stabilization of the presynaptic membrane. The indications are partial and generalized seizures and worsening severe myoclonic epilepsy. Lamotrigine causes less dysequilibrium than does CBZ in older people on monotherapy for epilepsy [17].

### Levetiracetam

Levetiracetam (LVT) selectively inhibits high-voltage–activated calcium channels and reduces calcium release from intraneuronal stores. It also binds to a specific target in the brain, the synaptic vesicle protein 2A (SV2A), an integral membrane glycoprotein, which is involved in the control of vesicle fusion and exocytosis. There is no substantial evidence that LVT can induce ataxia. However, in a single case report Chayasirisobhon et al. [18] comment on a patient with epilepsy who took an overdose of 63 grams of LVT, resulting in mild ADRs, including mild blurred vision and mild ataxia that rapidly subsided one day after drug discontinuation. However, a metaanalysis evaluating the risk of balance disorders in patients under treatment with second generation AEDs (LVT, GBP, LMT, OXC, pregabalin, tiagabine, topiramate, or zonisamide) at standard therapeutic doses revealed that LVT did not increase imbalance risk at any dose, while the other drugs included in this metaanalysis were found to increase the risk of imbalance in a dose-response fashion [19].

### Zonisamide

Zonisamide (ZNS) is a sulphonamide derivative, a broad spectrum AED that acts through multiple actions: facilitation of dopaminergic and serotoninergic neurotransmission through the blockade of T-type calcium channels, prolongation of sodium channel inactivation, and as a weak inhibitor of carbonic anhydrase. It is approved for use as an adjunctive therapy in adults with partial-onset seizures, IS, mixed seizure types of Lennox-Gastaut syndrome (LGS), myoclonic, and generalized tonic clonic seizure. Neurological side effects include ataxia, in addition to somnolence, agitation, and anorexia [20].

### Rufinamide

Rufinamide (RUF) is an AED that was approved in the European Union in January 2007 as an orphan drug for the adjunctive treatment of seizures associated with LGS. Its mechanism of action is not completely understood but it is believed to work by prolonging the inactive state of sodium channels and therefore limiting excessive firing of sodium-dependent action potentials. The common ADRs with RUF are consistent with the typical profile of AEDs, mainly involving the CNS and gastrointestinal systems. In a placebo-controlled trial [21] of RUF (n: 156) at therapeutic levels (400 mg twice daily, titrated up to 1600 mg twice daily) versus placebo (n: 157) for the adjunctive treatment of partial seizures in adults and adolescents, the incidence of ataxia versus placebo was 13.5 versus 0.6; they occurred primarily during the titration phase.

### Lacosamide

Lacosamide (LCS) is a functionalized amino acid that selectively enhances slow inactivation of voltage-gated sodium channels, increasing the proportion of sodium channels unavailable for depolarization. In a double blind, placebo-controlled, randomized trial, the most common ADRs which occurred in at least 10% of patients in any randomized treatment group were in the CNS and gastrointestinal system (dizziness, headache, nausea, fatigue, ataxia, abnormal vision, vomiting, diplopia, somnolence, and nystagmus). In their 2007 review Ben-Menachem et al. [22], reported that of 421 patients exposed to LCS, ataxia as an ADR was observed in 42 patients, corresponding to13% of the total population under analysis. Ataxia appeared to be related to LCS dose (600 mg/day), although data on serum levels of the drug was unavailable.

## Antineoplastics

Neurologic complications of chemotherapy have been reported with increasing frequency in cancer patients as a result of increasingly aggressive antineoplastic therapy with neurotoxic agents and prolonged patient survival. These complications may result from the direct toxic effects of the drug on the CNS or indirectly from metabolic derangements or cerebrovascular disorders induced by the drugs. The drugs that are most frequently associated with a cerebellar syndrome are: 5-fluorouracil (5-FU), cytosine arabinoside (Ara-C), methotrexate (MTX), and epothilone D.

### 5-Fluorouracil

Fluorouracil (5-FU) is a fluorinated pyrimidine that disrupts DNA synthesis by inhibiting thymidylate synthetase. It is used to treat many cancers, including colonic and breast neoplasms, as well as head and neck malignant tumors. 5-FU can cause both acute and delayed neurotoxicity. An acute cerebellar syndrome occurs in approximately 5% of patients [23, 24]. This usually begins weeks or months after oral dose treatment and is characterized by the acute onset of ataxia, dysmetria, dysarthria, and nystagmus. Acute neurotoxicity, either during or just after infusion of

5FU, is dose-related and generally self-limiting The drug should be discontinued in any patient who develops a cerebellar syndrome. With time, these symptoms usually resolve completely. The development of a cerebellar syndrome may be explained partly by the fact that 5-FU readily crosses the blood-brain barrier.

### Cytosine arabinoside or cytarabine (Ara-C)

This is a pyrimidine analog used in the treatment of leukemias, lymphomas, and neoplastic meningitis. High doses (1 to 3 $g/m^2$ every 12 to 24 hours) can cause an acute cerebellar syndrome in 10% to 25% of patients [25, 26]. Severity of ataxia can range from mild to severe truncal ataxia with inability to sit or walk unassisted [27]. Although it has been shown that Ara-C is preferentially toxic to cerebellar Purkinje cells and cerebellar granule neurons [28, 29], more recent data suggest that Ara-C targets both lineage-committed progenitor cell populations and nondividing oligodendrocytes, which are the myelin-forming cells in the CNS [30]. Thus, some of the neurotoxic ADRs and symptoms seen in patients, may, therefore, be a direct consequence of both oligodendrocyte toxicity and impairment of progenitor self-renewal in the germinal zones of the CNS. In a review published in 1987 by Sylvester et al. [31], the neurotoxicity seen with high-dose Ara-C was dose-related and occurred in up to 60% of treated patients. The incidence of cerebellar toxicity approached 30%, with irreversible ataxia reported in up to 16.7% of the cases. Because the cerebellar toxicity may be worsened by continuation of therapy after initial onset of symptoms, prompt termination of high-dose Ara-C is recommended. Patient's age (greater than 60 years) appears to be the most important risk factor, but drug dose/schedule, cumulative drug dose, renal and hepatic dysfunction, and concomitant use of neurotropic antiemetic agents may also influence the risk of neurotoxicity [27].

### Capecitabine

This is a pyrimidine analog used in the treatment of breast and gastrointestinal malignancies. Neurologic complications are uncommon, but some patients experience paresthesias, headaches, and cerebellar symptoms. There are only a few reported cases of cerebellar syndromes secondary to capecitabine, all of which improved after withdrawal of the drug [32, 33, 34].

## Methotrexate

Methotrexate (MTX) is an effective antimetabolite treatment for various oncological disorders including those affecting the CNS, in widespread leukemia, and CNS lymphoma. The degree of neurotoxicity is related to the dosage, its route of administration, and the concomitant use of other therapeutic modalities with overlapping neurotoxicities, including chemotherapeutic agents and irradiation. Neurotoxicity is characterized by dysarthria, gait dysfunction, dysmetria, and weakness, and has also been described after low-dose subcutaneous methotrexate administration for rheumatoid arthritis. Symptoms have been reported to be usually reversible, and resolved after discontinuation of treatment [35].

## Platinum (cisplatin, oxaliplatin, paclitaxel)

Peripheral axonal neuropathy is probably the most frequent and clinically relevant ADR associated with the use of platinum-derived drugs. Platinum neurotoxicity is first characterized by transient, acute, cold-induced painful paresthesias and numbness, which typically occur during the first few drug cycles. Loss of vibration sense, paresthesias, and ataxia can become apparent after several treatment cycles. In this case, ataxia may be due to the neuropathy (peripheral sensory ataxia) and may be misdiagnosed as cerebellar ataxia [2].

## Epothilone D

Epothilone D is a second-line chemotherapy agent used in the treatment of androgen-independent prostate cancer. In a review of this drug, it was established that ataxia may occur in almost 8% of patients under treatment [36].

# Antiarrhythmics

## Amiodarone

Amiodarone is commonly used for the treatment of ventricular arrhythmias and atrial fibrillation. Neurological ADRs, including ataxia and neuropathy, may occur, and may be dose-dependent. They are more prevalent in older patients [37]. These ADRs are reversible after cessation of amiodarone. The onset of neurologic symptoms may be anywhere from 12 days to 12 months after initiation of amiodarone, and improvement of symptoms has been seen from one week to four months after drug discontinuation [38, 39]. The reported prevalence of neurologic toxicity due to amiodarone has been variable, perhaps as a consequence of variable drug dosing, with a range of 3%–35% [40]. The exact mechanism of neurotoxicity is unknown. However, amiodarone has been shown to cross the blood-brain barrier, and amiodarone and its active metabolite, desethyl-amiodarone, are measurable in the CNS [39].

## Procainamide

Procainamide is used in cardiac arrhythmias. There is a single report in which high doses of the drug were thought to be responsible for the development of ataxia. This was associated with a marked increase in the serum drug level. Resolution occurred within days after drug therapy was discontinued [41].

## Propafenone

Propafenone is an effective antiarrhythmic drug used widely for the treatment of supraventricular and ventricular arrhythmias. Ataxia is an uncommon ADR. In a review, evaluating its safety, three elderly patients were reported to have developed moderate to severe ataxia [42].

# Antibiotics

## Metronidazole

Metronidazole is a commonly used antimicrobial agent. Although it is generally well tolerated with minimal side effects, there are a host of still under-recognized neurologic complications[43]. The most serious side effects of metronidazole involve the CNS. These include acute encephalopathy, seizures, headache, dizziness, syncope, ataxia, dysarthria, hallucinations, agitation, disorientation, and insomnia. Aseptic meningitis and optic neuropathy are also described. Prolonged oral administration of metronidazole has been associated with peripheral neuropathy, which probably is related to the dose and duration of therapy. Woodruff [44] described two cases of new onset ataxia and dysarthria associated with the use of metronidazole. Abnormalities were seen in the dentate nucleus on MRI. Symptoms and imaging abnormalities resolved after discontinuation of the drug.

## Polymyxins (polymyxin B, colistin)

Both drugs have acquired renewed relevance, particularly in the treatment of nosocomial infections. Neurologic side effects have been reported with an incidence as high as 7% to 27%. These typically consist of paresthesias and ataxia, and less commonly, diplopia, ptosis, and nystagmus [45].

### Isoniazid

Isoniazid is used for the treatment of tuberculosis, including tuberculous meningitis [2]. Because isoniazid interferes with pyridoxine (vitamin B6) metabolism, mild neurologic complications can occur. Peripheral neuropathy may occur with daily doses of 6 mg/kg. At higher doses, seizures, dizziness, ataxia, and slurred speech have been reported [46].

## Other drugs

### Lithium

Lithium is the archetypal mood stabilizing drug. It is used to treat mania in patients with bipolar disorders. Lithium can have toxic effects on the CNS that are both acute and chronic. Neurologic ADRs induced by lithium can often be seen with normal lithium levels, and in these cases the symptoms are frequently reversible. There is growing evidence that lithium can induce long-lasting neurological sequelae. Patients may exhibit a severe cerebellar syndrome with scanning speech, tremor, and ataxic gait [47]. These ADRs appear to be multifactorial in their cause, resulting mainly from overdosage, concomitant neuroleptic treatment, and hyperthermia. As regards the few pathological data available, there is a striking loss of cerebellar Purkinje cells, noted in all published neuropathological reports on this condition [48]. The pathological data available involved patients with supratherapeutic serum levels.

### Calcineurin inhibitors (cyclosporine, pimecrolimus, and tacrolimus)

Calcineurin inhibitors are potent immunosuppressants, and neurological complications with the use of this class of drugs are frequently observed after transplantation, their most common indication [49]. Neurological signs are tremor, behavioral disorders, aphasia, seizures, cerebellar ataxia, vestibular deficits, motor spinal cord syndrome, and paresthesia. Factors that may promote the development of serious complications include advanced liver failure, hypertension, hypocholesterolemia, elevated cyclosporine or tacrolimus blood levels, hypomagnesemia, and concomitant treatment with methylprednisolone. Although clinical deficits may be potentially

reversible after drug withdrawal, cerebellar atrophy may slowly develop even after cessation of the drug. Interestingly, in some patients the ataxia reversed despite the presence of signs of structural damage [50].

### Bismuth

A derivative of salicylic acid, bismuth salicylate displays antiinflammatory, bactericidal action and also acts as an antacid. Bismuth is usually used to treat temporary discomforts of the gastrointestinal tract such as diarrhea, indigestion, heartburn, and nausea. Neurotoxicity with high doses after long periods (greater than 6 weeks), from either unintentional or intentional overdose, causes delirium, psychosis, ataxia, myoclonus, and seizures, and is reversible over several weeks or months, after bismuth intake is stopped [51]. Single cases of bismuth-induced ataxia in the context of an encephalopathic syndrome have been reported [52, 53].

### Statins

Statins, or HMG-CoA reductase inhibitors, are cholesterol-lowering drugs. The most common complication of statin use is myopathy, ranging from painless creatine kinase elevations and myalgias to rhabdomyolysis. Teive et al. [54] described a patient who developed cerebellar ataxia following statin use. Coenzyme Q10 deficiency is associated with cerebellar ataxia and could be a possible link between statin use and the development of this condition [55].

## Management

Supportive treatment is the mainstay of therapy for acute or chronic drug-induced ataxia. Dose reduction or withdrawal of the drug is the most important therapeutic measure for symptom reversibility, although neurologic damage may persist in some cases even after drug discontinuation. In severe or acute ADRs, the first step is discontinuation of the offending drug. Symptomatic treatment may be indicated mainly for concomitant manifestations, other than ataxia, if they persist after the drug has been stopped. Specific therapeutic measures should be instituted based on the knowledge of the pathomechanism of the drug-induced neurologic disorder. At present, there are no specific antiataxic drugs.

Prevention is the most important approach to reduce the incidence of ADRs. Whenever several therapeutic alternatives are available, the one with the least neurotoxicity should be selected, particularly in susceptible patients with risk factors. Dose-related adverse effects may be reduced by stepwise dose increase over a longer period, allowing the patient to develop tolerance to the drug. The dosage should be titrated to a clearly defined clinical or biochemical therapeutic goal starting from a low initial dose.

## Conclusions

One of the main difficulties in addressing the issue of drug-induced ataxia is the variety of drugs involved, and the number of isolated or anecdotal reports found in the literature involving drugs that rarely or infrequently cause ataxia, which often make it difficult to unequivocally find a causative relationship, and even harder at times to provide a rational explanation for their occurrence, in terms of pathophysiological mechanisms. The occurrence of ataxia in the context of an antiepileptic treatment with drugs having a well-documented risk is often an expected event, and the treating physician should be vigilant and closely monitor the patient for the development of symptoms of cerebellar involvement. In other instances the ADR is unexpected, mostly due to its rare occurrence with the drugs involved or even an unknown consequence, as yet unreported. It is in these last instances where strict adherence to the steps involved in causality assessment may help the treating physician in ascertaining the responsibility of a given drug in the symptomatology exhibited by the patient.

## References

1. Factor S, Lang A, Weiner W (Eds). *Drug induced movement disorders*. Wiley-Blackwell; 2nd edition, 2005.
2. Manto M. Toxic agents causing cerebellar ataxias. *Handb Clin Neurol*. 2012;103:201–13.
3. Naranjo CA, Busto U, Sellers EM, Sandor P, Ruiz I, et al. A method for estimating the probability of adverse drug reactions. *Clin Pharacol Ther*. 1981; 30:239–45.
4. Gilman S, Bloedel JR, Lechtenberg R. *Disorders of the cerebellum*. Philadelphia: FA Davis Co (Ed), 1981.
5. Mariotti C, Fancellu R, Di Donato S. An overview of the patient with ataxia. *J Neurol*. 2005; 252(5):511–8.
6. Curtis DL, Piibe R, Ellenhorn MJ, Wasserberger J, Ordog G. Phenytoin toxicity: a review of 94 cases. *Vet Hum Toxicol*. 1989; 31(2):164–5.
7. Ghatak NR, Santoso RA, McKinney WM. Cerebellar degeneration following long term phenytoin therapy. *Neurology*. 1976; 26:818–820.
8. McLain LW Jr, Martin JT, Allen JH. Cerebellar degeneration due to chronic phenytoin therapy. *Ann Neurol*. 1980; 7:18–23.
9. Baier WK, Beck U, Doose H, Klinge H, Hirsch W. Cerebellar atrophy following diphenylhydantoin intoxication. *Neuropediatrics*. 1984;15(2):76–81.
10. Ney GC, Lantos G, Barr WB, Schaul N. Cerebellar atrophy in patients with long-term phenytoin exposure and epilepsy. *Arch Neurol*. 1994; 51:767–71.
11. Alioğlu Z, Sari A, Velioğlu SK, Cerebellar atrophy following acute phenytoin intoxication. *J Neuroradiol*. 2000; 27(1):52–5.
12. Seymour JF. Carbamazepine overdose. Features of 33 cases. *Drug Saf*. 1993; 8:81–88.
13. Specht U, May TW, Rohde M, et al. Cerebellar atrophy decreases the threshold of carbamazepine toxicity in patients with chronic focal epilepsy. *Arch Neurol*. 1997; 54:427–431.
14. Zaccara G, Giovannelli F, Maratea D, Fadda V, Verrotti A. Neurological adverse events of new generation sodium blocker antiepileptic drugs. Meta-analysis of randomized, double-blinded studies with eslicarbazepine acetate, lacosamide and oxcarbazepine. *Seizure*. 2013; 22(7):528–36.
15. Steinhoff BJ, Herrendorf G, Bittermann HJ, Kurth C. Isolated ataxia as an idiosyncratic side-effect under gabapentin. *Seizure*. 1997; 6(6):503–4.
16. Sander JW, Hart YM, Trimble MR, Shorvon SD. Vigabatrin and psychosis. *J Neurol Neurosurg Psychiatry*. 1991; 54(5):435–9.
17. Fife TD, Blum D, Fisher RS. Measuring the effects of antiepileptic medications on balance in older people. *Epilepsy Res*. 2006; 70(2–3):103–9.
18. Chayasirisobhon S, Chayasirisobhon WV, Tsay CC. Acute levetiracetam overdose presented with mild adverse events. *Acta Neurol Taiwan*. 2010; 19(4):292–5.
19. Sirven JI, Fife TD, Wingerchuk DM, Drazkowski JF. Second-generation antiepileptic drugs' impact on balance: a meta-analysis. *Mayo Clin Proc*. 2007; 82(1):40–7.
20. Carmichael K, Pulman J, Lakhan SE, Parikh P, Marson AG. Zonisamide add-on for drug-resistant partial epilepsy. *Cochrane Database Syst Rev*. 2013; 12.
21. Brodie MJ, Rosenfeld WE, Vazquez B, Sachdeo R, Perdomo C, Mann A, et al. Rufinamide for the adjunctive treatment of partial seizures in adults and adolescents: a randomized placebo-controlled trial. *Epilepsia*. 2009; 50(8):1899–909.
22. Ben-Menachem E, Biton V, Jatuzis D, Abou-Khalil B, Doty P, Rudd GD. Efficacy and safety of oral lacosamide as adjunctive therapy in adults with partial-onset seizures. *Epilepsia*. 2007; 48(7):1308–17.

23. Riehl J, Brown WJ. Acute cerebellar syndrome secondary to 5-fluorouracil therapy. *Neurology.* 1964; **14**:961–7.

24. Phillips PC, Reinhard CS. Antipyrimidene neurotoxicity: cytosine arabinoside and 5-fluorouracil. In: Rottenberg DA, editor. *Neurological complications of cancer treatment.* Boston: Butterworth-Heinemann, 1991:97–114.

25. Herzig RH, Hines JD, Herzig GP, et al. Cerebellar toxicity with high dose cytosine arabinoside. *J Clin Oncol.* 1987; **5**:927–32.

26. Hwang TL, Yung A, Estey EH, et al. Central nervous system toxicity with high dose Ara-C. *Neurology.* 1985; **35**:1475–7.

27. Baker WJ, Royer GL Jr, Weiss RB. Cytarabine and neurologic toxicity. *J Clin Oncol* 1991; **9**:679–93.

28. Courtney MJ, Coffey ET. The mechanism of Ara-C-induced apoptosis of differentiating cerebellar granule neurons. *Eur J Neurosci.* 1999; **11**(3):1073–84.

29. Dworkin LA, Goldman RD, Zivin LS, Fuchs PC. Cerebellar toxicity following high-dose cytosine arabinoside. *J Clin Oncol.* 1985;**3**(5):613–6.

30. Dietrich J, Han R, Yang Y, Mayer-Proschel M, Noble M. CNS progenitor cells and oligodendrocytes are targets of chemotherapeutic agents in vitro and in vivo. *J Biol.* 2006; **5**(7):22.

31. Sylvester RK, Fisher AJ, Lobell M. Cytarabine-induced cerebellar syndrome: case report and literature review. *Drug Intell Clin Pharm.* 1987; **21**(2):177–80.

32. Renouf D, Gill S. Capecitabine-induced cerebellar toxicity. *Clin Colorectal Cancer.* 2006; **6**(1):70–1.

33. Lam MS, Kaufman DA, Russin MP. Capecitabine-associated cerebellar ataxia. *Am J Health Syst Pharm.* 2008; **65**(21):2032–5.

34. Gounaris I, Ahmad A. Capecitabine-induced cerebellar toxicity in a patient with metastatic colorectal cancer. *J Oncol Pharm Pract.* 2010; **16**(4):277–9.

35. Masterson K, Merlini L, Lovblad KO. Coexistence of reversible cerebral neurotoxicity and irreversible cerebellar atrophy following an intrathecal methotrexate chemotherapy: two case reports. *J Neuroradiol.* 2008; **36**(2):112–4.

36. Beer TM, Higano CS, Saleh M, Dreicer R, Hudes G, Picus J, Rarick M, Fehrenbacher L, Hannah AL. Phase II study of KOS-862 in patients with metastatic androgen independent prostate cancer previously treated with docetaxel. *Invest New Drugs.* 2007; **25**(6):565–70.

37. Hindle JV, Ibrahim A, Ramaraj R. Ataxia caused by amiodarone in older people. *Age Ageing.* 2008; **37**:347–8.

38. Charness ME, Morady F, Scheinman MM. Frequent neurologic toxicity associated with amiodarone therapy. *Neurology.*1984; **34**:669–71.

39. Palakurthy PR, Iyer V, Meckler RJ. Unusual neurotoxicity associated with amiodarone therapy. *Arch Intern Med.* 1987; **147**:881–4.

40. Krauser DG, Segal AZ, Kligfield P. Severe ataxia caused by amiodarone. *Am J Cardiol.* 2005; **96**:1463–4.

41. Schwartz AB, Klausner SC, Yee S, Turchyn M. Cerebellar ataxia due to procainamide toxicity. *Arch Intern Med.* 1984; **144**(11):2260–1.

42. Odeh M, Seligmann H, Oliven A. Propafenone-induced ataxia: report of three cases. *Am J Med Sci.* 2000; **320**(2):151–3.

43. Sarna JR, Furtado S, Brownell AK. Neurologic complications of metronidazole. *Can J Neurol Sci.* 2013; **40**(6):768–76.

44. Woodruff BK, Wijdicks EF, Marshall WF. Reversible metronidazole-induced lesions of the cerebellar dentate nuclei. *N Engl J Med.* 2002; **346**(1):68–9.

45. Wolinsky E, Hines JD. Neurotoxic and nephrotoxic effects of colistin in patients with renal disease. *N Engl J Med.* 1972; **266**: 759–62.

46. Lewin PK, McGreal D. Isoniazid toxicity with cerebellar ataxia in a child. *CMAJ.* 1993; **148**(1):49–50.

47. Manto M, Godaux E, Jacquy J, Hildebrand JG. Analysis of cerebellar dysmetria associated with lithium intoxication. *Neurol Res.* 1996; **18**(5):416–24.

48. Grignon S, Bruguerolle B. Cerebellar lithium toxicity: a review of recent literature and tentative pathophysiology. *Therapie.* 1996; **51**(2):101–6.

49. Yamaguchi I, Ichikawa T, Nakao K, Hamasaki K, Hirano K, Eguchi S, Takatsuki M, Kawasita Y, Kanematsu T, Eguchi K. Cerebellar ataxia in a patient receiving calcineurin inhibitors after living donor liver transplantation: a case report. *Transplant Proc.* 2007; **39**(10):3495–7.

50. Kaleyias J, Faerber E, Kothare SV. Tacrolimus induced subacute cerebellar ataxia. *Eur J Paediatr Neurol.* 2006; **10**(2):86–9.

51. Gordon MF, Abrams RI, Rubin DB, Barr WB, Correa DD. Bismuth subsalicylate toxicity as a cause of prolonged encephalopathy with myoclonus. *Mov Disord.* 1995; **10**(2):220–2.

52. Masannat Y, Nazer E. Pepto bismuth associated neurotoxicity: A rare side effect of a commonly used medication. *W V Med J.* 2013; **109**(3):32–4.

53. Playford RJ, Matthews CH, Campbell MJ, Delves HT, Hla KK, Hodgson HJ, Calam J. Bismuth induced encephalopathy caused by tri potassium dicitrato bismuthate in a patient with chronic renal failure. *Gut.* 1990; **31**(3):359–60.

54. Teive HA, Munhoz RP, Werneck LC. Acquired cerebellar ataxia due to statin use. *Arq Neuropsiquiatr.* 2012; **70**(2):152.

55. Musumeci O, Naini A, Slonim AE, Skavin N, Hadjigeorgiou GL, Krawiecki N, et al. Familial cerebellar ataxia with muscle coenzyme Q10 deficiency. *Neurology.* 2001; **56**:849–855.

56. Awada AA, Al-Mezem S, Amene PC. Phenytoin intoxication: burden and risk factors. *Neurosciences (Riyadh).* 2001; **6**(3):166–8.

57. Pirzada NA, Ali II, Dafer RM. Fluorouracil-induced neurotoxicity. *Ann Pharmacother.* 2000; **34**(1):35–8.

58. Noguerón E, Berrocal A, Albert A, Camps C, Vicent JM. [Acute cerebellar syndrome due to 5-fluorouracil]. *Rev Neurol.* 1997; **25**(148):2053–4.

59. Barbieux C, Patri B, Cerf I, de Parades V. [Acute cerebellar syndrome after treatment with 5-fluorouracil]. *Bull Cancer.* 1996; **83**(1):77–80.

60. Friedman JH, Shetty N. Permanent cerebellar toxicity of cytosine arabinoside (Ara C) in a young woman. *Mov Disord.* 2001 May; **16**(3):575–7.

61. Yeshurun M, Marsot Dupuch K. Acute cerebellar syndrome following intermediate-dose cytarabine. *Br J Haematol.* 2001; **113**(4):846.

62. Hasle H. Cerebellar toxicity during cytarabine therapy associated with renal insufficiency. *Cancer Chemother Pharmacol.* 1990;**27**(1):76–8.

63. Ferhanoglu B, Ongören S, Ar CM, Uzel B, Forta H, Necioglu D. Intrathecal methotrexate-induced acute cerebellar syndrome. *Ann Hematol.* 2003;**82**(4):241–3.

64. Kobrinsky B, Joseph SO, Muggia F, Liebes L, Beric A, Malankar A, Ivy P, Hochster H. A phase I and pharmacokinetic study of oxaliplatin and bortezomib: activity, but dose-limiting neurotoxicity. *Cancer Chemother Pharmacol.* 2013; **72**(5):1073–8.

65. Chaubey VK, Chhabra L, Kapila A. Ataxia: a diagnostic perplexity and management dilemma. *BMJ Case Rep.* 2013; 2013.

66. Willis MS, Lugo AM. Amiodarone-induced neurotoxicity. *Am J Health Syst Pharm.* 2009; **66**(6):567–9.

67. Garretto NS, Rey RD, Kohler G, Cocorullo S, Monteverde DA, Ravera BI, Sica RE. Cerebellar syndrome caused by amiodarone. *Arq Neuropsiquiatr.* 1994; **52**(4):575–7.

68. Arnaud A, Neau JP, Rivasseau-Jonveaux T, Marechaud R, Gil R. [Neurological toxicity of amiodarone. 5 case reports]. *Rev Med Interne.* 1992; **13**(6):419–22.

69. Kuriyama A, Jackson JL, Doi A, Kamiya T. Metronidazole-induced central nervous system toxicity: a systematic review. *Clin Neuropharmacol.* 2011; **34**(6):241–7.

70. Niethammer M, Ford B. Permanent lithium-induced cerebellar toxicity: three cases and review of literature. *Mov Disord.* 2007; **22**(4):570–3.

71. Kaczmarek I, Schmauss D, Sodian R, Beiras-Fernandez A, Oberhoffer M, Daebritz S, Schoenberg SO, Reichart B. Late-onset tacrolimus-associated cerebellar atrophia in a heart transplant recipient. *J Heart Lung Transplant.* 2007; **26**(1):89–92.

# Chapter 15

# Myoclonus and asterixis

P.D. Thompson, T.J. Kleinig, and T.E. Kimber

Myoclonus is defined as an involuntary, brief, shock-like muscle jerk or a sudden, sharp movement. The brisk, sudden movements of myoclonus may be caused by muscle contraction (positive myoclonus) or a pause in muscle contraction leading to a lapse in limb posture (negative myoclonus or asterixis). The abrupt onset and offset of the brief jerky movements distinguishes myoclonus from chorea, dystonia, spasms, tics, tremor, and fasciculation. The clinical characteristics and distribution of myoclonus provide some clues to the site of origin. Cortical myoclonus is often multifocal, action-induced, reflex or stimulus sensitive, and associated with asterixis. Brainstem myoclonus is bilateral, synchronous, and induced by auditory stimuli or cutaneous stimulation of the upper body and face. Spinal myoclonus is segmental, involving the upper or lower limbs and adjacent trunk. In some cases the site of origin of myoclonus is unclear and designated "subcortical." Asterixis is typically subcortical in origin, notably in diffuse encephalopathies and thalamic lesions, but may arise from the cortex in association with cortical myoclonus.

Many examples of drug-induced myoclonus and asterixis are transient and occur in the setting of diffuse encephalopathy associated with drug toxicity, acute metabolic derangements, or infectious illness. In these situations it is not practical to conduct detailed investigation such as physiological studies to determine the precise mechanisms or site of origin in the majority of cases. Some clues may be obtained on clinical examination from the distribution of myoclonus, the pattern of any stimulus sensitivity, and electroencephalography (EEG). A cortical origin is often assumed without supportive evidence. For these reasons the following discussion is organized according to the classes of drug reported to cause myoclonus. A critical review of the potential pathophysiology or mechanism of myoclonus is included where the information allows.

## Antibiotics

The penicillins and cephalosporins are recognized causes of generalized, multifocal or segmental myoclonus, asterixis, and seizures. These signs typically occur in the setting of an encephalopathy with confusion, hallucinations, drowsiness or coma, and hyperreflexia. The majority of cases are recorded in the setting of severe illness, systemic and central nervous system sepsis (especially meningitis). Renal failure and advancing age are risk factors for penicillin and cephalosporin encephalopathy. The administration of penicillin in high doses, a reduction of urinary excretion due to renal failure, and increased permeability of the blood brain barrier as the result of meningitis lead to very high concentrations of the drugs within the central nervous system [1,2]. Antibiotic myoclonic encephalopathies subside with a reduction in dose of the offending drug. In experimental studies the myoclonic effect of penicillin has been observed following topical application of penicillin to the cortex and spinal cord and after intravenous administration in spinal and brainstem preparations, indicating that penicillin enhances neural excitability at cortical, subcortical, and spinal levels [2, 3]. Penicillin-induced myoclonus has been demonstrated in experimental spinal preparations [3] and observed after electrocerebral silence in humans [4]. The mechanism of action may be related to reducing gamma aminobutyric acid (GABA)–mediated inhibition by blocking GABA release or

---

*Medication-Induced Movement Disorders*, ed. Joseph H. Friedman. Published by Cambridge University Press.
© Cambridge University Press 2015.

blocking GABA receptors. Cephalosporins may have a similar mechanism. Other antibiotics including aminoglycosides (gentamicin), quinolones (ciprofloxacin), and sulphonamides (trimethoprim-sulfamethoxazole) have also been reported to produce a myoclonic encephalopathy in the setting of sepsis and renal failure. Truncal myoclonus, with the characteristics of propriospinal myoclonus [5], and multifocal stimulus sensitive myoclonus have been reported after ciprofloxacin administration [6].

## Anticonvulsants

Carbamazepine, lamotrigine, phenytoin, and vigabatrin may exacerbate idiopathic generalized epilepsy syndromes, particularly juvenile myoclonic epilepsy, resulting in myoclonic status epilepticus [7]. Carbamazepine has been reported to induce myoclonus, asterixis, and tics in children and adults with partial seizures. Myoclonus and tics were described in an 11-year-old boy with benign occipital lobe epilepsy with therapeutic doses of carbamazepine [8]. Focal upper limb myoclonus and tics were reported in a 31-year-old man with a history of generalized seizures beginning at age 10 and who had been seizure-free since age 15 on long-term carbamazepine at therapeutic levels [9]. The myoclonic bursts were of long duration [8], and there was no EEG correlate during the limb myoclonus [8,9], suggesting a subcortical origin. The movements stopped after withdrawal of carbamazepine. Oxcarbazepine-induced myoclonic status epilepticus was reported in a 44-year-old man with a 31-year history of juvenile myoclonic epilepsy. Repetitive generalized polyspike and wave discharges on EEG were associated with positive and negative myoclonus that resolved following withdrawal of the drug [10]. Serum levels were not recorded and the case was reported as an example of oxcarbazepine-induced exacerbation of an idiopathic generalized epilepsy syndrome [10]. Myoclonus complicating lamotrigine treatment (in combination with valproate) was reported in two young adult patients with generalized epilepsy and mental retardation since childhood (one with Lennox Gastaut and the other with absence seizures and epileptic drop attacks) [11]. Lamotrigine levels were elevated and both patients experienced an increase in positive myoclonus that was not correlated with spike and wave discharge on EEG [11]. Lamotrigine toxicity was also found to be associated with hyperreflexia

and myoclonus when administered in combination with lithium, antipsychotics, anticonvulsants, and a benzodiazepine for psychiatric indications [12]. A combination of lamotrigine, valproate, and olanzapine induced head and upper limb myoclonus in a woman with bipolar disorder associated with diaphoresis and psychomotor retardation [13]. These cases may have been due to serotonin syndrome, reflecting interactions of multiple drugs and the complex actions of lamotrigine that include inhibition of serotonin and dopamine reuptake and the anticonvulsant effect of reducing glutamate release.

Gabapentin may exacerbate preexisting myoclonus in epilepsy and induce focal myoclonus in patients with focal seizures, particularly in symptomatic epilepsy due to brain injury [14]. Mental slowing, dysarthria, and positive and negative myoclonus resulting in falls were reported in a patient with neuropathic pain, impaired renal function, and levels of gabapentin that exceeded the upper limit of the therapeutic range [15]. Symptoms resolved after stopping gabapentin, and the serum levels fell [15].

Pregabalin has also been associated with myoclonus when used as add-on therapy in epilepsy [16] and in the treatment of neuropathic pain [17]. Healy et al. [17] reported the case of a man with diabetic renal failure who developed myoclonus and an acute encephalopathy with confusion and formed visual hallucinations when treated with gabapentin then pregabalin for neuropathic pain. Cortical correlates preceding myoclonus have not been detected on EEG in either gabapentin- or pregabalin-induced myoclonus [14, 16, 17]. Since gabapentin and pregabalin are excreted via the kidney, toxic levels may accumulate in patients with renal failure [15,17].

Topiramate, prescribed for migraine prophylaxis, has been reported to precipitate an acute psychosis with tremor and multifocal, stimulus-sensitive myoclonus in association with preexisting brain injury [18] and in combination with fluvoxamine [19].

The origin of myoclonus induced by anticonvulsants in myoclonic epilepsy syndromes is not clear, since EEG cortical correlates preceding myoclonus are not found. This highlights the pathophysiological differences in the mechanisms of epileptic myoclonus and that of cortical (reflex and action) myoclonus associated with cerebellar disease, where there is clear electrophysiological evidence of a cortical origin. Pharmacological differences also are evident.

Myoclonus responds to treatment with anticonvulsants such as clonazepam, valproate, levetiracetam, and topiramate that promote GABAergic inhibition, while those that block neuronal excitation such as carbamazepine, lamotrigine, gabapentin, and pregabalin may cause or exacerbate preexisting myoclonus [17].

## Antidepressants

All classes of antidepressants at both therapeutic and toxic doses have been reported to cause myoclonus. Tricyclic antidepressants such as imipramine, amitriptyline, nortriptyline, and clomipramine may cause multifocal or generalized action myoclonus [20]. In many cases this not clinically significant and resolves with reduction in dose [20]. Selective serotonin reuptake inhibitors [SSRI] and noradrenaline reuptake inhibitors may produce generalized, small amplitude myoclonus ("polymyoclonus") [21], generalized action and reflex myoclonus without cortical correlates on EEG [22], or myoclonus as part of a mixed movement disorder with stereotypies [23]. A more dramatic myoclonic syndrome is seen when SSRIs are combined with other antidepressants (especially nonspecific monoamine oxidase inhibitors) and medications such as opiates, antipsychotics, and over-the-counter medications or recreational drugs with sympathomimetic or aminergic properties. Myoclonus in this situation occurs as one component of the serotonin syndrome comprising flushed facies, agitation, wakeful mutism, varying mental state, shivering, tremor, hyperreflexia, ataxia, diarrhea, diaphoresis, and fever [24]. Perioral and facial myoclonus is a characteristic feature, perhaps reflecting the excitatory effects of serotonin on facial motoneurons [25]. Pharmacokinetic interactions, especially involving drugs metabolized by cytochrome P450, also play a role in precipitating the serotonin syndrome.

Advanced age and coexisting neurological illness such as neurodegenerations causing dementia confer susceptibility to myoclonus with SSRI medications [26]. Escitalopram [27] and venlafaxine [28] have been reported to produce action myoclonus in patients with dementia. The combination of escitalopram and lamotrigine in a patient with epilepsy and anxiety resulted in nocturnal myoclonus [29].

Stuttering speech with jaw myoclonus has been reported in association with tricyclic antidepressants [20], fluoxetine [30], desipramine [31], and bupropion [32].

The physiology of myoclonus in these cases remains unclear. However, the serotonergic properties of the tricyclic and SSRI antidepressants and experimental models of myoclonus indicate involvement of the serotonin system. Increasing serotonin levels by administration of 5-hydroxytryptophan, the precursor of serotonin, in experimental models induces myoclonus [33]. Drugs such as imipramine and clomipramine potentiate this effect [34]. Anatomical studies of this model suggest a brainstem origin for the myoclonus [35].

Reversible enlargement of cortical somatosensory evoked potentials has been reported in patients treated with tricyclics who developed myoclonus, seizures, and spike discharges on EEG [36], indicating a cerebral cortical origin for the myoclonus.

In many reports of myoclonus induced by antidepressants, the movements were repetitive and occurred during sleep or involved the legs when relaxing in the evening [20]. This raises the possibility the myoclonic movements were in fact periodic limb movements during drowsiness and sleep [37]. Periodic movements are a side effect of many antidepressants including amitriptyline, clomipramine, fluoxetine, venlafaxine, paroxetine, sertraline, citalopram, and mirtazapine. Amitriptyline and mirtazapine have been shown to induce periodic leg movements during sleep in normal subjects [38, 39]. The mechanism of this effect is postulated to involve enhanced serotonergic and noradrenergic neurotransmission interfering with or reducing dopaminergic activity. Phenelzine, a monoamine oxidase inhibitor, was associated with regular leg movements occurring at sleep onset and waking that were relieved by the serotonin antagonist methysergide [40]. Repetitive jerky leg and trunk movements when recumbent are occasionally encountered in patients taking SSRIs. Such focal and segmental movements are often thought to represent "spinal myoclonus," though it is probable in many cases these also represent periodic leg movements (personal observations).

## Dopaminergic agonists

Levodopa induced myoclonus in Parkinson's disease was described by Klawans et al. [41]. The movements were bilateral and symmetrical or unilateral affecting the arm and leg on one side and occurred as single or repetitive jerks. Movements appeared only during sleep or drowsiness, were not associated with awakening, and increased in frequency when the dose of levodopa was increased. This pattern of movement in levodopa-induced myoclonus is similar to that of periodic limb movements of sleep [37]. Methysergide, a serotonin antagonist chosen because serotonin induced myoclonus in an animal model, abolished the myoclonus in all cases without other changes in parkinsonian signs [34]. In a subsequent study of patients with Parkinson's disease receiving long-term levodopa therapy, episodic nocturnal vocalization and myoclonus were observed to cause a significant disruption of sleep [34]. Nocturnal vocalization and movements during sleep are now recognized as characteristic of rapid eye movement sleep behavior disorder.

As observed in the case of antidepressants, altered serotonergic transmission may be important in the development of this form of nocturnal myoclonus. The effects of levodopa on the 5-HTP model of induced myoclonus were complex, with acute administration depressing the myoclonic response and chronic administration augmenting myoclonus [34]. In this experimental model tricyclic antidepressants and levodopa acted synergistically to augment 5-HTP induced myoclonus [34].

Levodopa-induced dyskinesias may have myoclonic characteristics [42], particularly at the onset of the levodopa effect, before the motor benefit is fully established [43].

Amantadine, an agent with antiglutamatergic, anticholinergic, and dopaminergic properties, has been reported to produce "vocal myoclonus" with stuttering speech and myoclonic jaw and laryngeal movements on attempting to speak in Parkinson's disease [44]. A similar phenomenon described as "cranial myoclonus" was observed in a patient with presumed progressive supranuclear palsy [32]. Limb myoclonus was reported in a patient with progressive supranuclear palsy receiving amantadine [45]. Generalized and multifocal myoclonus with the electrophysiological characteristics of cortical reflex myoclonus was reported in three patients with Parkinson's disease, two of whom had renal failure and an associated encephalopathy [46].

## Dopamine antagonists (antipsychotics)

Postural myoclonus of the arms and action myoclonus of the fingers were reported in 38% of a cohort of chronic schizophrenics receiving neuroleptics (most were taking haloperidol or propericiazine) [47]. Tardive myoclonus of the head and neck, drug-induced parkinsonism, and tardive buccolingual dyskinesia were reported in a patient treated with loxapine [48]. The atypical antipsychotics clozapine and olanzapine are associated with dose-dependent seizures and myoclonus. Several case reports describe multifocal or generalized myoclonus in patients receiving clozapine [49, 50]. Positive and presumably negative myoclonus (asterixis) of the legs and trunk may interfere with standing, causing "leg folding" and falls [51]. Olanzapine was associated with myoclonus and spike discharges on EEG in two patients with Alzheimer's disease, one taking citalopram and donepezil [52] and the other taking gabapentin [53]. The combination of olanzapine and clomipramine in a man with schizophrenia was complicated by myoclonus followed by a generalized seizure with spike wave discharges on EEG [54]. Spike discharges on routine EEG have been observed with clozapine [55], olanzapine, and haloperidol [56]. Such electrophysiological changes are less common with quetiapine [56], but myoclonus has been reported at high doses of quetiapine and following overdose [57, 58, 59, 60].

## Opiates

The oral, intramuscular, intravenous, and intrathecal administration of morphine and other opiate derivatives have been associated with generalized and multifocal myoclonus. This usually occurs in the setting of high doses, though the occurrence of myoclonus does not necessarily correlate with plasma opiate concentration and may be induced by excitatory opiate metabolites [61, 62]. Where tolerance has occurred in long-term opiate administration, the role of coadministration of other drugs precipitating myoclonus has been emphasized [63]. The addition of antipsychotic, antiemetic, antidepressant, and nonsteroidal antiinflammatory drugs may cause myoclonus in previously stable long-term opiate treatment. The myoclonus resolves following withdrawal of the additional drugs or lowering the opiate dose. Patients with renal failure receiving meperidine may be susceptible to developing myoclonus and seizures [62, 64, 65].

The site of origin of opiate-induced myoclonus is not known. In a personally observed case, auditory and somaesthetic stimulation elicited bilateral leg and trunk myoclonus, suggesting a brainstem origin and reticular reflex myoclonus. This is consistent with the findings in an animal model of morphine myoclonus of acoustic stimulus sensitivity and the requirement of an intact spinal cord for the expression of myoclonus, indicating involvement of supraspinal structures in generating myoclonus [66].

## Miscellaneous

### Bismuth

Bismuth-containing preparations are widely available as over-the-counter treatments for various gastrointestinal symptoms. Bismuth encephalopathy, comprising confusion, hallucinations, myoclonus, postural tremor, and gait ataxia was first described in patients following abdominoperitoneal resection for colon carcinoma [67]. Subsequent reports confirmed the association of bismuth and a reversible myoclonic encephalopathy [68].

### Lithium

A myoclonic encephalopathy with seizures, depressed conscious state, and spike discharges on EEG has been described in patients receiving combinations of lithium and antidepressants or neuroleptics [69, 70, 71], but appears less common in lithium intoxication than tremor or ataxia. Action myoclonus with an encephalopathy and paroxysmal spike discharges on EEG were reported after a lithium overdose [69]. Multifocal action cortical myoclonus was described in four patients taking lithium alone and one in combination with sertraline and nefazodone, with electrophysiological studies revealing a cortical EEG correlate preceding the myoclonus and confirming a cortical origin [72].

### Cardiovascular drugs

There are scattered single case reports of calcium channel blockers associated with myoclonus. Nifedipine was associated with myoclonus and dysarthria [73]. Verapamil was associated with myoclonic dystonia [74] and in overdose with bradycardia and hypotension [75]. Amlodipine-induced myoclonus was reported in the setting of stable chronic renal failure [76]. Diltiazem, in therapeutic doses and in combination with citalopram, was considered responsible for myoclonus while recumbent and in response to startle [77]. The mechanism of these effects is not known, nor is the origin of myoclonus, though parkinsonism has also been reported with several calcium channel blocking agents and attributed to effects on

dopamine metabolism. Carvedilol, a nonselective beta adrenergic blocker, was reported to cause multifocal myoclonus without other clinical signs [78].

## Summary

Combinations of drugs appear a significant risk factor for the development of myoclonus. Neurological comorbidities, such as epilepsy, neurodegenerations and meningoencephalitis, and severe systemic illness with an encephalopathy, constitute further risk factors, particularly when there is organ failure that interferes with normal drug metabolism. Some drugs alter neuronal excitability and are capable of generating myoclonus at many levels within the central nervous system, including the cortex (penicillin, lithium) and spinal cord (penicillin). The commonest class of contemporary drugs causing myoclonus are those affecting serotonergic neurotransmission, particularly when used in combination with other antidepressants, opiates, and drugs affecting the dopamine system. Serotonergic drugs also generate myoclonus at multiple levels of the nervous system, including the brainstem, as one element of the serotonin syndrome; or in isolation, when the movements may have the characteristics of periodic limb movements.

## References

1. Conway N, Beck E, Somerville J. Penicillin encephalopathy. *Postgrad Med J* 1968; **44**: 891–897.

2. Lerner PI, Smith H, Weinstein L. Penicillin neurotoxicity. *Ann NY Acad Sci* 1967; **145**: 310–318.

3. Lothman EW, Somjen GG. Motor and electrical signs of epileptiform activity induced by penicillin in the spinal cord of decapitate cats. *Electroenceph Clin Neurophysiol* 1976; **41**: 237–252.

4. Sackellares JC, Smith DB. Myoclonus with electrocerebral silence in a patient receiving penicillin. *Arch Neurol* 1979; **36**: 857–858.

5. Post B, Koelman HTM, Tijssen MAJ. Propriospinal myoclonus after treatment with ciprofloxacin. *Mov Disord* 2004; **19**: 595–597.

6. Striano P, Zara F, Coppola A, Ciampa C, Pezzella M, Striano S. Epileptic myoclonus as ciprafloxacin adverse effect. *Mov Disord* 2007; **22**:1675–1676.

7. Thomas P, Valton L, Genton P. Absence and myoclonic status epilepticus precipitated by antiepileptic drugs in idiopathic generalized epilepsy. *Brain* 2006, **129**, 1281–1292.

8. Aguglia U, Zappia M, Quattrone A. Carbamazepine-nonepileptic myoclonus in a child with benign epilepsy. *Epilepsia* 1987; **28**: 515–518.

9.  Maggaudda A, Di Rosa G. Carbamazepine induced nonepileptic myoclonus and tic like movements. *Epileptic Disord* 2012; **14**: 172–173.

10. Fanella M, Egeo G, Fattouch J, et al. Oxcarbazepine-induced myoclonic status epilepticus in juvenile myoclonic epilepsy *Epileptic Disord* 2013; **15**: 181–187.

11. Janszky J, Rasonyi G, Halasz P, et al. Disabling erratic myoclonus during lamotrigine therapy with high serum level - report of two cases. *Clin Neuropharmacol* 2000; **23**, 86–89.

12. Moore PW, Donovan JW, Burkhart KK, Haggerty D. A case series of patients with lamotrigine toxicity at one center from 2003 to 2012. *Clin Toxicol* 2013; **51**: 545–549.

13. Corcuera PF, Pomarol E, Amann B, McKenna P. Myoclonus provoked by lamotrigine in a bipolar patient. *J Clin Psychopharmacol* 2008; **28**: 248–249.

14. Asconape J, Diedrich A, DellaBadia J. Myoclonus associated with the use of gabapentin. *Epilepsia* 2000; **41**: 479–481.

15. Holtkamp M, Halle A, Meierkord H, Masuhr F. Gabapentin induced severe myoclonus in a patient with impaired renal function. *J Neurol* 2006; **253**: 382–383.

16. Huppertz H-J, Feuerstein TJ, Schulze Bonhage A. Myoclonus in epilepsy patients with anticonvulsive add-on therapy with pregabalin. *Epilepsia* 2001; **42**: 790–792.

17. Healy DG, Ingle GT, Brown P. Pregabalin and gabapentin associated myoclonus in a patient with chronic renal failure. *Mov Disord* 2009; **24**: 2028–2029.

18. Miller AD, Prost VM, Bookstaver PB, Gaines KJ. Topirimate induced myoclonus and psychosis during migraine prophylaxis. *Am J Health Syst Pharm* 2010; **67**: 1178–1180.

19. Oulis P, Potagas C, Masdrakis VG, et al. Reversible tremor and myoclonus associated with topiramate-fluvoxamine coadministration. *Clin Neuropharmacol* 2008; **31**: 366–367.

20. Garvey MJ, Tollefson GD. Occurrence of myoclonus in patients treated with cyclic antidepressants. *Arch Gen Psychiatry* 1987; **44**: 269–272.

21. McKeon A, Pittock SJ, Glass GA, et al. Whole body tremulousness: isolated generalised polymyoclonus. *Arch Neurol* 2007; **64**: 1318–1322.

22. Ghika Schmid F, Ghika J, Vuadens P, et al. Acute reversible myoclonic encephalopathy associated with fluoxetine therapy. *Mov Disord* 1997; **12**: 622–623.

23. Bharucha KJ, Sethi KD. Complex movement disorders induced by fluoxetine. *Move Disord* 1996; **11**: 324–326.

24. Sternbach H. The serotonin syndrome. *Am J Psychiatry* 1991; **148**: 705–713.

25. McCall RB, Aghajanian GK. Serotonergic facilitation of facial motor neuron excitation. *Brain Res* 1979; **169**: 11–28.

26. Lauterbach EC. Reversible intermittent rhythmic myoclonus with fluoxetine in presumed Pick's disease. *Mov Disord* 1994; **3**: 343–346.

27. Tremelizzo L, Fermi S, Fusco ML, et al. Generalized action myoclonus associated with escitalopram in a patient with mixed dementia. *J Clin Psychopharmacol* 2011; **31**: 394–395.

28. Dutra LA, Pedroso JL, Felix EP, et al. Venlafaxine induced myoclonus in a patient with mixed dementia. *Arq Neuropsiquiatr* 2008; **66**: 894–895.

29. Rosenhagen MC, Schmidt U, Weber F, Steiger A. Combination therapy of lamotrigine and escitalopram may cause myoclonus. *J Clin Psychopharmacol* 2006; **26**: 346–347.

30. Guthrie S, Grunhaus L. Fluoxetine induced stuttering. *J Clin Psychiatry* 1990; **51**: 85.

31. Masand P. Desipramine induced oral-pharyngeal disturbances: stuttering and jaw myoclonus. *J Clin Psychopharmacol* 1992; **12**: 444–445.

32. Gupta A, Lang AE. Drug induced cranial myoclonus. *Mov Disord* 2010; **25**: 2264–2265.

33. Klawans HL, Goetz C, Weiner WJ. 5-Hydroxytryptophan induced myoclonus in guinea pigs and the possible role of serotonin in infantile myoclonus. *Neurology* 1973; **23**: 1234–1240.

34. Klawans HL, Carvey PM, Tanner CM, Goetz CG. Drug induced myoclonus. *Adv Neurol* 1986; **43**: 251–264.

35. Chadwick D, Hallett M, Jenner P, Marsden CD. 5-hydroxytryptophan-induced myoclonus in guinea pigs: a physiological and pharmacological investigation. *J Neurol Sci* 1978; **35**: 157–165.

36. Forstl H, Zagorski A, Pohlmann-Eden B. Somatosensory evoked potentials as indicators of altered cerebral excitability during psychotropic drug treatment. *Biol Psychiatry* 1991; **29**: 397–402.

37. Coleman RM, Pollach CP, Weitzman ED. Periodic movements in sleep [nocturnal myoclonus]: relation to sleep disorders. *Ann Neurol* 1980; **8**: 416–421.

38. Goerke M, Rodenbeck A, Cohrs S, Kunz D. The influence of the tricyclic antidepressant amitriptyline on periodic limb movements during sleep. *Pharmacopsychiatry* 2013; **46**: 108–113.

39. Fulda S, Kloiber S, Dose T, Lucae S. Mirtazapine provokes periodic leg movements during sleep in young healthy men. *Sleep* 2013; **36**: 661–669.

40. Askenasy JJM, Yahr MD. Is monoamine oxidase inhibitor induced myoclonus serotonergically mediated? *J Neural Transm* 1988; **72**: 67–76.

41. Klawans HL, Goetz C, Bergen D. Levodopa induced myoclonus. *Arch Neurol* 1975; **32**: 331–334.

42. Luquin MR, Scipioni O, Vaamonde J, Gershanik O, Obeso JA. Levodopa induced dyskinesias in Parkinson's disease: clinical and pharmacological classification. *Mov Disord* 1992; **7**: 117–124.

43. Marconi R, Lefebvre-Caparros D, Bonnet AM, et al. Levodopa induced dyskinesias in Parkinson's disease phenomenology and pathophysiology. *Mov Disord* 1994; **9**: 2–12.

44. Pfeiffer RF. Amantadine induced vocal myoclonus. *Mov Disord* 1996; **11**: 104–106.

45. Yarnell AJ, Burn DJ. Amantadine induced myoclonus in a patient with progressive supranuclear palsy. *Age Aging* 2012; **41**: 695–696.

46. Matsunaga K, Uozumi T, Qingrui L, Hashimoto T, Tsuji S. Amantadine induced cortical myoclonus. *Neurology* 2001; **56**: 279–280.

47. Fukuzako H, Tominaga H, Izumi K, et al. Postural myoclonus associated with long term administration of neuroleptics in schizophrenic patients. *Biol Psychiatry* 1990; **27**: 1116–1126.

48. Little JT, Jankovic J. Tardive myoclonus. *Mov Disord* 1987; **2**: 307–311.

49. Bak TH, Bauer M, Schaub RT, Hellweg R, Reischies FM. Myoclonus in patients treated with clozapine: a case series. *J Clin Psychiatry* 1995; **56**: 418–422.

50. Sajatovic M, Meltzer HY. Clozapine induced myoclonus and generalized seizures. *Biol Psychiatry* 1996; **39**: 367–370.

51. Antelo RE, Stanilla JK, Martin Llonch N. Myoclonic seizures and "leg folding" phenomena with clozapine therapy. Report of two cases. *Biol Psychiatry* 1994; **36**: 759–762.

52. Camaco A, Garcia-Navarro M, Martinez B, Villarejo A, Pomares E. Olanzapine induced myoclonic status. *Clin Neuropharmacol* 2005; **28**: 145–147.

53. Rosen JB, Milstein MJ, Haut SR. Olanzapine associated myoclonus. *Epilepsy Res* 2012; **98**: 247–250.

54. Deshauer D, Albuquerqu J, Alda M, Grof P. Seizures caused by possible interaction between olanzapine and clomipramine. *J Clin Psychopharmacol* 2012; **20**: 283–284.

55. Malow BA, Reese KB, Sato S, Bogard PJ, Malhotra AK, Su TP, Pickar D. Spectrum of EEG abnormalities during clozapine treatment. *Electroencephalogr Clin Neurophysiol* 1994; **91**: 205–211.

56. Amann BL, Pogarell O, Mergl R, et al. EEG abnormalities associated with antipsychotics: a comparison of quetiapine, olanzapine, haloperidol and healthy subjects. *Hum Psychopharmacol* 2003; **18**: 641–646.

57. Velayudhan L, Kirchner V. Quetiapine induced myoclonus. *Int Clin Psychopharmacol* 2005; **20**: 119–120.

58. Aggarwal A, Jiloha RC. Quetiapine induced myoclonus. *Indian J Med Sci* 2008; **62**: 422–423.

59. George M, Haasz M, Coronado A, et al. Acute dyskinesia, myoclonus, and akathisia in an adolescent male abusing quetiapine via nasal insufflation: a case study. *BMC Pediatr* 2013; **13**: 187.

60. Strachan PM, Benoff BA. Mental status change, myoclonus, electrocardiographic changes, and acute respiratory distress syndrome induced by quetiapine overdose. *Pharmacotherapy* 2006; **26**: 578–582.

61. Smith MT. Neuroexcitatory effects of morphine and hydromorphine: evidence implicating the 3-glucuronide metabolites. *Clin Exp Pharmacol Physiol* 2000; **27**: 524–528.

62. Kaiko RF, Foley KM, Grabinski PY, et al. Central nervous system excitatory effects of meperidine in cancer patients. *Ann Neurol* 1983; **13**: 180–185.

63. Potter JM, Reid DB, Shaw RJ, Hackett P, Hickman PE. Myoclonus associated with treatment with high doses of morphine: the role of supplemental drugs. *Br Med J* 1989; **299**: 150–153.

64. Hochman MS. Meperidine associated myoclonus and seizures in long term hemodialysis patients. *Ann Neurol* 1983; **14**: 593.

65. Reutens DC, Stewart-Wynne EG. Norpethidine induced myoclonus in a patient with renal failure. *J Neurol Neurosurg Psychiatry* 1989; **52**: 1250–1451.

66. Shohami E, Evron S, Weinstock M, Soffer D, Carmon A. A new animal model for action myoclonus. *Adv Neurol* 1986; **43**: 545–552.

67. Burns RJ, Thomas DW, Barron VI. Reversible encephalopathy possibly associated with bismuth subgallate ingestion. *Br Med J* 1974; **1**: 220–223.

68. Gordon MF, Abrams RI, Rubin DB, Barr WI, Correa DD. Bismuth subsalicylate toxicity as a cause of prolonged encephalopathy with myoclonus. *Mov Disord* 1995; **10**: 220–222.

69. Rosen PB, Stevens R. Action myoclonus in lithium toxicity. *Ann Neurol* 1983; **13**: 221–222.

70. Julius SC, Brenner RP. Myoclonic seizures with lithium. *Biol Psychiatry* 1987; **22**: 1184–1190.

71. Devanand DP, Sackeim HA, Brown RP. Myoclonus during combined tricyclic antidepressant and lithium treatment. *J Clin Psychopharmacol* 1988; **8**: 446–447.

72. Caviness JN, Evidente VG. Cortical myoclonus during lithium exposure. *Arch Neurol* 2003; **60**: 4011–404.

73. Pedro-Botet ML, Bonal J, Caralps. Nifedipine and myoclonic disorders. *Nephron* 1989; **51**: 281.

74. Hicks CB, Abraham K. Verapamil and myoclonic dystonia. *Ann Int Med* 1985; **103**: 154.

75. Vadlamudi L, Wijdicks EF. Multifocal myoclonus due to verapamil overdose. *Neurology* 2002; **58**: 984.

76. Wallace EL, Lingle K, Pierce D, Satko S. Amlodipine induced myoclonus. *Am J Med* 2009; **122**: e7.

77. Swanowski MT, Chen JS, Monson MH. Myoclonus associated with long term use of diltiazem. *Am J Health Syst Pharm* 2011; **68**: 1707–1710.

78. Fernandez HH, Friedman JH. Carvedilol induced myoclonus. *Move Disord* 1999; **14**: 703.

# Chapter 16

# Imaging in medication-induced parkinsonism

Danna Jennings

## Introduction

Drug-induced parkinsonism (DIP) represents one of the most prevailing diagnostic dilemmas in movement disorders clinics and is the second most common cause of parkinsonism (1, 2). While there may be clinical clues to help differentiate DIP from Parkinson's disease (PD) or other forms of degenerative parkinsonian syndromes, in many patients DIP is clinically indistinguishable (3, 4). Age is a primary risk factor for DIP, which may be in part related to the loss of dopaminergic neurons with increasing age (5). It is estimated that approximately 18% of the population presenting with parkinsonism have a drug-induced disorder (6) and about 7% of patients initially diagnosed with PD are later reclassified as having DIP, thus underscoring the difficulties in accurately diagnosing DIP (7). To add to the complexity, clinical differentiation usually requires withdrawal of the offending agent for several months, which is often difficult, and in some cases impossible, in the setting of active psychiatric symptoms. In addition, drug-induced extrapyramidal symptoms are one of the main causes of treatment noncompliance in psychiatric patients, often leading to hospital admission and ultimately a poorer prognosis (8).

Patients with suspected drug-induced parkinsonism (DIP) should be considered a unique population with regard to assessing diagnostic accuracy for parkinsonism. The key driver in clarifying the diagnosis of DIP versus an underlying degenerative parkinsonian syndrome is the potential impact on treatment decisions and prognosis. While DIP is mainly related to striatal D2 receptor blockade (9), a distinctive feature of patients with suspected DIP is that evidence of subclinical drug-exacerbated parkinsonism may become apparent in some patients. After drug withdrawal, 60%–70% have resolution of parkinsonian features in seven weeks, although some can take up to 12 months (10). In a subset of patients, the symptoms persist beyond 12 months, suggesting that the offending drug exacerbated or unmasked a neurodegenerative parkinsonian syndrome earlier than would have otherwise been expected. There are also reports of patients with initial improvement upon discontinuation of the drug who again develop parkinsonian symptoms 1–2 years later, suggesting that the drug had unmasked a subclinical parkinsonian syndrome (3, 11). Further evidence supporting this phenomenon comes from a report by Rajput (12) in which two cases of DIP, in the setting of neuroleptic treatment with complete recovery upon drug withdrawal, were found on postmortem to have pathology revealing nigral degeneration and Lewy bodies. The data from this report suggests that preclinical PD in these cases was unmasked by the neuroleptic treatment. Treatment with levodopa in patients with suspected subclinical parkinsonism that has been unmasked by dopamine blocking agents has been shown to be useful, thus underscoring the benefit of making an accurate diagnosis of subclinical parkinsonism, as it can often influence therapeutic decisions (13, 14). Therefore, the relevance of learning whether there is an underlying neurodegenerative process is that in patients with evidence of a degenerative process based on either imaging markers or lack of clinical improvement following drug withdrawal, the treatment should be carefully considered. Specifically, if neuroleptic treatment is necessary, use of atypical neuroleptics to minimize the severity of extrapyramidal symptoms should be prescribed. In addition, a trial of dopaminergic replacement may also be warranted.

DIP usually occurs secondary to the use of a broad range of substances including dopaminergic blocking agents (neuroleptics), antidepressants, and calcium channel blocking agents (15, 16). Neuroleptics are the most common offending drugs and act by blocking the dopaminergic D2 receptors, located primarily on the postsynaptic neurons. DIP has been shown to occur in 15%–60% of neuroleptic treated patients (12, 17–20). The onset of DIP appears to be dose-dependent, and one report suggests an expectation for DIP in patients on doses of dopamine receptor blocking agents that reach a level of 80% blockade of D2 receptors (21). In neuroleptic-induced parkinsonism, there is blockade of the D2 receptors located on the postsynaptic membrane, while the presynaptic terminals remain unaffected. Therefore in pure DIP it is anticipated that there is normal uptake of DAT SPECT tracers and [18F]-Dopa in the striatum, thus differentiating these patients from neurodegenerative forms of parkinsonism (20).

Access to diagnostic markers for degenerative parkinsonian syndromes offers the possibility of making this differentiation between DIP and a subclinical drug-exacerbated degenerative parkinsonism in a more objective fashion and at an earlier stage of the condition. DIP has been reported as the second most common form of parkinsonism; however, there are a relatively limited number of studies investigating the utility of the imaging modalities as potential tools to improve diagnostic accuracy. This chapter will provide a review of the current literature investigating the imaging modalities that play a potential role in clarifying the diagnosis of DIP.

## Nuclear medicine imaging in the diagnosis of DIP

## Presynaptic dopaminergic imaging in the brain

Advances in nuclear medicine imaging have led to the development of several radioligands relevant to DIP targeting the presynaptic dopaminergic terminal. The availability and application of these imaging techniques as diagnostic tools has resulted in an improvement in our ability to establish a more accurate diagnosis in cases where the clinical evaluation may be unclear. The presynaptic dopamine transporters (DAT) can be evaluated with several positron emission tomography (PET) and single-photon emission tomography (SPECT) ligands

including [123]I-(2)-2β-carboxymethoxy-3b-(4-iodophenyl)tropane ([123I]-β-CIT) (Dopascan; Guilford Pharmaceuticals Inc.); [123]I-N-3-fluoropropyl-2b-carboxymethoxy-3b-(4-iodophenyl)tropane ([123I]-FP-CIT) (DaTSCAN; GE Healthcare); and [123]I-altropane. The PET ligand, [18]F-3,4-dihydroxyphenylalanine ([18F]-Dopa), provides a marker of the presynaptic dopaminergic function through measuring terminal dopamine decarboxylase activity and dopamine turnover. In addition, radioligands targeting vesicular monoamine transporter (VMAT2) available in the research setting, including 9-[18F]fluoropropyl(+)-dihydrotetrabenazine ([18F]-AV-133) and [11]C-or [18]F-dihydrotetrabenazine, provide another means for evaluating the integrity of presynaptic dopaminergic neurons. Using DAT imaging, early parkinsonian patients show a bilateral reduction in putaminal uptake, with a more pronounced reduction in the putamen contralateral to the most affected limbs (22), while the uptake in the region of the caudate is relatively preserved. Early PD patients have a loss of approximately 40%–50% of putaminal uptake when observed at the time of initial clinical symptoms (22, 23).

There are imaging studies reported in the literature comparing clinically probable PD and other conditions that mimic PD clinically, but without degeneration of the presynaptic dopaminergic neurons. In a study comparing striatal DAT imaging with [123I]-FP-CIT SPECT in probable PD and essential tremor patients, a sensitivity and specificity of greater than 90% has been shown (24). In cases for which the diagnosis is uncertain, DAT imaging performance has been evaluated through three main clinical trials: the Query study comparing clinical diagnosis to DAT imaging over a 6-month period in patients with an uncertain diagnosis (25); the Clinically Uncertain Parkinsonian Syndromes (CUPS)(26), and the European multicenter study in which the clinical diagnosis was prospectively compared to DAT imaging over a 3-year period (27). These studies have consistently demonstrated that clinicians have high sensitivity and low specificity (as low as 30% in some studies) in identifying the correct diagnosis, whereas DAT imaging offers high specificity in differentiating PD from nondegenerative forms of parkinsonism, including DIP (25, 28). The long-term impact of having a normal DAT scan has been studied by Marshall and colleagues (28), who followed 150 patients with normal [123I]-FP-CIT imaging obtained for diagnostic purposes. Approximately

20 of these subjects were ultimately given a clinical diagnosis of DIP after 2-year clinical follow-up. Although 4/120 subjects (3%) demonstrated clinical progression consistent with PD, none of these cases were suspected of having DIP at baseline.

While DIP represents one of the best indications for a $[^{18}F]$-Dopa PET or DAT SPECT imaging, there are relatively few published studies evaluating the role of dopaminergic imaging in this setting. $[^{123}I]$-FP-CIT SPECT is the only approved imaging procedure to aid in establishing a diagnosis of PD, and the indication is limited to differentiating PD from other conditions presenting with tremor, encompassing only a subset of individuals with DIP. Studies specifically aimed at evaluating the diagnostic accuracy of $[^{123}I]$-FP-CIT as a useful tool in differentiating PD from DIP provide support for the role of DAT imaging in cases of suspected DIP, which are summarized below. Given that $[^{123}I]$-FP-CIT is more widely available than the other imaging agents, most studies to date have been conducted with this ligand; however, other radioligands interrogating the presynaptic dopaminergic terminal, available primarily in research settings, would be expected to be equally effective in establishing an accurate diagnosis in suspected DIP cases.

It should be noted that drugs known to cause parkinsonism, including dopamine receptor binding agents, have been shown to have negligible affinity for DAT (29, 30). Imaging the presynaptic dopaminergic neuronal integrity with DAT radioligands demonstrates normal symmetric uptake in pure DIP cases, even for those exhibiting significant parkinsonism clinically. Whereas in cases of a reduction DAT uptake in the striatum, particularly when the reduction is asymmetrical, a diagnosis of subclinical drug-exacerbated PD or other degenerative parkinsonian syndrome needs to be considered.

Romero and Padillo (31) conducted a prospective study evaluating 19 DIP patients completing $[^{123}I]$-FP-CIT SPECT at the time of discontinuation of the offending drug, which was most frequently a neuroleptic (39%), and at a mean follow-up of 8.8 (range 6–34) months. The final clinical diagnosis was subclinical drug-exacerbated PD in 31% (6/19 subjects), 4 subjects with a reduction in $[^{123}I]$-FP-CIT uptake, and 2 with normal uptake. In this study, $[^{123}I]$-FP-CIT SPECT demonstrated a sensitivity of 66.7% and specificity of 100% (negative predictive value 86.7%) using the clinical diagnosis as the "gold standard." There may be an underrepresentation of patients with subclinical parkinsonism unmasked by a medication, given that only subjects capable of withdrawal from the medication were included in the study.

Lorberboym and colleagues (32) studied 20 patients who had developed parkinsonism while on neuroleptic agents and ten age-matched healthy controls using $[^{123}I]$FP-CIT SPECT. Nine (45%) of the patients had normal scans and 11 (55%) showed a reduction in striatal binding, supporting the prescribed concept (3, 4, 11) that a significant proportion of patients have evidence of subclinical degenerative changes based on imaging predisposing the onset of parkinsonism when dopamine receptor blocking agents are administered. This study is also particularly instructive in demonstrating that DIP was clinically indistinguishable from PD, including significant asymmetry of symptoms, even in the patients with normal imaging. In addition, gait freezing, a symptom usually present in more advanced PD, was noted in two patients with normal imaging. The authors concluded that DAT SPECT imaging is effective in determining whether these conditions are entirely drug-induced or an exacerbation of subclinical PD (32).

A key to understanding the accuracy of DAT imaging in differentiating DIP from a subclinical degenerative parkinsonian syndrome is through determining the most accurate clinical diagnosis with longitudinal follow-up. In the first prospective, longitudinal study evaluating suspected DIP patients, 32 patients who had developed parkinsonism on neuroleptic treatment were consecutively recruited for $[^{123}I]$FP-CIT imaging (33). There was normal putaminal $[^{123}I]$FP-CIT binding in 18 (55%) patients and reduced binding in 14 (45%) patients. Clinically, the groups were similar, with the exception of more frequent symmetrical and oral-buccal dyskinetic cases in the group with normal binding. Nineteen of the 32 patients (ten with normal $[^{123}I]$FP-CIT uptake and nine with reduced uptake) were reassessed clinically and with $[^{123}I]$FP-CIT SPECT imaging at 9–13 months following initial evaluation (14). Patients in the normal $[^{123}I]$FP-CIT group also had normal uptake on follow-up imaging and no substantial change in UPDRS scores from their baseline. For patients with a reduction in $[^{123}I]$FP-CIT, the uptake remained abnormal at follow-up and UPDRS motor scores were higher than at baseline. This longitudinal study provides critical evidence that DAT imaging with $[^{123}I]$FP-CIT SPECT at baseline is a sensitive marker for identifying patients with pure DIP compared to those with a subclinical degenerative parkinsonian syndrome at follow-up. In addition, all patients in this study underwent a 3-month trial of levodopa treatment (400–800 mg/day), resulting in improvement of motor symptoms in 3/10 patients with normal [123I]FP-CIT uptake and 8/9 patients with reduced [123I]FP-CIT uptake, which was a novel finding in this study. Interestingly, there were no psychiatric side effects reported as a result of the dopaminergic treatment.

Given the relatively high percentage of DIP cases with a reduction in DAT binding (43%–55%) (14, 32, 33), Tinazzi and colleagues (19) designed a study in a large population of schizophrenic subjects aimed at evaluating the prevalence of DIP and rate of DAT deficit in this population. Schizophrenic patients treated with neuroleptics for at least 6 months were eligible for participation in the clinical and [123I]FP-CIT SPECT imaging. Parkinsonian signs were present in 149/448 (33%) patients and 97 agreed to undergo imaging, 41 (42%) of whom showed a reduction in [123I]FP-CIT uptake. Two-year clinical follow-up of this cohort was completed in 60 (33 with normal [123I] FP-CIT uptake and 27 with reduced uptake) patients. The UPDRS scores showed significant worsening in the patients with reduced [123I]FP-CIT uptake at baseline, while there was no difference in those with normal imaging. In addition, only the patients with reduced [123I]FP-CIT uptake demonstrated an improvement in motor symptoms with levodopa treatment. The results of these studies suggest that parkinsonism in patients with neuroleptic exposure has at least two etiologies: in patients with normal [123I]FP-CIT uptake parkinsonism is likely to be pure DIP and related to neuroleptic-induced D2 receptor blocking activity, whereas in patients with a reduction in [123I]FP-CIT uptake, blocking of the D2 receptors occurs in the setting of a subclinical degeneration of presynaptic dopaminergic neurons.

The only published study utilizing [18F]-Dopa PET imaging to distinguish DIP from presynaptic dopaminergic neuronal degeneration included a cohort of 13 patients classified as relatively severe DIP, warranting referral to a movement disorders clinic (20). All cases were willing and able to withdraw from the offending medication(s) and 12/13 were followed clinically for a median of 23.5 months. Putaminal [18F]-Dopa uptake was normal in 8/9 patients with longitudinal follow-up, which was

predictive of an improvement in the clinical signs of parkinsonism in all cases and resolution in 3 cases. In patients with a reduction in [18F]-Dopa, 3/4 (75%) had a progression in clinical parkinsonian symptoms despite discontinuation of the dopamine receptor blocking agent(s). While the authors claim that 31% (4/13) of cases demonstrating a reduction in [18F]-Dopa was higher than expected, it is consistent with the prevalence in more recently conducted studies (19, 32). Nevertheless, they attribute the higher than expected number of cases with reduced [18F]-Dopa uptake to the severity of the cases. The results from this study indicate that normal [18F]-Dopa PET imaging is well correlated with improvement in parkinsonian signs in DIP, while the majority of patients with a reduction in [18F]-Dopa uptake show worsening parkinsonian signs off medications at follow-up. There is data to support the notion that chronic treatment with dopamine receptor blocking agents may in fact result in a compensatory increase in presynaptic dopamine metabolism (34, 35), which would be expected to result in increased [18F]-Dopa uptake and be inconsistent with the result of this study.

A retrospective analysis was performed by Diaz-Corrales et al. (36) involving 32 patients clinically diagnosed with DIP, 25 patients with PD unmasked by neuroleptic treatment, and 22 patients with PD with no history of neuroleptic treatment. Clinical diagnosis was determined during a follow-up period after withdrawal of the neuroleptic. [123I]-FP-CIT SPECT images obtained at symptom onset were analyzed by nuclear medicine experts blinded to the clinical information. The [123I]-FP-CIT SPECT was normal in 90.6% (29/32) patients diagnosed with DIP, while all patients diagnosed with PD or PD unmasked by neuroleptic treatment showed a reduction in [123I]-FP-CIT SPECT uptake.

In a study aimed at elucidating the influence of neuroleptics on DAT binding using [123I]FP-CIT SPECT in schizophrenic patients (10 drug naïve, 8 previously treated with neuroleptics and now drug-free, and 15 treated with olanzapine or risperidone), no difference in [123I]FP-CIT binding was found between any of the groups and the ten age-matched healthy subjects (29). These findings are consistent with a study using [123I]β-CIT SPECT demonstrating no difference in striatal dopamine transporter density in schizophrenic patients compared to healthy subjects (37), and with postmortem pathological studies showing no change in dopamine transporter density in schizophrenic patients compared to those without schizophrenia (38, 39). In contrast, another study to understand if schizophrenic patients are at increased risk for a degenerative parkinsonian syndrome was conducted by Mateos and colleagues (40) and evaluated first-episode schizophrenic subjects (ten with DIP and ten without DIP) and ten age-matched healthy subjects using [$^{123}$I]FP-CIT SPECT 4 weeks after initial treatment with risperidone (6 mg/day ± 2 mg). While there was no significant difference in the uptake of striatal [$^{123}$I]FP-CIT among the schizophrenic patients with and without DIP, this study showed a significant reduction in uptake when comparing all schizophrenic subjects and healthy subjects. The authors suggest there may be a dysfunction in the presynaptic dopamine pathway in schizophrenic patients, which could explain the increase in the higher prevalence of observed parkinsonism in response to administration of neuroleptic therapies in this population. Based on the data presented in this study, there is a fair amount of overlap in striatal uptake in the schizophrenic patients and healthy subjects; and while the difference reaches statistical significance, there may be a specific population of schizophrenic subjects who are at increased risk for dysfunction in the presynaptic dopamine pathway, requiring further evaluation.

## PET and SPECT brain imaging in receptor occupancy studies

While PET and SPECT imaging techniques have proven to be useful diagnostic tools in parkinsonism and other extrapyramidal disorders, in recent years the utility of these imaging techniques for measuring brain receptor occupancy has come to the forefront. Specifically, D2 receptor ligands [$^{123}$I]iodobenzamide ($^{123}$I-IBZM) with SPECT and [$^{11}$C]-raclopride used with PET have been shown to be useful in evaluating the occupancy of dopamine receptors by neuroleptic agents in human trials (41, 42). PET studies have shown that D2 receptor occupancy at levels greater than 80% invariably results in extrapyramidal side effects including, but not limited to, parkinsonian symptoms. Using imaging techniques to elucidate the occupancy of specific receptors offers the possibility of developing medications with therapeutic effect while minimizing the occurrence of extrapyramidal side effects.

Dose occupancy studies performed over the past several years have informed researchers regarding the doses required to reach adequate efficacy with reducing the risk for side effects. A result of these studies is that, in general, lower doses of antipsychotic medications are being recommended. An example of data to support the use of lower doses is a study evaluating 5 and 20 mg of olanzapine which showed a higher D2 receptor occupancy at 20 mg (60 vs. 83%, respectively), demonstrating no difference in clinical efficacy at these doses (43). Another direct application of imaging informing neuroleptic doses is a PET study showing that a 4 mg dose of risperidone results in 70%–80% occupancy, therefore making this the highest recommended dose (44). As a result of D2 receptor occupancy imaging studies, both classical and atypical neuroleptic occupancy has been described as a saturation hyperbole. Specifically, by increasing low doses by small increments the result is a large increase in D2 occupancy, whereas the increase in higher doses showed a plateau or no further increase (45, 46). Several studies have demonstrated that lower doses of antipsychotic medications may provide equal efficacy than higher doses, with less risk for extrapyramidal symptoms, leading to the trend to use lower doses (47, 48).

Novel radioligands to evaluate the binding to other relevant receptor or enzyme targets in the brain, including serotonin receptor, phosphodiesterase 10(PDE10), the dopamine D1 receptor, and the muscarinic and GABA receptors, are under development, offering the ability to develop additional drugs with novel targets having the potential for fewer extrapyramidal side effects.

## The role of [123I]-MIBG cardiac imaging in DIP

Several studies have demonstrated a significant reduction in cardiac [$^{123}$I]-metaiodobenzylguanidine ([$^{123}$I]-MIBG) uptake in patients diagnosed with PD compared to healthy subjects. [$^{123}$I]-MIBG scintigraphy is an approved imaging technique to evaluate the integrity of the cardiac sympathetic nerve terminals. There is evidence that [$^{123}$I]-MIBG imaging may have the capability to differentiate PD from other atypical forms of degenerative parkinsonian syndrome (49). Based on this information, there is reason to expect that cardiac [$^{123}$I]-MIBG imaging may serve as a useful tool in differentiating DIP from degenerative parkinsonian syndromes.

The [$^{123}$I]-MIBG imaging literature describing studies directed at evaluating DIP cases is limited to three studies (50-52). The first reported trial assessed 20 DIP and 32 PD patients, finding a significant increase in the mediastinum ratio in the DIP cases (50). However, in 2/20 (10%) subjects, both of whom had no improvement in their parkinsonism with drug withdrawal and a favorable response to levodopa, demonstrated a reduced [123I]-MIBG uptake in the range of the PD subjects. In a second study, [123I]-MIBG was compared with Cross Cultural Smell Identification (CCSI) testing in 15 DIP, 24 PD, and 15 healthy subjects (51). Although the DIP subjects were not significantly different from the healthy controls on either test, one subject had both a reduced uptake in [123I]-MIBG and a low score on the CCSI, suggesting that olfactory testing may be a useful test in differentiating DIP from subclinical PD cases. The combination of [123I]-MIBG and [123I]FP-CIT SPECT was evaluated in 20 DIP patients and 16 subjects had normal DAT and MIBG uptake patterns (52). Two subjects had reduction in uptake on both modalities and showed no clinical improvement following drug withdrawal. The remaining two subjects had normal DAT uptake and a modest reduction in [123I]-MIBG, and clinically showed initial improvement with the reappearance of parkinsonian signs within 1–2 years later, raising the possibility that a reduction in [123I]-MIBG may predate DAT imaging abnormities. While the sample sizes for these studies are limited, the studies consistently suggest that in individuals with suspected DIP, an abnormality in cardiac [123I]-MIBG appears to be a reliable tool for predicting who may have a subclinical parkinsonian syndrome, and those subjects should be followed and treated accordingly for clinical deterioration.

## Transcranial ultrasound in the diagnosis of DIP

The results of various studies involving multiple patient groups suggest that transcranial B-mode sonography (TCS) is an imaging method that can serve as a marker to clarify the diagnosis in patients presenting with parkinsonism, even early in the disease process (53). TCS has been used for more than 10 years as a diagnostic marker for movement disorders, including PD. In patients with PD, the characteristic ultrasound finding is an area of echogenicity in the region of the substantia nigra (SN), which is likely associated with increased iron deposition (54). Identification of this echogenicity in the SN is highly

sensitive (90.7%) and specific (82.4%) for PD (53, 55–57). Specifically, patients with PD have an enlarged area of SN echogenicity (SN+) compared to patients with vascular parkinsonism (58), essential tremor, and DIP (31, 59), which have no enhancement of the echogenic signal in the SN (SN-).

The advantages of TCS over other diagnostic neuroimaging tools for PD include the noninvasive quality, broad availability, and relatively low cost of TCS. However, as with other neuroimaging approaches, TCS does not reach 100% accuracy for the differentiation of PD from other causes of parkinsonism.

Studies evaluating the accuracy of TCS as a tool to differentiate DIP from PD are quite limited. A prospective study performed by Bouwmans, et al. (59) included 196 subjects referred to neurology outpatient clinics based on a recent onset of parkinsonism of unclear etiology who underwent TCS and FP-CIT at enrollment. A final clinical diagnosis at 2-year follow-up was used as the surrogate gold standard for the study. The final clinical diagnosis was DIP in 7 subjects (mean age 63.1, 85.7% male, and mean duration of symptoms 6.5 years) and TCS accurately identified 86% (6/7 subjects) as SN negative. Interestingly for other diagnoses considered (idiopathic PD, atypical parkinsonian syndrome, vascular parkinsonism), the mean duration of symptoms at time of referral was between two and three years, underscoring the difficulty in clarifying the diagnosis in this subpopulation of parkinsonism.

In a larger prospective study, Romero et al. (31) evaluated 20 subjects with TCS at baseline and clinical examination at 6 months following discontinuation of the causative drug. At the 6-month follow-up, patients were diagnosed with DIP (n=15) if parkinsonian symptoms had resolved, and with subclinical drug-exacerbated parkinsonism (n=5) if parkinsonian symptoms persisted. In patients presenting with DIP, assessment of hyperechogenicity in the SN and/ or the lentiform nucleus by TCS had a sensitivity of 80% and negative predictive value of 87.5%. The authors describe one of the main limitations of conducting this study being the difficulty in discontinuing the offending drug. Many patients were not eligible for participation in this study given that discontinuation of the neuroleptic treatment would result in a decline in their level of function, further highlighting the need for a diagnostic tool to eliminate the need for drug withdrawal.

# Summary

The clinical differentiation between pure DIP and a subclinical degenerative parkinsonian syndrome unmasked by an antidopaminergic drug is often quite challenging based on clinical evaluation alone. Clarifying the diagnosis can have significant implications on treatment decisions and prognosis. Access to diagnostic markers for degenerative parkinsonism offers the possibility of more objectively making this differentiation. PET and SPECT brain imaging studies have provided evidence that identification of an abnormality in presynaptic dopaminergic neuronal integrity appears to be predictive of a subclinical degenerative parkinsonian syndrome, and ultimately, clinical progression of motor signs. While the studies conducted thus far are limited, cardiac [$^{123}$I]-MIBG appears to be another tool for predicting those who may have a subclinical parkinsonian syndrome and warrant clinical observation for potential clinical deterioration. With regard to TCS, additional studies are needed to clarify if this might be a useful tool for differentiating DIP from subclinical parkinsonian syndrome. In addition, a few studies have shown levodopa treatment to be particularly beneficial in the patients with DAT deficit on imaging, though this finding needs further investigation through larger, placebo-controlled studies specifically designed to address efficacy in this population.

# References

1. Barbosa M, Caramelli P, Maia D, Cunningham M, Guerra H, Lima-Costa M, et al. Parkinsonism and Parkinson's disease in the elderly: a community-based survey in Brazil (the Bambui study). *Mov Disord.* 2006;21:800–8.

2. Benito-Leon J, Bermejo-Paraja F, Morales-Gonzales J, Porta-Etessam J, Trincado R, Vega S, et al. Incidence of Parkinson disease and parkinsonism in three elderly populations of central Spain. *Neurology.* 2004;62:734–41.

3. Stephen P, Williamson J. Drug-induced parkinsonism in the elderly. *Lancet* 1984;2:1082–10–83.

4. Hardie R, Lees A. Neuroleptic-induced Parkinson's syndrome: clincal features and results of treatment with levodopa. *J Neurol Neurosurg Psychiatry.* 1988;51:850–4.

5. Volkow N, Ding Y, Fowler J, Wang G, Logan J, Gatley S, et al. Evaluation of the human brain dopamine system with PET. *J Nucl Med.* 1996;37:1242–56.

6. Mutch W, Strudwick A, Roy S, Downie A. Parkinson's disease: disability, review and management. *Br Med J.* 1986;13(293):675–7.

7. Esper C, Factor S. Failure of recognition of drug-induced parkinsonism in the elderly. *Mov Disord.* 2007;23:401–4.

8. Corrigan P, Liberman R, Engel J. From noncompliance to collaboration in the treatment of schizophrenia. *Hosp Community Psychiatry.* 1990;41:1203–11.

9. Jibson M, Tandon R. New atypical antipsychotic medications. *J Psychiatry Res.* 1998;32:215–28.

10. Melamed E, Achiron A, Shapira A, Davidovicz S. Persistent and progressive parkinsonism after discontinuation of chronic neuroleptic therapy: an additional tardive syndrome? *Clin Neuropharmacol.* 1991;14:273–8.

11. Goetz C. Drug-induced parkinsonism and idiopathic Parkinson's disease. *Arch Neurol.* 1983;40:325–6.

12. Rajput A, Rozdilsky B, Hornykiewicz O, et al. Reversible drug-induced parkinsonism: clinicopathologic study of two cases. *Arch Neurol.* 1982;39:644–6.

13. Hambye A, Vervat A, Dethy S. FP-CIT SPECT in clinically inconclusive Parkinsonian syndrome during amiodarone treatment: a study with follow-up. *Nucl Med Comm.* 2010;31:583–89.

14. Tinazzi M, Antonini A, Bovi T, et al. Clinical and [123I] FP-CIT SPET imaging follow-up in patients with drug-induced parkinsonism. *J Neurol.* 2009;256:910–15.

15. Lopez-Sendon J, Mena M, deYebenes J. Drug-induced parkinsonism in the elderly: incidence, management and prevention. *Drugs Aging.* 2012;29:105–18.

16. Bondon-Guitton E, Perez-Lloret S, Bagheri H, Brefel C, Rascol O, Monstrastruc J. Drug-induced parkinsonism: a review of 17 years' experience in a regional pharmacovigilance center in France. *Mov Disord.* 2011;26:2226–31.

17. Chakos M, Mayerhoff D, Loebel A, Alvir J, Lieberman J. Incidence and correlates of acute extrapyramidal symptoms in first episode of schizophrenia. *Psychopharm Bull.* 1992;28:81–6.

18. Korczyn A, Goldberg G. Extrapyramidal effects of neuroleptics. *J Neurol Neurosurg Psychiatry.* 1976;39:866–9.

19. Tinazzi M, Cipriani A, Matinella A, Cannas A, Solla P, Nicoletti A, et al. [18F]FP-CIT single photon emission computed tomography findings in drug-induced parkinsonism. *Schizophrenia Research.* 2012;139:40–5.

20. Burn D, Brooks D. Nigral dysfunction in drug-induced parkinsonism: an 18F-dopa PET study. *Neurology.* 1993;43:552–6.

21. Farde L, Wiesel F, Halldin C, Sedvall G. D2-dopamine receptor occupancy in schizophrenic patients treated with antipsychotic drugs. *Arch Gen Psychiatry.* 1988;45:71–6.

22. Marek K, Seibyl J, Zoghbi S, et al. [123I]b-CIT/SPECT imaging demonstrates bilateral loss of dopamine transporters in hemi-Parkinson's disease. *Neurology.* 1996;**46**:231–7.

23. Morrish P, Sawle G, Brooks D. Clinical and [18 F]Dopa PET findings in early Parkinson's disease. *J Neurol Neurosurg Psychiatry.* 1995;**59**:597–600.

24. Benamer H, Patterson J, Grosset D, Booij J, de Bruin K, van Royen E, et al. Accurate differentiation of parkinsonism and essential tremor using visual assessment of [123I]-FP-CIT SPECT imaging: the [123I]-FP-CIT study group. *Mov Disord.* 2000;**15**:503–10.

25. Jennings D, JP S, Oakes D, S E, Murphy J, Marek K. [123I]beta-CIT and single-photon emission computed tomographic imaging vs. clinical evaluation in parkinsonian syndrome: unmasking an early diagnosis. *Arch Neurol.* 2004;**61**(8):1224–9.

26. Catafu A, Tolosa E. The impact of dopamine transporter SPECT using [123I]-ioflupane on diagnosis and management of patients with clinically uncertain parkinsonian syndromes. *Mov Disord.* 2004;**1**:1175–82.

27. Marshall V, Renininger C, Marquardt M, Patterson J, Hadley D, Oertel W, et al. Parkinson's disease is overdiagnosed clinically at baseline in diagnostically uncertain cases: a 3-year European multicenter study with repeat [123I]FP-CIT SPECT. *Mov Disord.* 2009(24):**4**.

28. Marshall V, Patterson J, Hadley D, Grosset K, Grosset D. Two-year follow-up in 150 consecutive cases with normal dopamine transporter imaging. *Nuc Med Commun.* 2006;**27**(12):933–7.

29. Lavalaye J, Linszen D, Booij J, Dingermans P, Renerman L, Habraken J, et al. Dopamine transporter density in young patients with schizophrenia assessed with [123I] FP-CIT SPECT. *Schizopren Res.* 2001;**47**:59–67.

30. Tolosa E, Coelho M, Gallardo M. DAT imaging in drug-induced and psychogenic parkinsonism. *Mov Disord.* 2003;**18** Suppl 7:S28-S33.

31. Romero J, Padillo A, FJB H, MM G, Extremera B. Utility of transcranial sonography in the diagnosis of drug-induced parkinsonism: a prospective study. *Eur J Neurol.* 2013;**20**:1451–58.

32. Lorberboym M, Treves T, E M, Y L, Hellmann M, Djaldetti R. [123I]-FP/CIT SPECT imaging for distinguishing drug-induced parkinsonism from Parkinson's disease. *Mov Disord.* 2006;**21**(4):510–4.

33. Tinazzi M, Ottaviani S, Isaias I, Pasquin I, Steinmayr M, Vampini C, et al. [18F]FP-CIT SPET imaging in drug-induced parkinsonism. *Mov Disord.* 2008;**23**(13):1825–9.

34. Marsden C, Jenner P. The pathophysiology of extrapyramidal side-effects of neuroleptic drugs. *Psychol Med.* 1980;**10**:55–72.

35. Patterson T, Schenk J. Effects of acute and chronic systemic administration of some typical antipsychotic drugs on turnover of dopamine and potassium ion-induced release of dopamine in the striatum of the rat in vivo. *Neuropsychopharmacology.* 1991;**30**:943–52.

36. Diaz-Corrales F, Sanz-Viedma S, Garcia-Solis D, Escobar-Delgado T, Mir P. Clinical features and 123I-FP-CIT SPECT imaging in drug-induced parkinsonism and Parkinson's disease. *Eur J Nucl Med Mol Imaging.* 2010;**37**:556–64.

37. Laruelle M, Abi-Dargham A, Gil R, D'Souza C, Zoghbi S, Baldwin R, et al. SPECT measurements of dopamine transporters in schizophrenia. *J Nucl Med.* 1996;**37**:33.

38. Knable M, Hyde T, Herman M, Carter J, Bigelow L, Kleinman J. Quantitative autoradiography of dopamine-D1 receptors, D2 receptors, and dopamine uptake sites in postmortem striatal specimens from schizophrenic patients. *Biol Psychiatry.* 1994;**36**(12):827–35.

39. Czudek C, Reynolds G. [3H] GBR 12935 binding to the dopamine uptake site in post-mortem brain tissue in schizophrenia. *J Neurol Transm.* 1989; **77** (2–3): 227–30.

40. Mateos J, Lomena F, Parellada E, Font M, Fernandez E, Pavia J, et al. Decreased striatal dopamine transporter binding assessed with [123I]FP-CIT in first-episode schizophrenic patients with and without short-term antipsychotic-induced parkinsonism. *Psychopharmacology.* 2005;**181**:401–6.

41. Dresel S, Mager T, Rossmuller B, Meisenzahl E, Hahn K, Moller H, et al. In vivo effects of olanzapine on striatal dopamine D(2)/D(3) receptor binding in schizophrenic patients: an iodine-123 iodobenzamide single-photon emission tomography study. *Eur J Nucl Med* 1999;**26**:862–8.

42. Nordstrom A, Nyberg S, Olsson H, Farde L. Positron emission tomography finding of a high striatal D2 receptor occupancy in olanzapine-treated patients. *Arch Gen Psychiatry.* 1998;**55**:283–4.

43. Raedler T, Knable M, Lafargue T, Urbina R, Egan M, Pickar D, et al. In vivo determination of striatal dopamine D-2 receptor occupancy in patients treated with olanzapine. *Psychiatry Res: Neuroimaging.* 1999;**90**:81–90.

44. Nyberg S, Eriksson B, Oxenstiema G, Halldin C, Farde L. Suggested minimal effective dose of risperidone based on PET-measured D2 and 5HT-2A receptor occupancy in schizophrenic patients. *Am J Psychiatry.* 1999;**156**:869–75.

45. Nordstrom A, Farde L, Wiesel F, Forslund K, Halldin C, Uppfeldt G. Central D2-dopamine receptor occupancy in relation to antipsychotic drug effect: a double-blind PET study of schizophrenic patients. *Biol Psychiatry.* 1993;**33**:227–35.

46. Kapur S, Zipursky R, Remington G. Clinical and theoretical implications of 5-HT2 and D2 receptor occupancy of clozapine, risperidone, and olanzapine in schizophrenia. *Am J Psychiatry.* 1999;**156**:286–93.

47. Heinz A, Knable M, Weinberger D. Dopamine D2 receptor imaging and neuroleptic drug response. *J Clin Psychiatry.* 1996;**57**(Suppl 11):84–8.

48. de Haan L, Maksmovic I. Subjective experience and striatal dopamine D2 receptor occupancy in patients with schizophrenia stabilized on olanzapine or risperidone. *Am J Psychiatry.* 1999;**157**:1019–20.

49. Rascol O. 123I-metaiodobenzylguanidine scintigraphy in Parkinson's disease and related disorders. *Mov Disord.* 2009;**24**(Suppl 2):S732–41.

50. Lee P, Kim J, Shin D, Yoon S, Huh K. Cardiac 123I-MIBG scintigraphy in patients with drug induced parkinsonism. *J Neurol Neurosurg Psychiatry.* 2006;**77**:372–4.

51. Lee P, Yeo S, Yong S, Kim Y. Odour identification test and its relation to cardiac [123]I-metaiodobenzylguanidine in patients with drug induced parkinsonism. *J Neurol Neurosurg Psychiatry.* 2007;**78**:1250–2.

52. Kim J, Oh Y, Kim Y, Yang D, Chung Y, You I, et al. Combined use of 123I-metaiodobenzlguanidine (MIBG) scintigraphy and dopamine transporter (DAT) positron emission tomography (PET predicts prognosis in drug-induced parkinsonism (DIP): A 2-year follow-up study. *Arch Gerontol Geriat.* 2013;**56**:124–8.

53. Gaenslen A, Unmuth B, Godau J, Liepelt I, SiSanto A, Schweitzer K, et al. The specificity and sensitivity of transcranial ultrasound in the differential diagnosis of Parkinson's disease: a prospective blinded study. *Lancet Neurol.* 2008;**7**:417–24.

54. Berg D, Roggendorf W, Schroder U, et al. Echogenicity of the substantia nigra: association with increased iron contect and marker for susceptibility to nigrostriatal injury. *Arch Neurol.* 2002;**59**:999–1005.

55. Berg D, Siefker C, Becker G. Echogenicity of the substantia nigra in Parkinson's disease and its relation to clinical findings. *J Neurol.* 2001;**248**:684–89.

56. Walter U, Wittstock M, Benecke R, Dressler D. Sustantia nigra echogenicity is normal in non-extrapyramidal cerebral disorders but increased in Parkinson's disease. *J Neural Transm.* 2002;**109**:191–96.

57. Becker G, Sueufert J, Bogdahn U, Reichmann H, Reiners K. Degeneration of substantia nigra in chronic Parkinson's disease visualized by transcranial color-coded real time sonography. *Neurology.* 1995;**45**:182–84.

58. Tsai C, Wu R, Huang Y, et al. Transcranial color-coded sonography helps differentiation of Parkinson's disease and vascular parkinsonism. *J Neurol.* 2007;**254**:501–7.

59. Bouwmans A, Vlaar A, Mess W, Kessels A, Weber W. Specificity and sensitivity of transcranial sonography of the substantia nigra in the diagnosis of Parkinson's disease: prospective cohort study in 196 patients. *BMJ Open.* 2013;**3**:e002613 doi:10.1136.

# Chapter 7

# Deep brain stimulation for tardive disorders

Bernardo Rodrigues and Kelvin L. Chou

## Introduction

Deep brain stimulation (DBS) is a procedure in which electrical wires are inserted into precise areas of the brain. These wires are then connected to a pacemaker-like device implanted subcutaneously in the chest. When the device is turned on, electrical stimulation is delivered to the brain and can improve the symptoms of certain conditions. DBS is an established therapy for Parkinson's disease (PD) and essential tremor (ET), but has also been successfully used to treat patients with other movement disorders, such as dystonia and tics [1].

Tardive disorders are characterized by the presence of abnormal involuntary movements that occur after prolonged exposure to dopamine receptor blocking compounds, such as antipsychotic or antiemetic medications. The tardive disorders include tardive dyskinesia (typically a choreoathetoid or stereotypic movement involving the orobuccolingual region, but may involve other body parts), tardive dystonia (sustained contractions of agonist and antagonist muscles causing abnormal postures), tardive tremor (regular oscillation of a body part, such as the hand), tardive tics (sudden, jerky movements preceded by urges or sensations), tardive myoclonus (sudden muscle contractions producing a brief muscle twitch or movement), and tardive akathisia (subjective and observed restlessness) [2, 3].

Clinicians have been reluctant to use DBS for tardive disorders for at least three reasons. First, DBS for tardive disorders has not been tested in randomized controlled trials; only case reports and case series exist. Second, psychiatric side effects from DBS have been reported in other populations. PD patients treated with subthalamic nucleus (STN) DBS may develop depression, suicidality, mania,

and impulse-control problems after electrode implantation [4, 5]. Thirdly, patients may develop psychotic delusions such as thought control, thought broadcasting, and thoughts of being controlled. Because the majority of patients who develop tardive disorders have underlying psychiatric disease (the exception is patients whose tardive syndrome is caused by a drug given for nonpsychiatric reasons), there is limited experience and evidence for DBS in tardive syndromes.

In recent years, several case reports and case series have demonstrated that DBS may improve tardive dyskinesia and dystonia in patients with and without psychiatric disease [6–30]. To date, DBS results have not been published for other tardive syndromes (akathisia, tics, tremors, myoclonus). Tardive dyskinesia affects 15% to 20% of patients treated with neuroleptics [31], while dystonia is present in 1% to 4% of patients exposed to dopamine receptor blockers [32]. However, tardive dystonia often coexists with other tardive movements, so it is not uncommon to see patients with both tardive dystonia and the classic orobuccolingual movements of tardive dyskinesia [11, 14, 16], or patients with tardive dyskinesia and akathisia [15] or even blepharospasm [6]. Because of this considerable overlap, and because the criteria for the diagnoses of tardive dystonia or dyskinesia are not always presented in these case reports, we will use the expression "tardive dyskinesia and dystonia" (TDD) in this chapter when the type of tardive syndrome is unclear or when reports are grouped together.

This chapter will discuss what is known about the mechanism of DBS, clinical outcomes from DBS, stimulation side effects, and surgical complications from DBS in patients with TDD.

*Medication-Induced Movement Disorders*, ed. Joseph H. Friedman. Published by Cambridge University Press.
© Cambridge University Press 2015.

## How does DBS work and how did it come to be used for tardive disorders?

The mechanism by which DBS is effective in controlling the involuntary movements of TDD remains unknown. In broad terms, there is abnormal signaling in the basal ganglia in patients with dystonia, and DBS somehow removes this abnormal signal, allowing better function of the basal ganglia [33]. However, it still is not clear if DBS inhibits or activates the target nucleus. Some evidence supports activation of target nuclei [34, 35], while others show suppression or interruption of abnormal firing patterns [36].

Attempts to treat primary dystonia through neurosurgical interventions began in the 1950s. Initially, lesions were made, and though many different sites were tried, the GPi and especially the thalamus appeared to be the most frequent targets. Unfortunately, the effectiveness of these lesions varied markedly, and there were high rates of complication. The first report of DBS on dystonia was published by Mundinger in 1977 [37], when he used a thalamic target for cervical dystonia, but thalamotomies continued to be performed despite Mundinger's good short-term results with stimulation. The success of pallidotomy for generalized dystonia in the 1990s switched attention back to the GPi, and several groups started successfully treating dystonia with GPi-DBS [38–40]. The efficacy and safety of GPi-DBS in primary dystonia is now well established [41], and in 2003, the US Food and Drug Administration (FDA) approved DBS for dystonia under a humanitarian device exemption. Because of this, and the decreased likelihood of behavioral side effects, the GPi has become the most common stimulation site for the treatment of TDD [42], though some cases of DBS in the thalamus and subthalamic nucleus have also been reported [28–30].

## DBS procedure

Prior to surgery, high-resolution volumetric magnetic resonance imaging (MRI) is usually performed. In many surgical centers, a stereotactic targeting frame is then placed on the patient's head, and specialized software is used to identify stereotactic coordinates [43, 44]. Other centers may use a frameless stereotactic approach [45]. Coordinates of the GPi target are typically around 20–22 mm lateral to midline, 2–3 mm anterior to the anterior commissure, and 4–6 mm below the bicommissural line [42]. The

DBS lead, impulse generator, and connecting wires are then implanted. Depending on the center, bilateral electrodes may be implanted on the same day, or the surgery may be performed in a staged fashion [46, 47]. The impulse generator and connecting wires may be implanted on the same day or later in a separate surgery.

Techniques such as microelectrode recording and macroelectrode stimulation may be used to enhance the accuracy of placement. Microelectrode recording identifies individual cell activity that may be unique to specific basal ganglia structures. This information can be used to map regions in order to generate a picture of the deep nuclei and their location. Techniques for microelectrode recording vary between groups. Some prefer to use a single microelectrode recording pass, whereas others use multiple simultaneous passes. As soon as a location for the lead is determined, the deep brain stimulation lead can be placed. Macrostimulation can then be performed to check for side effects. For example, with GPi placement, the lead might be too ventral if visual phosphenes occur with stimulation. If tonic motor contractions occur with GPi stimulation, the lead might be too posterior. The presence of side effects may lead the surgeon to move the lead [44]. Electrode placement can be confirmed with postoperative imaging (MRI or CT). The timing for initiating stimulation varies from center to center, and may range from the day after to a few weeks after implantation.

## Clinical outcomes of GPi-DBS for tardive disorders

Again, DBS has only been used to treat TDD, and the majority of cases have used the GPi as the target. The main criteria for undergoing DBS in these reports were 1) that TDD had to be disabling and refractory to medical management and 2) that the patient had to be stable psychiatrically and cognitively. The interval between exposure to neuroleptics and development of TDD varied from a few months to many years in the DBS cases, but in most cases, TDD had been present for many years before surgery [9].

Trottenberg et al. reported the first case of a tardive disorder being treated with DBS. This was a 70-year-old woman with a 6-year history of tardive dystonia, who had electrodes implanted in bilateral ventral intermediate thalamic nuclei (VIM) as well as bilateral GPi [10]. With bilateral pallidal stimulation, the patient's dystonia improved within hours.

Bilateral thalamic stimulation did not improve symptoms, and the combination of thalamic and pallidal stimulation was not better than pallidal stimulation alone. Since then, a total of 66 patients have been reported in the literature who have undergone GPi-DBS for TDD [42]. In general, patients have shown fairly consistent improvement in signs and symptoms based on standardized scales. It should be noted that all of these case reports were unblinded, with the exception of one report by the French Stimulation for Tardive Dyskinesia Study Group (STARDYS) [9]. In this study, ten patients with severe tardive dyskinesia underwent bilateral GPi-DBS surgery. At six months, patients were evaluated in the stimulation on and stimulation off conditions in a double blind fashion (i.e., both patients and evaluators were blinded as to whether DBS was on or off). With stimulation on, patients experienced a mean improvement of 50% (range, 30%–66%) in symptoms based on the Extrapyramidal Symptoms Rating Scale.

Some description of the scales used in these studies is provided to better understand the outcomes. Three main scales have been used: the Burke-Fahn-Marsden Dystonia Rating Scale (BFMDRS) [48], the Abnormal Involuntary Movement Scale (AIMS) [49], and the Extrapyramidal Symptoms Rating Scale (ESRS) [50].

The BFMDRS is composed of two subscales: a motor subscale (based on an examination) and a disability subscale (based on patient report) [48]. The motor subscale has nine components and assesses dystonia symptoms in the eyes, mouth, speech/swallowing, neck, arms, trunk, and legs. Both severity of dystonic symptoms and provoking factors for the dystonia in each body region are rated on a scale from 0 to 4. The score for each body region is obtained by multiplying the ratings of the severity and provoking factors, except for the eyes, mouth, and neck, where the product of the severity and provoking factors ratings is halved. Each body region score is then totaled, for a maximum score of 120. The disability subscale has seven items that assess speech, writing, feeding, eating, hygiene, dressing, and walking. All items are rated on a 5-point scale except walking, which is rated on a 7-point scale. The maximum disability subscore is 30. In general, the 12 patients in the literature who were evaluated with the BFMDRS total (motor plus disability) score showed a mean improvement that ranged from 6% to 100% and averaged 62.1% [42]. A total of 42 patients also had the individual motor and disability subscores of

the BFMDRS reported. These patients had a mean improvement of 71% in motor and 65% in disability subscore with GPi-DBS [42]. The BFMDRS motor subscore can improve substantially, up to 87%, at 6 months after GPi-DBS [11], but there also have been cases of no response [21].

The AIMS is composed of seven items that rate the severity of involuntary movements from 0 (none) to 4 (severe) in the face, lips, jaw, tongue, extremities, and trunk [49]. Tremor is excluded from the ratings. Items 8–10 refer to the patient's global judgment of severity of symptoms, incapacitation due to abnormal movements and awareness of the abnormal movements. There are also two "yes/no" questions about dental status. The maximum possible score is 42. Spindler et al. [42] reported a man with severe tardive dyskinesia who experienced 71% improvement in the AIMS score after GPi-DBS, sustained for over 5 years with small adjustments to his stimulator voltage and medications. This level of response in the AIMS score with GPi-DBS is similar to that reported by a systematic review showing a mean improvement in the AIMS score by 71.5% (95% CI, 62.6%–79.3% [p<0.0001]) with GPi-DBS [51]. In the double blind assessment by Damier et al. [9], the mean AIMS score improved by 56% (33%–69%) 6 months after GPI-DBS.

The ESRS is a scale that was specifically developed to rate drug-induced movement disorders [50]. The questionnaire includes four subscales: 7 items assessing the patient's subjective impression of their drug-induced movement disorder (I), 17 items based on examination of parkinsonism and akathisia (II), 10 items based on examination of dystonia (III), and 10 items based on examination of dyskinesia (IV). There are also four clinical global-impression-of-severity questions of parkinsonism, akathisia, dystonia, and dyskinesia (V–VIII) for a total of 45 items. In a systematic review, TDD improved by a mean of 67.2% (95% CI, 55.5%–77.2%) when assessed with the ESRS after GPi-DBS [51]. A double blind evaluation of ten patients reported a similar (50%) improvement in the ESRS at the 6-month evaluation after GPi-DBS [9].

Though TDD overall seems to be responsive to GPi-DBS, different symptoms may respond differently. Fixed dystonic postures appear to be the least responsive to GPi-DBS [11, 16, 18, 20]. Phasic dystonic movements and orobuccolingual dyskinesias are quite responsive and tend to improve similarly [11, 18, 20]. Dystonic symptoms in different regions may also respond differently to DBS. Franzini et al.

**Table 17.1** Follow-up after GPi-DBS for tardive dyskinesia.

| Author | Year | # of patients with follow-up | | | Evaluation time points | Last f/u |
|---|---|---|---|---|---|---|
| | | <6mo | 6mo | >6mo | | |
| Trottenberg | 2001 | | 1 | | 6mo | 6mo |
| Eltahawy | 2004 | | | 1 | 6mo | 18mo |
| Schrader | 2004 | 1 | | | 5mo | 5mo |
| Franzini | 2005 | | | 2 | 12mo | 12mo |
| Trottenberg | 2005 | | 5 | | 1w/3mo/6mo | 6mo |
| Cohen | 2007 | | | 2 | 7mo–13mo | 13mo |
| Damier | 2007 | | 10 | | 6mo | 6mo |
| Kosel | 2007 | | | 1 | 18mo | 18mo |
| Sako | 2008 | 1 | 1 | 4 | 3–6–13–15–39–48mo | 48mo |
| Gruber | 2009 | | | 9 | 1 w/3–6mo/18–80mo | 80mo |
| Kefalopoulou | 2009 | | | 1 | 3mo/6mo | 6mo |
| Capelle | 2010 | | | 4 | 12mo | 36mo |
| Chang | 2010 | | | 5 | 6mo/12mo | 76mo |
| Spindler | 2013 | | | 1 | 6mo | 60mo |
| Total cases | | 2 | 17 | 30 | | |

reported two cases where the tardive cervical dystonia appeared to have more improvement than orobucco-lingual dystonia [16], while other investigators have reported that the degree of motor improvement appears to be equal in all anatomic regions (orobuc-colingual, axial, and limb dystonia) [17, 19]. The response of axial vs. appendicular dyskinesias to GPi-DBS appears to be quite variable [7, 8, 15].

The time from stimulation initiation to benefit also varies. Some TDD cases have reported improvement within a few seconds after starting stimulation, while others may take months. The immediate response to stimulation was achieved in two cases of tardive dyskinesia who were unblinded as to whether the stimulation was on or off [6, 8]. For other cases of tardive dyskinesia, 10 patients improved within days, but the rest improved gradually over 3 to 6 months [7, 9, 15]. For those patients with tardive dystonia, phasic dystonic movements seem to respond more promptly to GPi-DBS, with improvement within days of stimulation, while tonic abnormal postures can take months to achieve significant improvement [12].

Long-term follow-up in patients undergoing DBS for tardive disorders is limited. From the 49 cases reviewed here, 29 patients were followed for more than 6 months and experienced sustained benefit as follow-up continued [7, 12–18, 42], in some cases for more than 6 years [13, 17]. See Table 17.1 for more details regarding follow-up.

## Clinical outcomes of STN and thalamic DBS for tardive disorders

The number of TDD cases treated with thalamic or subthalamic DBS in the literature is small. As mentioned earlier in this chapter, in the first case of DBS for tardive dystonia, Trottenberg et al. implanted electrodes to both GPi and VIM bilaterally. VIM stimulation did not result in improvement of clinical symptoms and it did not add benefit when paired with GPi stimulation [10].

Five cases of STN DBS for TDD have been reported. Zhang et al. presented a series of nine patients who received STN DBS for secondary dystonia, 2 of whom had tardive dystonia [30]. In one case, the dystonia was due to neuroleptic treatment and improved by 91.9% on the total BFMDRS 3 months postoperatively. The other tardive dystonia case was secondary to antiemetics and experienced 90.6% improvement on the total BFMDRS at 3 months. Another report of STN DBS for 12 primary and 2 tardive dystonia showed improvement on the BFMDRS ranging from 76% to 100% [29]. These results were achieved within hours in 90% of patients and sustained at last follow-up ranging from 6 months to 42 months, with no side effects. Johnsen reported a patient with tardive dyskinesia treated with left thalamotomy and right STN DBS with partial control of hyperkinetic movements, who later achieved complete remission suddenly after general anesthesia [28]. They did not administer any standardized motor rating scales, and the sudden remission raises a concern for the accuracy of the underlying diagnosis. Though the number of cases has been small, the limited data suggest that STN DBS could potentially be used safely for treatment of TDD. Quick and sustained clinical responses in these early reports allowed faster programming and lower stimulator settings, which may ultimately result in longer battery life.

## Side effects of stimulation

Much concern has been dedicated to potential psychiatric and cognitive side effects of GPi-DBS. This concern is based on early reports of psychiatric side effects after STN implantation of DBS, and has been added as exclusion criteria to most DBS protocols. Since most patients with tardive dyskinesia and tardive dystonia have ongoing psychiatric disease and require continued use of antipsychotics, it is important to monitor psychiatric function. Unfortunately, very few of the case reports assessed depression systematically before and after DBS. Damier et al. assessed mood using the Montgomery Asberg Depression Rating Scale (MADRS). Of their 10 cases, 1 patient had mood improvement while 3 had transient worsening of their mood, which resolved spontaneously or with medication within 6 months [9]. In 9 patients with tardive dystonia who underwent GPi-DBS, Gruber et al. reported an improvement of 59% in the mean MADRS score at their long-term follow-up (range 18–80 months) [17]. Kosel et al. reported a reduction in the Hamilton Rating Scale for Depression (HRSD) from 26 to 13 (50%) and a reduction in the Beck Depression Inventory (BDI) from 22 to 16 (27.2%) in a patient suffering from major depression, 18 months after surgery [7].

Of the other 44 patients in the literature undergoing GPi-DBS who had a psychiatric diagnosis before DBS, 2 (5%) were reported to have a transient exacerbation of their symptoms, and none were reported to have new psychiatric symptoms [51]. Moreover, marked subjective improvement in mood has been reported after surgery in isolated cases [18]. There have not been any cognitive sequelae from GPi-DBS in patients with TDD reported thus far in the literature.

In the case reports of STN DBS for tardive dystonia, 2 patients had stimulation side effects with persistent laughter and lethargy, respectively. These symptoms resolved with reprogramming [30]. No other mention of psychiatric side effects was reported, so future studies of STN DBS for TDD with rigorous ascertainment of depression and psychosis are needed.

## Surgical complications

Complications from GPi-DBS surgery for TDD include painful traction of the cable connection in one patient, requiring fixation of the stimulator to the clavicle [9]. In another report, one patient developed local infection of the chest after a battery replacement surgery, requiring two weeks of antibiotics, while another patient suffered a venous infarct in the premotor area [13]. One patient was reported to have had the electrode removed due to infection [21]. One patient reportedly suffered a left frontal hemorrhage secondary to venous infarct 2 days postoperatively, causing aphasia and hemiparesis with full recovery within 3 months [24].

No surgical complications were reported in patients undergoing STN DBS [29, 30]. One patient had a lead fracture 16 months after implantation and required evacuation [30].

## Deep brain stimulation settings

Most of the GPi-DBS patients reported were given monopolar stimulation, either with one or two cathodes [42], but bipolar mode was used for some [12, 25]. Three stimulation parameters can be adjusted with the DBS device: amplitude, pulse width, and frequency. Stimulation amplitudes in these patients ranged from 1.0 V to 6.5 V [42]. Most studies typically started with amplitude of 1.0 V and slowly increased it over time as tolerated. Pulse widths used in the literature varied widely (60μs to 450μs) as well, though higher pulse widths (≥120 μs) were preferred at most centers [6, 8, 9, 11–13, 16–18, 42]. Some studies used a stable frequency while others allowed adjustments to frequency depending on clinical response. In general,

**Table 17.2** GPi-DBS settings commonly used to treat tardive dyskinesia and tardive dystonia

| Author | Year | N | Age (mean) | Amplitude | Pulse width | Frequency |
|---|---|---|---|---|---|---|
| Trottenberg et al. | 2001 | 1 | 70 | 3V | 210µs | 150Hz |
| Eltahawy et al. | 2004 | 1 | 53 | 2.6V | 210µs | 40Hz |
| Schrader et al. | 2004 | 1 | 64 | 3 – 5.5V | 60µs | 30 – 180Hz |
| Franzini et al. | 2005 | 2 | 31.5 | 1V | 90µs | 130Hz |
| Trottenberg et al. | 2005 | 5 | 56.2 | 2.7±0.8V | 111±57µs | 144±22 |
| Cohen et al. | 2007 | 2 | 47 | 3.4 – 4V | 90 – 120µs | 130Hz |
| Damier et al. | 2007 | 10 | 45.1 | 3.5±0.2 | 150µs | 130Hz |
| Kosel et al. | 2007 | 1 | 62 | 3.5 – 3.8V | 90µs | 130Hz |
| Sako et al. | 2008 | 6 | 44.5 | 1.3 – 3.8V | 450µs | 60 – 135Hz |
| Gruber et al. | 2009 | 9 | 63.2 | 2.8 – 3V | 83.3±13.2µs | 154±25.1Hz |
| Kefalopoulou et al. | 2009 | 1 | 42 | 2.5 – 3.6V | 250 – 450µs | 185Hz |
| Capelle et al. | 2010 | 4 | 46 | 3 – 6.5V | 90 – 210µs | 130 – 160Hz |
| Chang et al. | 2010 | 5 | 41.2 | 2.5 – 3.6V | 180 – 210µs | 60 – 185Hz |
| Spindler et al. | 2013 | 1 | 42 | 1.5 – 3.6V | 90µs | 185Hz |
| Range | | | 26 – 76 | 1 – 7V | 60 – 450µs | 40 – 250Hz |

frequencies ranged from 40Hz to 185Hz [6, 15]. The most commonly used frequency was 130Hz [9, 12, 14, 16, 21]. Table 17.2 presents a summary of commonly used GPi-DBS settings for the treatment of tardive dyskinesia and tardive dystonia.

For STN DBS cases, only Sun et al. reported the stimulation parameters [29] and found that bipolar settings produced the best clinical effect. Amplitude was typically between 2 and 3 V, pulse width between 90 and 120 µs, and frequency between 135 and 185 Hz.

## Conclusions

Deep brain stimulation seems to be safe and effective for TDD, although the data are limited. The GPi has been targeted the most, with only a few reports of TDD being treated with STN DBS. The orobuccolingual dyskinesias common in tardive dyskinesia, as well as choreiform movements of the limbs appear to respond similarly to tardive dystonia, though phasic dystonic movements seem to respond faster and more consistently than fixed abnormal postures. Once obtained, motor improvement tended to be sustained.

Although not assessed systematically, clear deterioration of psychiatric disease was not seen in these patients. Improvement of mood was seen in some cases of GPi-DBS, which allowed reduction of psychiatric medication. GPi-DBS thus appears to be a viable option for patients with disabling choreiform or dystonic movements secondary to dopamine blocking agents. Future randomized, controlled trials of DBS for tardive dyskinesia and tardive dystonia will be necessary in order to be certain that the improvement seen thus far in the literature is not due solely to a placebo effect. It also remains to be seen if improvement in these tardive symptoms can be sustained long term.

## References

1. Hamani C, Moro E. Surgery for other movement disorders: dystonia, tics. *Curr Opin Neurol* 2007 Aug;**20**(4):470–6.

2. Fernandez HH, Friedman JH. Classification and treatment of tardive syndromes. *Neurologist* 2003 Jan;**9**(1):16–27.

3. Chou KL, Friedman JH. Tardive syndromes in the elderly. *Clin Geriatr Med* 2006 Nov;**22**(4):915–33, viii.

4. Voon V, Kubu C, Krack P, Houeto JL, Troster AI. Deep brain stimulation: neuropsychological and neuropsychiatric issues. *Mov Disord* 2006 Jun;**21** Suppl 14:S305–27.

5. Chou KL, Friedman JH. Treatment-induced mental changes in Parkinson's disease. *Handb Clin Neurol* 2007;**84**:219–40.

6. Kefalopoulou Z, Paschali A, Markaki E, Vassilakos P, Ellul J, Constantoyannis C. A double-blind study on a patient with tardive dyskinesia treated with pallidal deep brain stimulation. *Acta Neurol Scand* 2009 Apr;**119**(4):269–73.

7. Kosel M, Sturm V, Frick C, Lenartz D, Zeidler G, Brodesser D, et al. Mood improvement after deep brain stimulation of the internal globus pallidus for tardive dyskinesia in a patient suffering from major depression. *J Psychiatr Res* 2007 Nov;**41**(9):801–3.

8. Schrader C, Peschel T, Petermeyer M, Dengler R, Hellwig D. Unilateral deep brain stimulation of the internal globus pallidus alleviates tardive dyskinesia. *Mov Disord* 2004 May;**19**(5):583–5.

9. Damier P, Thobois S, Witjas T, Cuny E, Derost P, Raoul S, et al. Bilateral deep brain stimulation of the globus pallidus to treat tardive dyskinesia. *Arch Gen Psychiatry* 2007 Feb;**64**(2):170–6.

10. Trottenberg T, Paul G, Meissner W, Maier-Hauff K, Taschner C, Kupsch A. Pallidal and thalamic neurostimulation in severe tardive dystonia. *J Neurol Neurosurg Psychiatry* 2001 Apr;**70**(4):557–9.

11. Trottenberg T, Volkmann J, Deuschl G, Kuhn AA, Schneider GH, Muller J, et al. Treatment of severe tardive dystonia with pallidal deep brain stimulation. *Neurology* 2005 Jan 25;**64**(2):344–6.

12. Capelle HH, Blahak C, Schrader C, Baezner H, Kinfe TM, Herzog J, et al. Chronic deep brain stimulation in patients with tardive dystonia without a history of major psychosis. *Mov Disord* 2010 Jul 30;**25**(10):1477–81.

13. Chang EF, Schrock LE, Starr PA, Ostrem JL. Long-term benefit sustained after bilateral pallidal deep brain stimulation in patients with refractory tardive dystonia. *Stereotact Funct Neurosurg* 2010;**88**(5):304–10.

14. Cohen OS, Hassin-Baer S, Spiegelmann R. Deep brain stimulation of the internal globus pallidus for refractory tardive dystonia. *Parkinsonism Relat Disord* 2007 Dec;**13**(8):541–4.

15. Eltahawy HA, Feinstein A, Khan F, Saint-Cyr J, Lang AE, Lozano AM. Bilateral globus pallidus internus deep brain stimulation in tardive dyskinesia: a case report. *Mov Disord* 2004 Aug;**19**(8):969–72.

16. Franzini A, Marras C, Ferroli P, Zorzi G, Bugiani O, Romito L, et al. Long-term high-frequency bilateral pallidal stimulation for neuroleptic-induced tardive dystonia. Report of two cases. *J Neurosurg* 2005 Apr;**102**(4):721–5.

17. Gruber D, Trottenberg T, Kivi A, Schoenecker T, Kopp UA, Hoffmann KT, et al. Long-term effects of pallidal deep brain stimulation in tardive dystonia. *Neurology* 2009 Jul 7;**73**(1):53–8.

18. Sako W, Goto S, Shimazu H, Murase N, Matsuzaki K, Tamura T, et al. Bilateral deep brain stimulation of the globus pallidus internus in tardive dystonia. *Mov Disord* 2008 Oct 15;**23**(13):1929–31.

19. Egidi M, Franzini A, Marras C, Cavallo M, Mondani M, Lavano A, et al. A survey of Italian cases of dystonia treated by deep brain stimulation. *J Neurosurg Sci* 2007 Dec;**51**(4):153–8.

20. Katsakiori PF, Kefalopoulou Z, Markaki E, Paschali A, Ellul J, Kagadis GC, et al. Deep brain stimulation for secondary dystonia: results in 8 patients. *Acta Neurochir (Wien)* 2009 May;**151**(5):473–8;discussion 8.

21. Krause M, Fogel W, Kloss M, Rasche D, Volkmann J, Tronnier V. Pallidal stimulation for dystonia. *Neurosurgery* 2004 Dec;**55**(6):1361–8; discussion 8–70.

22. Magarinos-Ascone CM, Regidor I, Gomez-Galan M, Cabanes-Martinez L, Figueiras-Mendez R. Deep brain stimulation in the globus pallidus to treat dystonia: electrophysiological characteristics and 2 years' follow-up in 10 patients. *Neuroscience* 2008 Mar 18;**152**(2):558–71.

23. Pretto TE, Dalvi A, Kang UJ, Penn RD. A prospective blinded evaluation of deep brain stimulation for the treatment of secondary dystonia and primary torticollis syndromes. *J Neurosurg* 2008 Sep;**109**(3):405–9.

24. Starr PA, Turner RS, Rau G, Lindsey N, Heath S, Volz M, et al. Microelectrode-guided implantation of deep brain stimulators into the globus pallidus internus for dystonia: techniques, electrode locations, and outcomes. *Neurosurg Focus* 2004 Jul 15;**17**(1):E4.

25. Yianni J, Bain P, Giladi N, Auca M, Gregory R, Joint C, et al. Globus pallidus internus deep brain stimulation for dystonic conditions: a prospective audit. *Mov Disord* 2003 Apr;**18**(4):436–42.

26. Halbig TD, Gruber D, Kopp UA, Schneider GH, Trottenberg T, Kupsch A. Pallidal stimulation in dystonia: effects on cognition, mood, and quality of life. *J Neurol Neurosurg Psychiatry* 2005 Dec;**76**(12):1713–6.

27. Kim JP, Chang WS, Chang JW. Treatment of secondary dystonia with a combined stereotactic procedure: long-term surgical outcomes. *Acta Neurochir (Wien)* 2011 Dec;**153**(12):2319–27; discussion 28.

28. Johnsen M, Wester K. Full remission of tardive dyskinesia following general anaesthesia. *J Neurol* 2002 May;**249**(5):622–5.

29. Sun B, Chen S, Zhan S, Le W, Krahl SE. Subthalamic nucleus stimulation for primary dystonia and tardive dystonia. *Acta Neurochir Suppl* 2007;**97** (Pt 2):207–14.

30. Zhang JG, Zhang K, Wang ZC, Ge M, Ma Y. Deep brain stimulation in the treatment of secondary

dystonia. *Chin Med J (Engl)* 2006 Dec 20;**119**(24):2069–74.

31. Raja M. Tardive dystonia. Prevalence, risk factors, and comparison with tardive dyskinesia in a population of 200 acute psychiatric inpatients. *Eur Arch Psychiatry Clin Neurosci* 1995;**245**(3):145–51.

32. Adityanjee, Aderibigbe YA, Jampala VC, Mathews T. The current status of tardive dystonia. *Biol Psychiatry* 1999 Mar 15;**45**(6):715–30.

33. Capelle HH, Krauss JK. Neuromodulation in dystonia: current aspects of deep brain stimulation. *Neuromodulation* 2009 Jan;**12**(1):8–21.

34. Anderson ME, Postupna N, Ruffo M. Effects of high-frequency stimulation in the internal globus pallidus on the activity of thalamic neurons in the awake monkey. *J Neurophysiol* 2003 Feb;**89**(2):1150–60.

35. Perlmutter JS, Mink JW, Bastian AJ, Zackowski K, Hershey T, Miyawaki E, et al. Blood flow responses to deep brain stimulation of thalamus. *Neurology* 2002 May 14;**58**(9):1388–94.

36. Liu Y, Postupna N, Falkenberg J, Anderson ME. High frequency deep brain stimulation: what are the therapeutic mechanisms? *Neurosci Biobehav Rev* 2008;**32**(3):343–51.

37. Mundinger F. [New stereotactic treatment of spasmodic torticollis with a brain stimulation system (author's transl)]. *Med Klin* 1977 Nov 18;**72**(46):1982–6.

38. Coubes P, Echenne B, Roubertie A, Vayssiere N, Tuffery S, Humbertclaude V, et al. [Treatment of early-onset generalized dystonia by chronic bilateral stimulation of the internal globus pallidus. *Apropos of a case*. J. Neurochirurgie 1999 May;**45**(2):139–44.

39. Krauss JK, Pohle T, Weber S, Ozdoba C, Burgunder JM. Bilateral stimulation of globus pallidus internus for treatment of cervical dystonia. *Lancet* 1999 Sep 4;**354**(9181):837–8.

40. Kumar R, Dagher A, Hutchison WD, Lang AE, Lozano AM. Globus pallidus deep brain stimulation for generalized dystonia: clinical and PET investigation. *Neurology* 1999 Sep 11;**53**(4):871–4.

41. Vidailhet M, Vercueil L, Houeto JL, Krystkowiak P, Benabid AL, Cornu P, et al. Bilateral deep-brain stimulation of the globus pallidus in primary generalized dystonia. *N Engl J Med* 2005 Feb 3;**352**(5):459–67.

42. Spindler MA, Galifianakis NB, Wilkinson JR, Duda JE. Globus pallidus internal deep brain stimulation for tardive dyskinesia: case report and review of the literature. *Parkinsonism Relat Disord* 2013 Feb;**19**(2):141–7.

43. Gibson V, Peifer J, Gandy M, Robertson S, Mewes K. 3D visualization methods to guide surgery for Parkinson's disease. *Stud Health Technol Inform* 2003;**94**:86–92.

44. Machado A, Rezai AR, Kopell BH, Gross RE, Sharan AD, Benabid AL. Deep brain stimulation for Parkinson's disease: surgical technique and perioperative management. *Mov Disord* 2006 Jun;**21** Suppl 14:S247–58.

45. Tai CH, Wu RM, Lin CH, Pan MK, Chen YF, Liu HM, et al. Deep brain stimulation therapy for Parkinson's disease using frameless stereotaxy: comparison with frame-based surgery. *Eur J Neurol* 2010 Nov;**17**(11):1377–85.

46. Papapetropoulos S, Salcedo AG, Singer C, Gallo BV, Jagid JR. Staged unilateral or bilateral STN-DBS? *Mov Disord* 2008 Apr 15;**23**(5):775.

47. Samii A, Kelly VE, Slimp JC, Shumway-Cook A, Goodkin R. Staged unilateral versus bilateral subthalamic nucleus stimulator implantation in Parkinson disease. *Mov Disord* 2007 Jul 30;**22**(10):1476–81.

48. Burke RE, Fahn S, Marsden CD, Bressman SB, Moskowitz C, Friedman J. Validity and reliability of a rating scale for the primary torsion dystonias. *Neurology* 1985 Jan;**35**(1):73–7.

49. American Psychiatric Association. *Handbook of Psychiatric Measures*. Arlington/US: American Psychiatric Press, Inc.; 2000.

50. Chouinard G, Margolese HC. Manual for the Extrapyramidal Symptom Rating Scale (ESRS). *Schizophr Res* 2005 Jul 15; **76**(2–3): 247–65.

51. Mentzel CL, Tenback DE, Tijssen MA, Visser-Vandewalle VE, van Harten PN. Efficacy and safety of deep brain stimulation in patients with medication-induced tardive dyskinesia and/or dystonia: a systematic review. *J Clin Psychiatry* 2012 Nov;**73**(11):1434–8.

# Index

Printed in the United States
by Baker & Taylor Publisher Services